MATERIALS IN DENTISTRY

Principles and Applications

SECOND EDITION

MATERIALS IN DENTISTRY
Principles and Applications

SECOND EDITION

Jack L. Ferracane, MS, PhD, FADM
Professor and Chair
Department of Biomaterials and Biomechanics
Oregon Health Sciences University
School of Dentistry
Portland, Oregon

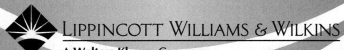

LIPPINCOTT WILLIAMS & WILKINS
A **Wolters Kluwer** Company
Philadelphia • Baltimore • New York • London
Buenos Aires • Hong Kong • Sydney • Tokyo

Publisher: Susan Katz
Managing Editor: Jacquelyn Merrell
Marketing Manager: Anne Smith
Production Editor: Bill Cady

Printed in the United States of America

First Edition, 1995

Library of Congress Cataloging-in-Publication Data

Ferracane, Jack L.
    Materials in dentistry : principles and applications / Jack L. Ferracane.—2nd ed.
        p. cm.
    Includes bibliographical references and index.
    ISBN 0-7817-2733-2
    1. Dental materials. I. Title.

    RK652.5 .F47 2001
    617.6'95—dc21

00-069159

03 04 05
2 3 4 5 6 7 8 9 10

Preface

Materials in Dentistry: Principles and Applications covers the basic science, clinical indications, manipulative variables and procedures, physical and mechanical characteristics, and clinical performance of the materials used in the general practice of dentistry. This text is written specifically for the dental assistant, but the information is also useful for the dental hygienist and beginning dental student.

This second edition provides an update and includes new information on materials introduced since the first edition, such as compomers, new ceramics, new adhesives, and packable, flowable, and fiber-reinforced composites. The new edition has expanded discussions of fluoride-containing materials, the application of different types of dentin adhesives, the placement of posterior composites, and the care of dental implants. Additional suggested readings have been included for each chapter.

The approach used in *Materials in Dentistry: Principles and Applications* is to present in detail those materials with which an assistant would have routine experience, while introducing, through an overview, those materials and procedures with which the dental auxiliary will have limited contact. This will allow the student to become familiar with all areas of dental materials while maximizing his or her exposure to those materials over whose characteristics and clinical success they have significant influence. Although this book is written primarily for the auxiliaries in a general dental practice, certain sections are useful for assistants of dental specialists.

Materials in Dentistry: Principles and Applications differs from other texts in the manner in which the material is organized. In this text, the science and the use of the various materials are discussed from the standpoint of applications and indications. Materials often are introduced together according to their use, rather than having each type discussed in isolation in its own chapter. For example, amalgams and composites are materials used for the restoration of posterior teeth and are covered in individual sections of one chapter that considers the general subject of direct posterior restoratives. Another example is the chapter on materials for cast restorations, which includes discussions of waxes, die materials, and investments, all of which are materials used in the production of cast restorations such as inlays, onlays, crowns, and bridges. It is believed that this approach will provide the necessary information to the student while highlighting the similarities and differences between materials. These similarities and differences are important because they influence the process by which a clinician selects a specific material for a specific dental procedure.

Another feature of this text is the inclusion of step-by-step instructions (complete with photographs or diagrams) for the mixing and use of certain materials, such as cements, impression materials, gypsum products, and acrylics. This approach often is seen in chapters on dental materials in complete texts on dental assisting but is used only rarely in complete texts on dental materials aimed at this audience. A unique feature is the manner in which the basic science information, required by the dental auxiliary to ensure the appropriate handling of materials, is integrated with the necessary "how-to" information. I firmly believe that it is not sufficient just to know the correct way to handle dental materials, but that a strong grounding in the reasons for doing so is critical for obtaining the most successful product. The student must have the background knowledge to know why the material behaves as it does and what alterations in handling can do to change its characteristics and, ultimately, its performance. This subject often is treated less completely in chapters on dental materials in texts on dental assisting but usually is given greater emphasis in complete texts on dental materials.

An additional feature of this text is the introduction of questions or comments within the chapters that the student may use as study guides. These questions, which appear in ***bold italicized print***, usually introduce the topic that follows. They have been included to encourage students to stop and think about what they have just read and how they can use that information. Usually, the student need only read on to the next paragraph or so for an answer to the question. This format is designed to encourage the student to read the text "actively" while constantly relating the material to the clinical situation, which is the ultimate goal. Similarly, certain important concepts or points have been highlighted by placing them in boxes and setting them apart from the rest of the text.

A glossary of terms is provided at the end of the text. Throughout the text, the words defined in the Glossary are highlighted in **bold type**. These usually are new terms, materials, or procedures that have been introduced in that chapter. The bold type enables their easy identification as the student reads along.

Each chapter begins with a list of study objectives that identify the most important concepts to be covered in the chapter. Each chapter ends with a short summary of these important points. Also at the end of most chapters are study questions designed to test the student's comprehension of important concepts and a list of selected readings. For the Selected Readings the author has chosen articles and texts that most likely would be available to the student in his or her school library.

Finally, two appendices have been included to help with product and manufacturer identification. A list of commonly used commercial materials is provided, as is a listing of manufacturers, complete with Internet website addresses and phone numbers. Each member of the dental team should find this information useful for reference purposes and, whenever questions arise about the use of a specific dental material, is encouraged to contact the individual manufacturer. Most manufacturers have toll-free phone numbers and maintain a staff able to answer technical and compositional questions.

Jack L. Ferracane, MS, PhD, FADM

Acknowledgments

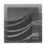

The author requested and received the help of many friends and colleagues in compiling the first and second editions of this text. Several people spent many hours to provide excellent reviews of the content and format, which was most helpful during the editing process. The author also is indebted to the many individuals who provided materials for the illustrations. Special thanks are given to Dr. Jack Mitchem and Dr. John Engle for their help in this area. The constant encouragement and advice from the publisher, specifically Andrew Allen and Jacqui Merrell, were of great help throughout the production of the first and second editions, respectively. Finally, the author would like to thank his wife Tricia and sons Lucas, Christopher, and Zachary for their patience and understanding during this entire process. The compilation of a manuscript such as this requires a tremendous amount of time and often came at their expense.

Contents

Chapter 4
Intermediary Materials and Cements 59

Chapter 5
Direct Esthetic Anterior Restoratives 85

Chapter *1*

Introduction

Goals
History of Dental Materials
The Oral Environment

Characteristics of the Ideal Dental Material
Quality Assurance Programs

Objectives

- Explain the overall goal of a course in dental materials and its importance in the current and future training of the oral health care provider.

- Describe specific conditions within the oral cavity that make it such a demanding environment for the placement and long-term performance of dental materials.

- List and explain the characteristics of the ideal dental material.

- Describe the programs that are in place to ensure that quality control is maintained during the manufacture of dental devices and that materials for intraoral use are safe and effective.

"What do you do for a living?" my new acquaintance asked me. I offered my standard reply, "I teach and do research in a dental school."

"Oh, you're a dentist," she responded.

"No, but I study the materials that dentists, dental assistants, and dental hygienists use to fix or replace teeth," I stated with pride.

"Oh, I see," she answered with a puzzled look. I'd seen it many times before. Can you really make a living doing that? She didn't really understand until I began to elaborate. I explained that a person in my field plays several roles. These include serving as an inventor or developer of new materials for use in dentistry; as a quality control engineer who evaluates existing products to ensure that they meet acceptable standards for use in the mouth; as a scientist who spends a tremendous number of hours trying to discover why certain materials behave the way they do and how to improve their strength, looks, or other characteristics; and as an educator who tries to relate this information to students and practicing dental personnel. I concluded by citing some specific examples of the ways in which dental materials are used. Then her eyes lit up. "Say, when are you guys going to make gold crowns that look like teeth?"

"We already have them," I said, and proceeded to describe composites and ceramics, porcelain bonded to metal, and other esthetically improved choices that have become an integral part of the dental practice.

"That sounds pretty interesting," she responded. She paused briefly and then looked at me and said, "Hey, take a look at this. What can you do about this tooth back here?" She immediately began to retract her cheek to enhance my view of a badly worn first molar. "No, I'm not a d . . . ." I began, but it was too late. Anyway, I really didn't mind. It is important to remember that the interesting material's questions are inextricably tied to "real-life" problems in "real" people.

■ *Goals*

Many materials and devices used in dentistry are mixed or produced at chairside. To a large extent, the ultimate success of a patient's dental work depends on the manner in which the materials from which it is made are manipulated. Thus, the dental assistant plays an important role for both the dentist and the patient. A thorough understanding of the nature of the various materials used, as well as the proper way to handle them in the clinical setting, cannot be overemphasized. This is the primary reason for a course in dental materials for dental personnel.

The ultimate concern for any health care provider is the welfare of the patient. The ideal material or procedure for a specific situation depends on the needs of the particular patient, and one must be aware of all of the factors that can influence the selection process. Therefore, providers should be competent clinicians, well-schooled biologists, and, in some cases, design engineers.

The science of **dental materials** encompasses the development, characterization, use, and evaluation of the materials used to repair or replace teeth. It represents a marriage between the basic and clinical sciences. Workers in the basic sciences provide expertise in engineering principles and design, as well as in many areas of biology. Contributions from the clinical sciences are made by both general and specialized practitioners. Every discipline within the field of dentistry depends to some extent on the materials available to repair, restore, or maintain the health of the oral tissues. The field has exploded in the past 10 to 20 years, with new materials and procedures introduced almost weekly. This keeps the discussion lively but also contributes to a great deal of confusion and uncertainty.

What makes today's material or technique better than yesterday's? What really constitutes an improvement in formulation or function? Educators and researchers spend a great deal of time trying to answer these questions for students and practitioners alike. Often the answer is found only after extensive testing or clinical use, which necessarily slows the development of products and the advancement of the state of the science in dental materials. A solid background in some of the basic principles on which the science is based can greatly facilitate the process, however, by improving one's chances of making truly educated decisions concerning the selection and handling of materials. Only through a process of informed decision making can the assistant, hygienist, or clinician ensure that the patient will realize the optimal characteristics of a particular **restoration** or **appliance**. Each procedure comprises many discrete steps that must be accomplished with care and attention to produce the best product.

Thus, the main goal of any course in dental materials must be to provide the basic information required to facilitate the optimal selection, handling, placement, and care of the materials used in dentistry. This is a challenging task, given the abundance of information written on the subject and the rate at which it continues to be generated. What is even more impressive is the fact that although the basic tenet of using foreign materials to repair or replace teeth predates Christianity by 400 to 500 years, all but a few of the materials in today's **armamentarium** were developed in the 20th or 21st century.

■ *History of Dental Materials*

The earliest known use of dental materials can be traced to approximately 500 B.C. and the Etruscans, who used gold to make the first dental bridges. The **pontic** for the first bridges was a tooth that had been extracted, probably from a deceased person. When these gold appliances were found 2000 or more years later, they were still gold colored and virtually free of **corrosion**, underscoring the durability of gold, one of its major benefits as a dental restorative.

In the first century A.D., carious teeth were filled with molten metal to facilitate extraction by keeping them intact during the procedure. It was not until approximately 1500 A.D. that very thin pieces of **gold foil** or leaf were used in Italy as a restorative material.

Not long afterward, wax was used to make **impressions** from which plaster **models** of the gums or teeth were formed. These models were then used to carve replacement dentition from ivory or animal bones. In France in the early 1700s, lead, tin, and gold were first used as filling materials because they could be adapted to the tooth with relative ease to replace missing portions. At the same time, sealing wax mixtures or metals with low melting temperatures were used like cement to fix ivory or natural teeth in place. The late 1700s are also associated with the first use of **porcelain** to make complete dentures or individual teeth. The ability to mimic natural dentition with smooth surfaces and various color shades was an important reason for considering porcelain as a dental material.

The first dental **amalgam**, or "silver filling," was produced in France in the early 1800s and found its way to the United States in approximately 1830. Porcelain teeth were introduced in America at about the same time. A version of amalgam containing high levels of copper, the so-called copper amalgam, was introduced circa 1850. Also at that time, plaster began to be used to make impressions, **gutta percha** appeared for the filling of root canals, metal mixtures based on gold and platinum came into use, the hard rubber material *vulcanite* was introduced as a replacement for ivory dentures, and a compound made of zinc oxychloride was developed as both a cementing agent and a restorative. In the late 1880s, zinc phosphate and silicate cements were introduced to secure circular gold **inlays** into prepared cavities. At the end of the 19th century, the father of modern dentistry, Dr. G. V. Black, perfected the formulation and use of dental amalgam in his laboratory at Northwestern University in Chicago, Illinois.

In 1910, a dentist named Taggert brought the **lost wax casting technique** to the dental field. This process would revolutionize dentistry because it made possible the accurate production of metal inlays, crowns, and bridges made of gold-containing **alloys**, similar to jeweler's gold. Possibly one of the greatest discoveries to benefit all of humankind, not just the dental industry, was the development of synthetic resins such as **acrylic**. This occurred around 1940. These **polymers**, or plastics, would eventually be used in almost every aspect of human life. Within a few years after these plastics were developed, virtually all dentures were made from them. After the 1950s, other important contributions included stainless steels for orthodontics, non-**noble metals** (i.e., gold "free") for the casting process, **elastic** impression materials, dental **composites** to be used with the **acid-etch technique**, new noble casting metals, pit and fissure sealants, and high-copper amalgams. In the 1970s, **glass ionomer** and **polycarboxylate cements** were developed, and a host of other materials were introduced, including new wires for orthodontics, new composites, **adhesives** that could bond to dentin, more accurate impression materials that enhanced **prosthodontic** treatment, and **ceramics** to be used by themselves as restoratives.

The 1980s brought further developments in dentin adhesives, composites, and ceramics. In addition was the introduction of light-cured **liners** and glass ionomers, sealants for the surfaces of restorations, and further alterations to orthodontic wires. The 1990s brought simplified dentin adhesives, reinforced ceramics for fixed bridges, resin-modified glass ionomers, **compomers**, fiber-reinforced composites, low-fusing porcelains, new root canal fillers, and modified impression materials. One can only expect that by the end of the first decade of the new millennium, many of our current materials will be outdated and replaced with improved versions or alternatives. Thus, the importance of keeping current is underscored once again, as is the need to establish a firm foundation of knowledge on which to evaluate new information.

■ *The Oral Environment*

The oral environment provides a unique opportunity for the **bioengineer** and oral health care provider, mainly because it presents such a harsh environment for materials. Consider the heterogeneous nature of the tissues that must be restored or replaced. The materials also must be inert and **biocompatible**, as well as durable, and be provided to the patient in a cost-effective manner. These demands must be met in an environment characterized by moisture, the presence of acids, tremendous grinding and impact forces, rapid alterations in temperature, and the frequent introduction of foreign objects of vastly differing chemistries and physical structure. Imagine yourself as a little person trapped in such an environment—a Tom Thumb of the oral cavity, if you will. Your day may start like this:

> I awoke to find myself in a huge cavern—a dark, damp, and musty-smelling place that gave every appearance of having been closed up or sealed for quite some length of time. Just as I began to arise to inspect my situation, the huge door to the cavern began to open, and within seconds, an orange solution came gushing in on me, burning my eyes and nostrils because it was very acidic and bitter and also quite cold. I raced behind a huge stone pillar to avoid the next surge of fluid, since the cavern door was once again opening. This time, however, a hot, steamy fluid, black in color and very strong and bitter, came pouring in. I could not escape it and I was all at once burned by it. Soon after, small boulders were introduced to the cavity on a huge metallic shovel. The shovel was removed and a huge racket ensued as the cavern began to seize and grind as if being undermined by an earthquake of magnificent proportions. The boulders were smashed to bits between the huge stone pillars that I attempted to hide behind. The grinding sent shivers up my spine as pieces of the ground-up rocks fell down between the pillars, pummeling me from all directions. All the while, my eyes, ears, nose, and mouth burned, for I was standing knee deep in salt water the entire time. Then, after several minutes of this most perilous activity, interrupted only by intermittent gushes of the hot, acidic, black fluid, there was silence. I prayed for it to last, but it did not. Soon the cave reopened and I was most abruptly introduced to a large white object containing many long, slender tubes, on top of which was spread a blue, paste-like substance. The huge object began a series of dragging and scraping movements across and over the huge stone pillars, sending me running for my life as the froth of the paste enveloped the entire cavern and choked me incessantly. This continued for what seemed to be an eternity, and just when I was sure that I would succumb to the froth, the mighty tool was retracted. Within seconds a cold stream of water poured in, ultimately carrying me out of the huge cavern, along with the remnants of the paste and ground-up boulders.

■ Characteristics of the Ideal Dental Material

The constraints of the oral environment necessitate that guidelines be set forth for the development of dental materials. Requirements for some materials differ from those for others, depending on their uses; however, a list of ideal characteristics can be generated for the materials to be used within the mouth to repair or replace oral tissues (Display 1-1). The characteristics are listed in order of importance, although the order may change depending on the requirements of a particular situation. Cost also is a primary concern when selecting a material.

As specific materials are discussed throughout the text, it would be helpful to keep this list in mind to compare the ideal with the actual characteristics. Dental personnel have appropriate materials for the many different situations that present, but no one material simultaneously meets all of the requirements. In other words, there is no universal restorative material. Many materials have been touted as such, but after extensive testing or evaluation, deficiencies usually are revealed. That is why it is important to identify products that have been proven to exceed some standard of quality. Although this is not always a requirement for the marketing of a new product, there are specifications for such evaluations, and it is the responsibility of oral health care providers to ensure that these materials are used in their practices when they are appropriate and available.

Characteristics of the Ideal Dental Material

1. **Biocompatible**—nontoxic; nonirritating; nonallergenic
2. **Mechanically Stable and Durable**—strong; fracture resistant; stiff
3. **Resistant to Corrosion or Chemicals**—does not deteriorate over time
4. **Dimensionally Stable**—minimally affected by temperature or solvents
5. **Minimally Conductive Both Thermally and Electrically**—insulators
6. **Esthetic**—oral tissue-like appearance
7. **Easy to Manipulate**—placement and finishing with reasonable time and effort
8. **Adherent to Tissues**—provide durable, tight union for retention and sealing
9. **Tasteless and Odorless**—not irritating or unpleasant
10. **Cleanable/Repairable**—can be maintained or fixed
11. **Cost-effective**—within the patient's budget

■ Quality Assurance Programs

The Food and Drug Administration (FDA) of the United States is the government regulatory body that has the authority to ensure the safety of medical devices—in other words, to protect the general population. Dental materials are called devices and include the instruments and implements used to diagnose, treat, or prevent oral disease. Dental devices are classified by panels of dental experts as class I, II, or III. Class I is a general classification given to all devices and simply implies that they are registered and made according to good manufacturing practices. If there is cause for further concern, the device may be classified as class II, which means that it must meet certain performance standards established by the FDA or some similar body, such as the American Dental Association (ADA). These standards address the composition and properties or characteristics of the device. Class III is more restrictive, requiring that data be provided that ensure the safety and **efficacy** of the device before it can be marketed. Implants fall into this category. Most dental materials are listed in class II because sufficient data existed to support their safe use before the 1976 law was enacted that gave the FDA the authority to regulate the industry. For many of these materials, specifications exist to evaluate them in the laboratory to ensure that they meet certain minimum requirements for quality. For new materials, the manufacturer must apply for FDA approval, usually by filing a 510K. This is designed for materials that are similar to currently approved products. A premarket approval (PMA) from the FDA is much more difficult to obtain and requires data from extensive testing to ensure the safety of the device. This approval is usually necessary for those products that will be permanently implanted in the body.

The ADA through its Council on Scientific Affairs has assumed the responsibility of establishing specifications by which the materials, instruments, and equipment used in dentistry can be evaluated to ensure a certain level of quality. This effort is coordinated through the ADA under the authority of the ANSI (American National Standards Institute). A committee (MD156) of this organization is composed of dental scientists, users, and manufacturers who propose for each material a battery of useful and, it is hoped, predictive tests. For example, dental composites must pass certain minimal standards for flexure strength, color stability, water sorption, etc. These tests can be carried out in the laboratory in a reasonable amount of time and with minimal cost to ensure that the product has sufficient strength and resistance to deterioration for use in the mouth. Following the successful completion of this evaluation, the ADA Seal of Acceptance is awarded, and a label can be affixed to the package informing the clinician that this is so.

A second program exists to evaluate products for which no specification currently exists. This acceptance program requires that the manufacturer provide proof of physical stability, data showing biologic safety, or clinical results that meet specific guidelines. One example of a material to which the acceptance program pertains is the dentin adhesive. For acceptance, a manufacturer of an adhesive must provide for review data from at least two independent clinical evaluations in which the material was used in class V restorations. Acceptable success is defined as 95% retention at 6 months and 90% retention at 18 months.

An international body, the ISO (International Standards Organization), also develops specifications and testing standards for all materials, including those used in dentistry. The development of the European Community in the 1990s has generated an effort to merge many of the ADA's programs with those of the ISO's TC106, the technical committee for dental materials, instruments, and equipment.

The ultimate goal for all of these agencies is to establish guidelines for some minimal level of evaluation that has been deemed sufficient to ensure the safe use of a particular device. Obviously, the final proving ground is the oral cavity. But because of the similarity in compositions, the cost and time involved in evaluations, and the long history of safe use for many existing products, it is not surprising that every device does not undergo a clinical "road test" before being marketed to oral health care providers. Therefore, as stated previously, it is the responsibility of the provider to use devices that are made by manufacturers who support the certification and acceptance programs by having their products evaluated before marketing.

SELECTED READINGS

ADA website: http://www.ada.org
This is the official website of the American Dental Association. It has information on the ADA standards and acceptance programs for new materials.

American Dental Association. Dentist's Desk Reference: Materials, Instruments and Equipment. 2nd ed. Chicago: American Dental Association, 1983.
Put out by the Council on Dental Materials, Instruments and Equipment, this book explains the specification program and provides a comprehensive list of dental materials, including those that are ADA certified.

Craig RG (ed). Dental Materials Review. Ann Arbor, MI: The University of Michigan School of Dentistry, 1977.
This book is a collection of manuscripts presented at a symposium to review the state of the art of dental materials in 1977. The first chapter provides a history of the development of dental materials.

FDA website: http://www.fda.org
This is the official website of the Food and Drug Administration and has information relating to the programs used for new product approval.

Ring ME. Dentistry. An Illustrated History. St. Louis: Mosby-Year Book, 1985, 319 pages.
This book presents a complete illustrated history of dentistry, including dental materials.

Chapter 2

Characteristics of Materials

Objectives

- Describe the four classes of materials and give dental examples of each.
- Define thermal conductivity and the coefficient of thermal expansion and discuss their importance in dentistry, using clinical examples.
- Explain the significance of achieving adhesion in dentistry and list physical and clinical factors that determine successful adhesion.
- Define color in terms of hue, value, and chroma and give appropriate values for natural teeth.
- Compare tarnish and corrosion in terms of the extent and nature of the degradation they produce on a metallic restoration.
- Identify a galvanic cell and discuss its impact in terms of biocompatibility and degradation of existing restorations.
- Define stress and strain and identify elastic modulus, ultimate strength, percent elongation, toughness, resilience, and elastic limit on a stress-strain curve; describe the clinical significance of each for a dental restorative.

- Define hardness, fatigue, creep, and fracture toughness and explain their importance to dental materials.

- Identify and explain the factors that contribute to secondary decay in terms of the placement of a dental restoration.

- Explain the hydrodynamic theory of pulp pain and identify possible causes for sensitivity, given a set of clinical observations.

An object can occupy one of three different states: solid, liquid, or gas. We make use of all three in dentistry, although dental materials exist primarily as solids or liquids. The state of a material is a function of temperature. The more energy that is put into a material by increasing its temperature, the more difficult it is to keep the atoms or molecules in close proximity to one another. Thus, the atoms or molecules of a solid tend to move apart and expand as heat is applied. The addition of sufficient heat causes a solid to melt and become liquid. Further addition of heat to a liquid causes it to vaporize and become gas. Therefore, increasing the energy within a given material through the application of heat can have a destabilizing effect on both its structure and dimensions. The temperature at which a given material loses its dimensional and structural stability depends on its composition—its atomic "makeup," in other words. In fact, every characteristic of the material is dictated by its chemistry. This chapter introduces materials according to their chemical classification and describes how this affects their physical and mechanical characteristics. As the limitations and benefits of each class of material are explained, it will become more apparent why certain classes of materials are more useful than others for specific dental applications.

■ Classes of Materials—Examples in Dentistry

There are four classes of materials: **metals**, **ceramics**, **polymers**, and **composites**. Composites are mixtures of two or more of the first three classes in which the different components remain distinct from one another in the final structure. A common example is fiberglass, a polymer reinforced with fine glass fibers that remain physically separate and uniformly distributed throughout the polymer matrix.

Metals

Metals are the oldest of the three major classes of materials that have been used as dental materials. A **metal** is often defined by a certain set of characteristics, including high **thermal** and **electrical conductivity**, **ductility** (they can be bent without breaking), **opacity** (they do not transmit light), and **luster** (they have a surface that strongly reflects light and appears bright and shiny). Another characteristic of metals is that elements classified as such tend to dissolve to some extent in water or other aqueous solutions, producing atoms with a positive charge (i.e., cations). Nearly 80% of the elements in the periodic table are classified as metals. All metals are white (actually, gray), except for gold, which is yellow, and copper, which is reddish. Metals solidify with their atoms in a regular or **crystalline** arrangement, often in the form of a cube. The high strength of the **metallic bond** that holds the atoms together causes metals to have high melting temperatures. One metal, mercury, is liquid at room temperature, however, and is used in den-

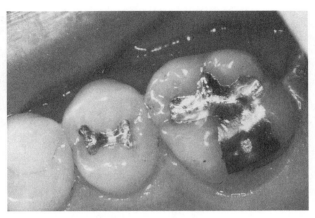

Figure 2–1 Small occlusal amalgam restoration in a premolar and larger amalgam restoration of a first molar.

tistry for the restoration of decayed teeth. Drops of mercury are mixed with particles of other metals, such as silver, tin, and copper, to produce a hard restorative material called **amalgam** (Fig. 2-1).

Because of their high strength and stability and the ease with which they can be formed or **cast** into many different shapes, metals are used extensively as structural components for the repair or replacement of tooth structure. They can be used as **crowns** to replace the outer coronal structure of a tooth (Fig. 2-2), specifically in the posterior region of the mouth where the metallic color is less objectionable. They can also be used more conservatively to replace portions of a tooth. When the portion of the tooth to be replaced is within the cusps, this type of restoration is called an **inlay** (Fig. 2-3). When one or more cusps is included in the restoration but the entire crown is not replaced, it is called an **onlay** (Fig. 2-4). Often a dentist must replace lost teeth. In these cases, he or she uses the remaining teeth as supports for metallic **bridges** that span the empty spaces to fill in the arch (Fig. 2-5). These bridges are permanently fixed on the teeth with a dental cement and, because they replace only a part of the dentition, are often called **fixed partials**. The missing teeth are replaced by metallic teeth, called **pontics**, which are

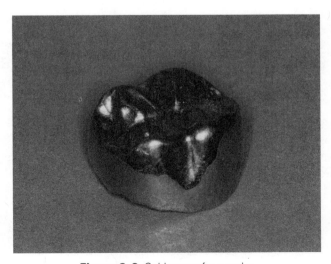

Figure 2–2 Gold crown for a molar.

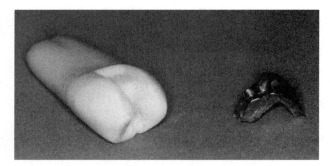

Figure 2–3 Gold inlay for a premolar and the die used to prepare it.

attached to the bridge either by casting it as one entire unit or by **soldering** the individual pieces together. In any case, it is the **rigidity** of the metal that allows it to be used in this way, similar to the manner in which it is used in bridges that span rivers and canyons. Because a dental bridge made entirely of metal is not esthetically satisfactory, it is common to **veneer** the surface of the metal with porcelain, producing a **PFM (porcelain-fused-to-metal)** restoration (Fig. 2-6). The porcelain must be baked onto the metal framework in an oven, just like pottery and dinnerware are produced. In this case, it is the high melting temperature of certain metals that allows them to be used for these applications without melting or deforming at the high firing temperatures used to bake the porcelain.

When a patient has several missing teeth, or when it is necessary to simulate lost gingival tissue with the dental **prosthesis** (often called a dental appliance), the dentist can make a **removable partial denture** (Fig. 2-7). A plastic is used to simulate the gums, and plastic or porcelain teeth are used to replace the missing natural teeth. The prosthesis is not permanently fixed to the teeth but instead is held in place by metal clasps that "hook" around existing teeth, thereby allowing it to be removed for cleaning. The metal clasps are an extension of the metal body or structural component of the removable partial denture, which provides it with strength and stability.

Most instruments and equipment used in dentistry are made of metals, usually stainless steel. Stainless steel is popular because it is abundant and economic.

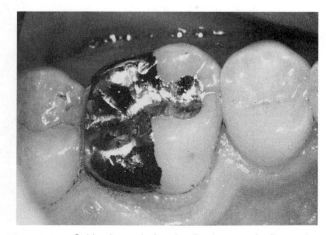

Figure 2–4 Gold onlay replacing the distal cusps of a first molar.

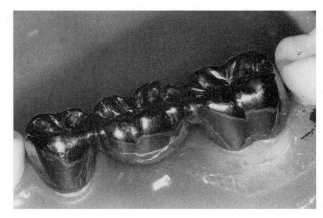

Figure 2–5 Three-unit gold bridge using the premolar and second molar as abutments, with a pontic replacing the first molar.

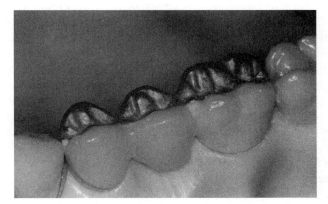

Figure 2–6 Facial view of a three-unit PFM bridge. The lingual cusps are metal, whereas the buccal cusps have been covered with porcelain for esthetic reasons.

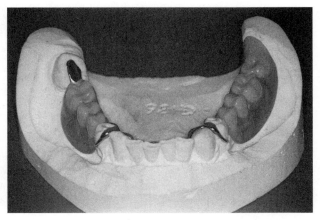

Figure 2–7 Removable partial denture mounted on a plaster cast.

In addition, steels are strong, corrosion resistant, biocompatible, cleanable, and easily sterilized and can be sharpened to produce cutting edges.

Ceramics

Although metals have many characteristics that make them useful in dentistry, they do not look like natural teeth. In contrast, a superb esthetic result can be achieved with **ceramics**. A ceramic is a compound formed by the union of a metallic and a nonmetallic element. Most of these materials are oxides, formed by the union of oxygen with metals such as silicon, aluminum, calcium, and magnesium. Glass, concrete, fine crystal, and gypsum are ceramics. **Porcelain** is a specific type of ceramic used extensively in dentistry and in other industries. Ceramics may be crystalline or noncrystalline (i.e., **amorphous**). The atoms that make up a ceramic may be bonded together by ionic or covalent bonds. Ceramics are generally very **brittle** materials, which means they cannot be bent or deformed to any extent without actually cracking and breaking. Everyone is aware of what happens when a ceramic dish or cup is dropped onto a hard floor; contrast that behavior with what happens when a metal fork or knife is dropped, and it is easy to understand the difference between brittle ceramics and ductile metals.

Ceramics are characterized by high melting points and low thermal and electrical conductivity. Therefore, they are used as **insulators** in many industries. Ceramics are manufactured by fusing oxide powders together in ovens at high temperatures. Most pigmenting agents used in dentistry are ceramic oxides. Their inclusion in appropriate ratios enables the ceramist to produce nearly any color imaginable. This quality also provides the dentist with the ability to match almost any tooth color with esthetic results that are unachievable with other materials. Finally, the fact that these materials are oxides means that they are **inert**, i.e., not very chemically reactive. This quality provides ceramics with an unequaled biologic compatibility, and sometimes the patient's body treats them as if they were actually the same as natural bone or tooth, which in essence are biologically produced ceramics.

Glass ceramics are used extensively as reinforcing agents, or fillers, for dental composites. They also are used in several dental cements and temporary restorative materials. As mentioned, ceramics have been used routinely as coatings or veneers to improve the esthetics of metallic dental restorations (Fig. 2-6) or as stand-alone veneers for anterior teeth (Fig. 2-8). The use of ceramics in dentistry has been some-

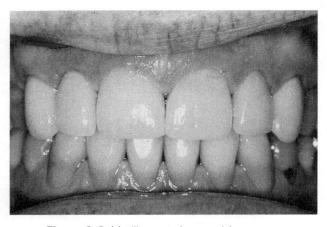

Figure 2–8 Maxillary anterior porcelain veneers.

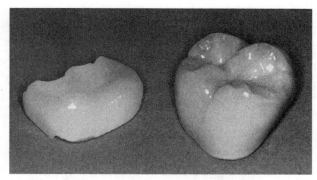

Figure 2–9 A cast ceramic onlay and a cast ceramic crown.

what limited to date, however, owing to their low fracture resistance as compared with that of metals. Recently, materials with improved fracture resistance have been developed for inlays, onlays, full crown restorations, and three-unit bridges (Fig. 2-9). Because of their excellent biologic properties, ceramics also are used extensively as implant materials, either alone or as coatings for metal substructures made from titanium that are placed directly into the mandible or maxilla.

Polymers

The last class of materials to be discussed is the newest addition to the series. Man-made **polymers** were first produced in the early to mid-1900s. Polymers are giant, long-chain organic molecules. Like ceramics, they are poor conductors of heat and electricity. Most are based on a structure containing thousands of carbon atoms linked together like beads on a string. Others, such as silicone polymers, are formed with silicon-oxygen bonds. Silicones are used in such diverse applications as caulking agents for bathrooms and as impression materials for dentistry (Fig. 2-10). Polymers are characterized by covalent bonds within each molecule, giving them tremendous strength in a single direction. This is demonstrated by the difficulty in trying to break a nylon fishing line by pulling on it. The interaction between each polymer chain is usually of a weaker nature, however, which reduces the structural and thermal stability of the materials in comparison with metals and ceramics.

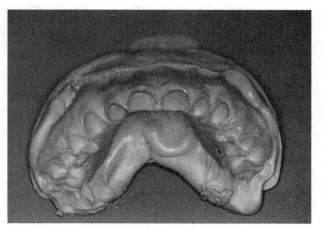

Figure 2–10 A full arch maxillary impression.

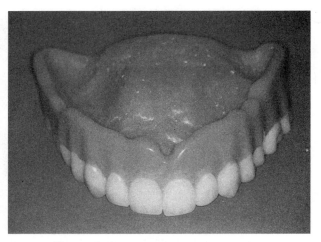

Figure 2–11 A full arch maxillary denture.

Because of their minimal stability and strength, polymers have not been used extensively in dentistry as permanent structural materials. They are used to make both the teeth and base of **dentures,** appliances that completely replace the teeth and gums of an edentulous person (Fig. 2-11). They are used extensively as temporary restorative materials for single restorations and bridges to be worn while the permanent metallic or ceramic restoration is being fabricated by a laboratory (Fig. 2-12). They are used as **adhesive** agents to enhance the bonding between various materials and tooth structure or as sealants of the pits and fissures present on the occlusal surfaces of permanent teeth (Fig. 2-13). When mixed with glass particles, polymers are formed into a dental composite that is used as an esthetic anterior restorative (Fig. 2-14) or as a posterior restorative material much in the same way as amalgam (Fig. 2-15). Their limited structural stability still restricts their use, but improvements in fracture and wear resistance have greatly expanded their applications.

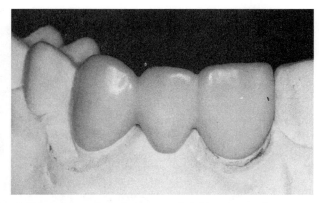

Figure 2–12 A three-unit temporary acrylic bridge mounted on a stone cast.

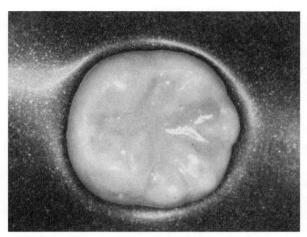

Figure 2–13 A pit and fissure sealant in a molar.

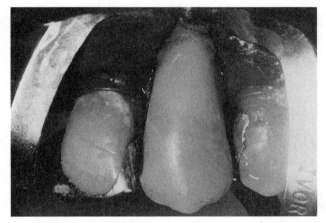

Figure 2–14 An esthetic class V composite restoration of a canine.

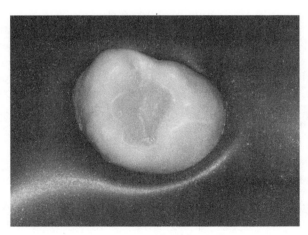

Figure 2–15 An esthetic composite restoration of a molar.

■ *Structure of Materials*

The structure of a material can be described on both a microscopic and a macroscopic level. On the microscopic level, we experience the material through the arrangement of its atoms and their bonding schemes. On the macroscopic level, we see a material as a solid, liquid, or gas that either has its own shape or takes on the shape of its container. It is beyond the scope of this text to address these issues in detail. It is appropriate, however, to review briefly the concepts of atomic bonding and microscopic structure with examples from dental materials.

Bonding

Primary atomic bonds provide the forces that hold solids together, whereas secondary bonds hold liquids together. Therefore, we associate the term "primary bond" with a certain amount of strength and stability. These bonds can take the form of **covalent**, **ionic**, or **metallic** interactions. A **covalent bond** is strong and stable and is the result of a sharing of electrons between two atoms. An example is the carbon-carbon bond that holds the backbone of the polymer chain together in a denture or dental composite. Another example is the strong silicon-oxygen bond that holds a porcelain inlay together. Strong bonds can also be generated by the interaction of a positive with a negative charge. One atom donates its electron to the other, and both atoms become stable through the linkage. This example of **ionic** bonding is characteristic of salts, such as sodium chloride table salt. These bonds are not relied on heavily in dentistry because they often are unstable in water. The bonding between **glass ionomer** or **polycarboxylate cements** and tooth structure, however, is an example of an ionic interaction between negatively charged atoms in the cement and positively charged atoms in the tooth structure. Finally, the **metallic bond** represents a different arrangement in which many atoms share all of their outer, or valence, electrons with their neighbors. The arrangement is very strong and stable, with the shared electrons free to move between and among the billions of atoms that make up the solid, never being tightly held to any specific atom. This accounts for the ability of a metal to conduct electricity and heat readily. All metals used in dentistry are held together by these bonds.

Secondary bonds are less stable than primary bonds because they involve weaker attractions of charge. Typical examples are van der Waals forces and hydrogen bonds. These interactions keep the molecules or atoms in a liquid from dispersing and becoming a gas, but they generally are not strong enough to keep the liquid confined without an external container. These bonds also are responsible for the adhesion between a liquid and a solid or between two solids that are not chemically attached. Secondary bonds are responsible for the limited strength of dental polymers because, although the long polymer chains contain internal covalent bonds, the bonds between individual chains are often of the secondary variety and, therefore, are much weaker and less stable. These interactions, however, are still important in dental materials.

Atomic Arrangements

When a material solidifies, it may do so in an irregular pattern or, conversely, with a regular arrangement of its atoms. When the arrangement is irregular, the material is described as **amorphous**. In other words, if one were to stand on an atom in the middle of the material and look out, it would appear different in every direction. To describe accurately this arrangement of atoms is not possible. Amorphous structures are best described as frozen liquids. Glass is an example. Most polymers used in dentistry also solidify in this manner. On a microscopic level, a polymer might be imagined as a bowl of spaghetti, with each noodle representing a separate polymer molecule and running off in a different, unpredictable direction.

When the atoms arrange themselves in a specific order during solidification, as occurs in metals, the view from any individual atom in the **crystal** appears the same no matter which way one looks. Picture a mound of stacked cannon balls, and then imagine standing on one cannon ball within the pile. The pile would look the same in any direction, simply appearing as another row or column of cannon balls. Each ball is equally spaced from the next in a regular arrangement, similar to the atoms within a crystalline solid. The usual arrangement in three dimensions is cubic, but more complicated crystals also are common. It is important to be able to identify the structure of a material because structure determines its physical and mechanical characteristics.

■ *Physical Characteristics*

The physical nature of a material is described by various properties, all of which play a role in defining its applications and limitations in dentistry. While reading these sections, keep in mind the list of ideal properties for a dental material presented in Display 1-1.

Thermal and Electrical Properties

Dental materials used intraorally do not need to be conductors of electricity. Those that do conduct electricity require the use of appropriate preventive measures to insulate them from the pulp, which contains the living cells in the tooth. Because of their atomic arrangement, in which the electrons are free, metals are good electrical conductors. It is possible to generate electrical currents and voltages in the oral cavity by a variety of means, one of the most common being the contact of metals of dissimilar composition. This can happen by touching a steel fork to an amalgam or by establishing contact between an amalgam in the maxilla and a gold restoration in the mandible during biting. The saliva facilitates the flow of electrons from one metal to the other, producing an electrical current. In a deep restoration in which there is little insulating dentin between the metallic restoration and the pulp, it is possible to generate sufficient current to flow through the tooth by this reaction to cause pain by stimulating the cells in the pulp chamber. *What can be done to prevent this?*

Because it is difficult to ensure that dissimilar metals never come into contact, a reasonable alternative is to insulate metallic restorations from the pulp. Normally, the remaining dentin in the cavity provides a natural insulator. When little dentin remains as a result of caries, however, cement bases can be used to perform the same role. Thus, an amalgam that is placed within approximately 1 mm of the pulp is often insulated with a *base*. Composite and ceramic restorations are nonconductive and do not need insulators.

The base under a metallic restoration serves another purpose, that of insulating the pulp from thermal insult. Heat and electricity are conducted the same way. Any tooth susceptible to electrically stimulated pain could also experience thermally stimulated pain. The thermal stimulus is far more frequent than the electrical one and is therefore of greater concern. **Thermal conductivity** is the characteristic that determines the rate at which heat flows through a material. It is a function of the composition, which determines the *heat capacity* (the amount of heat required to raise the temperature of an object by a certain amount), and of the magnitude of the temperature change and the thickness of the object. Consider the following example. A person with several large and deep amalgam restorations is chewing nachos, corn tortillas smothered in hot, melted cheese. Amalgam has a very low heat capacity—in other words, it readily warms up and quickly transmits the heat. The temperature change between the hot cheese at 55°C and the pulp at 37°C is large, thus providing a strong stimulus. If the amalgam is deep, the temperature below the amalgam may be raised to an unacceptable level while the cheese is in contact with the tooth. If the amalgam is shallow, however, the dentin below it, which has a high heat capacity, will absorb the heat instead of transmitting it to the pulp, thus minimizing the effect. *What can be done when the remaining dentin below the restoration is thin?*

Studies have shown that an insulating cement base of 0.75 to 1.0 mm is sufficient to minimize the effects of a rapid and extreme change in temperature at the surface of an amalgam during the ingestion of hot or cold foods and fluids (Fig. 2-16). Although many types of bases can be used, they appear to be of equivalent effectiveness. *If a base of 1 mm is helpful, why not use a base that is 2 to 3 mm thick to eliminate completely the potential for heat transfer through the restoration?*

Amalgams are brittle materials that must be applied in sufficient bulk to withstand the forces of mastication. Increasing the thickness of the base would reduce the bulk of the amalgam that could be used to fill the cavity, resulting in a shallow and weaker amalgam. Although the cavity could be made deeper, that would be unacceptable because it would require the removal of more tooth structure. Therefore, a compromise must be made, and the minimum amount of base is

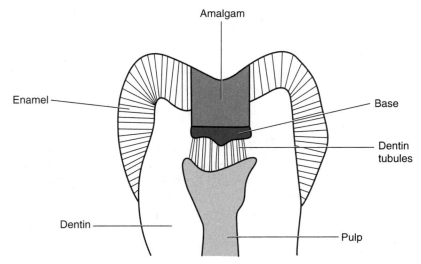

Figure 2-16 A base for thermal and mechanical insulation under an amalgam restoration.

TABLE 2–1. **Thermal Properties of Selective Dental Materials**

Material	Thermal Expansion $\alpha(\times 10^{-6}/°C)$	Thermal Conductivity k ([mcal · cm]/[cm^2 · sec · °C])
Tooth	8–11	1–2
Porcelain	6–15	2–3
Dental cement	10–12	1–3
Gold	14–16	710
Amalgam	22–28	55
Dental composite	20–50	1–3
Wax	250–400	1

used. Although metals do not meet the requirements of the ideal restorative materials in terms of their electrical and thermal properties, there are effective ways to offset this deficiency through the combined use of other materials that are similar to tooth structure in this regard. *Can you choose appropriate insulating base materials from the values for thermal conductivity provided in Table 2-1?*

Temperature also can have a profound effect on the dimensional accuracy of dental materials. A change in temperature can produce an immediate or delayed change in dimension. The magnitude of the change is determined by another thermal property, the *linear coefficient of thermal expansion*. This property describes the change in length of an object produced by a certain increase or decrease in its temperature. *What is the principle behind this property?*

Imagine this familiar example. If one were to place a balloon onto the neck of a soda bottle and then heat the bottle, what would happen? The air in the bottle expands during heating. Because the balloon can expand but the glass cannot, the expanding air fills the balloon. If the bottle were cooled down, assuming there were no leaks, the air would contract and the balloon would deflate. All matter behaves in this way. The application or removal of heat causes any object to expand or contract, respectively. The rate at which this occurs depends on the composition of the material. We can assume that objects with different coefficients of thermal expansion will expand and contract at different rates in response to temperature changes. Consider the example of a composite restoration. The seal between the composite and tooth may be compromised over time by the repeated temperature changes in the mouth, which cause different amounts of expansion and contraction of the composite and the tooth. This difference may create gaps between the two, which leads to leakage of salivary components into the tooth toward the pulp (Fig. 2-17). *Can you suggest which dental materials provide the most ideal match for the tooth, based on the table of thermal expansion coefficients (Table 2-1)?*

Thermal changes can also have an effect on the components of the tooth, specifically the fluid contents of the dentinal tubules. Expansion and contraction of these fluids under an unsealed restoration can cause tooth pain. This topic will be discussed later in this chapter.

Solubility and Sorption

One of the requirements for a dental restorative material is that it be stable in the oral environment. In other words, it should undergo a minimal amount of dimensional change and chemical alteration. All dental materials are **soluble** to some extent and dissolve in water. The least soluble of all dental materials are the

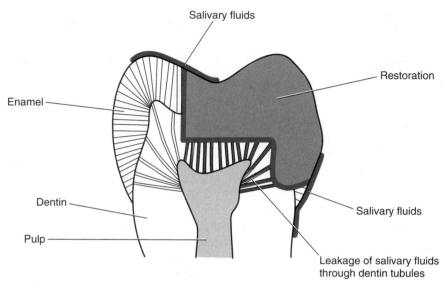

Salivary fluids

Restoration

Enamel

Dentin

Pulp

Salivary fluids

Leakage of salivary fluids through dentin tubules

Figure 2–17 Salivary microleakage along the margins of a tooth and restoration.

porcelains and ceramics, although even they dissolve elements into solution on a regular basis. In contrast, unreacted molecules in polymers may be readily extracted or dissolved into oral fluids. The loss of small organic molecules from soft tissue conditioners and denture liners is responsible for them hardening in the mouth and becoming irritating. Metallic ions are slowly released from cast restorations and amalgams. Although there are case reports of allergic reactions to amalgams, composites, orthodontic appliances, and the like, and people can be irritated by the residual molecules that dissolve from incompletely cured denture-base resins, there is no evidence to show that any compound or element can be extracted from any dental material in sufficient quantity to cause a systemic disease. In fact, the extraction of some agents, such as fluoride ions from glass ionomer restoratives, may have therapeutic effects. There is much interest in the further development of "timed-release" dental materials, restorations, or liners containing dental therapeutics that are released to the oral tissues as the material slowly dissolves over time. Future development of such materials may result in restoratives that inhibit further decay and perhaps even replace lost tooth structure through remineralization.

Certain materials will also absorb molecules. **Sorption** is the uptake of fluids or substances by a material. This process is usually confined to polymeric materials but can also occur at the union between two materials, such as the porcelain and metal interface on a PFM restoration. In the latter example, sorption may lead to a subtle discoloration of the porcelain. The result of sorption in a polymeric material is often a swelling or increase in dimension. It has been suggested that the uptake of fluids from saliva may cause a slow expansion of composite restorations that improves their adaptation to the tooth, thus enhancing the seal at the margin.

The uptake of foreign agents can also lead to chemical disintegration, such as that occurring in dental cements at the margin between the cast restoration and the tooth. This "washout" of cement is believed to be responsible for the eventual loosening of the restoration and possible decay of the supporting tooth structure. The latter is a result of the penetration of microorganisms and their by-products into the open space. Therefore, the ideal dental material would neither dissolve into nor take components up from its environment, unless specifically designed to do so (e.g., for the purpose of remineralization). The ceramics and metals would be most ideal by these guidelines, although some concerns have been expressed about the ions released from metallic materials.

Adhesion

Adhesion is defined as the force of attraction between the molecules or atoms on two different surfaces as they are brought into contact. Contrast this with **cohesion**, which is the force of attraction between the molecules or atoms within a given material (i.e., not on the surface). An example is useful to highlight the difference. An orthodontic bracket is adhered to an upper bicuspid with cement but within a few days falls off. By examination of the failed surfaces, the orthodontist can ascertain a potential cause for the failure. If the bracket is clean and contains no remnants of the cement, the failure was adhesive, occurring at the interface between the bracket and the cement (Fig. 2-18). This might suggest that the bracket had been contaminated before placement, ruining its adhesion with the cement. Failure of the interface between the cement and the tooth would be verified by the absence of cement on the tooth, probably as a result of poor tooth surface preparation or contamination of the tooth itself. Finally, if a cement layer remains on both the tooth and the bracket, it suggests that the adhesion to both surfaces was good but that the cohesive forces within the cement itself were exceeded, causing it to break.

Strong, durable adhesion between two materials can be achieved through chemical or mechanical means. Often the word *bonding* is used, even though no primary chemical bonds are formed between two surfaces.

> There are several reasons why it is desirable to produce primary chemical bonds between an adhesive and the substrate, or *adherend*, to which it will be attached. First, strong adhesion increases the likelihood that a given restoration or appliance will be retained on the teeth. Second, strong chemical adhesion eliminates the need for excessive removal of tooth structure to ensure retention through mechanical *undercuts*, sites at which the adhesive can be locked into and held in place by friction. Therefore, chemical adhesion conserves tooth structure. Third, adhesion promotes the sealing of a margin, minimizing the chance for penetration or leakage of bacterial microorganisms or their damaging by-products.

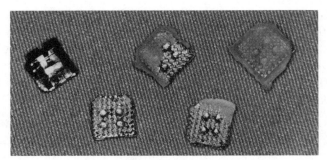

Figure 2–18 Orthodontic brackets that have been debonded from a tooth, showing evidence of complete adhesive failure from the bracket (second from left) to complete adhesive failure from the tooth (fifth from left).

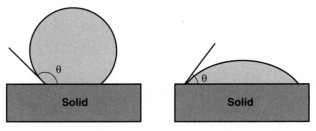

Figure 2–19 A liquid on two surfaces showing a high and low contact angle.

Many factors determine the effectiveness of the adhesion between two surfaces. The most important is probably the degree to which the adhesive wets the surface of the adherend. **Wetting** is characterized by the extent to which an adhesive will spread out on a surface. The angle made between the adhesive and the surface can be measured to give a value for wetting. This angle is called the **contact angle** (Fig. 2-19). Good wetting is characterized by contact angles below 90°, with the best spreading to an angle approaching 0°. Poor wetting occurs when the angle is obtuse. An example of the latter is the way water beads up on a car on the first rainy day after the car is waxed.

Adhesion also depends on achieving intimate contact between the two surfaces and is enhanced when the area of the contacting surfaces is large. Obviously, good wetting is a requirement for adhesion because in its absence it is not possible to put the two surfaces within the atomic and molecular distances required to achieve chemical interactions. Even in the absence of chemical bonding, it is important to have good wetting to increase the contact area between the two surfaces, thus maximizing the frictional forces that will keep them together. *What factors might be important for achieving good wetting and ultimately good adhesion?*

Essentially, anything that makes it difficult for the two surfaces to come into contact will compromise adhesion. A dirty or contaminated surface is a deterrent to wetting because it reduces the surface energy of the adherend. Surface atoms and molecules have higher energies than those in the interior because all of their potential chemical bonds are not satisfied. In other words, they have no neighbors above them to bond with, so they are unstable and prefer to be covered with something. This can be dirt or, in the mouth, plaque. That is why the enamel of the teeth normally is covered with a very thin layer of **pellicle**, an organic mixture of substances deposited from the saliva. To adhere a material to the enamel, it is necessary to clean the surface by removing the pellicle, thus increasing the enamel's **surface energy**. Similarly, the adhesive has a surface energy of its own. It is often referred to as **surface tension**, the attraction that atoms and molecules on the surface of a liquid have for one another. A high surface tension would mean that the surface atoms or molecules are strongly held together and do not want to be displaced. A liquid like this would "ball up" instead of spreading out. Mercury is a good example of a liquid with a high surface tension. *How desirable would a high surface tension be for a dental adhesive?*

As one might expect, a high surface tension would inhibit the spreading and, therefore, the wetting ability of an adhesive and would be undesirable for promoting adhesion. An adhesive with a low surface tension and an adherend with a high surface energy provide the best possible situation for good adhesion.

Because it is desirable for the adhesive to spread out onto the substrate, its **viscosity** is important. Viscosity is a measure of a liquid's resistance to forces that tend to cause it to flow. An adhesive with a high viscosity would have a high resistance to flow and would be less likely to spread out on a surface. Conversely, if the viscosity is too low, it may be hard to control the placement of the adhesive.

Finally, the dimensional change the adhesive undergoes after it is placed may dictate whether it remains attached or pulls away from the surface. Most dental adhesives are composed of polymeric materials that shrink during hardening. This shrinkage can pull them away from the cavity preparation, compromising adhesion. Obviously, the development of polymers that do not shrink during hardening would facilitate the placement and stability of dental composites and other restorations.

Color and Esthetics

Much of dentistry today is driven by the desire to have esthetically acceptable restorations in all areas of the mouth. It is possible to simulate a natural appearance only if one understands the factors that affect visual perception of these structures. A full description of these factors would encompass a text in itself. Basically, one must understand what light is and how it interacts with different structures. Start with the basic premise that color exists only if three conditions are satisfied. First, there must be an object, often called a "modifier" because it interacts with a light source. The second necessary condition is a light source; the next time you are stumbling around in near darkness, notice that the objects that you can see appear only in various shades of gray, essentially devoid of color. Last, there must be someone with the capacity to observe or receive the modified light coming from the object. ***Does color exist to totally color-blind persons?***

No, because they cannot perceive it, although they do see the object itself. It is not uncommon for people to have some form of color blindness, or color anomaly. The fact that different people perceive the same color somewhat differently is testimony to that fact. That is why it is important to have objective measures of color, such as with standardized paint chips or a color-measuring instrument like the spectrophotometer, to define a color without bias.

Several different color-measuring systems are available, with the most popular being the Munsell (a visual system) and the CIE (a spectrophotometric system). The CIE system uses somewhat expensive equipment to define how much red, blue, and yellow a certain object appears to contain. Red, blue, and yellow are referred to as the primary colors because any color can be made by adding the correct amounts of each primary. The Munsell system is based on a well-defined series of color tabs, like paint chips, that are precisely arranged. This practical system is composed of three indices defined as **hue**, **value**, and **chroma**. **Hue** refers to the dominant color of the object. In other words, is it red, yellow, or blue? Natural teeth do not vary much in terms of their hue, generally being in the yellow to yellow-red range. **Value** refers to the lightness of a color, on a scale from 1 to 10, with 1 = black and 10 = white. As you might expect, natural teeth are generally high in value, in the range of 6 to 8 for most people. **Chroma** refers to the intensity of the color on a scale from 1 to 10, where 10 means saturated. In other words, is the object rich in color or somewhat pale? Natural teeth are relatively low in chroma, in the range of 1 to 3. Dental personnel and technicians must be aware of these ranges to communicate effectively with one another.

Also, teeth are composed of layers of different structures. The appearance of the incisal edge is dictated by enamel, which is translucent. **Translucency** refers to the fact that light entering the tooth may be affected in several ways. Part of the light may be **transmitted** completely through the object, whereas part of it may be **reflected** from its surface and not penetrate at all. Still another part of the light may enter the object and be **scattered** and subsequently absorbed. If the tooth were clear, it would be **transparent**, like glass, and there would be virtually no absorption of the light. Conversely, if the tooth did not transmit any light, it would be **opaque**, and totally absorbing.

Because enamel is more transparent than dentin, one's perception of the incisal edges of anterior teeth is most influenced by the enamel (Fig. 2-20). These edges are the most translucent portions of the teeth and actually appear bluish in color. Light passing through the middle portion of the tooth is influenced by both the outer enamel shell and the inner dentin. Because the dentin is more opaque, less light passes through this portion of the tooth, and the tooth does not appear very translucent. If a tooth were replaced with a material of a uniform translucency, it would not appear natural. The gingival portion of the tooth usually appears more reddish than the rest of the tooth. The reason for this can easily be determined by looking in the mirror and smiling: The gums are reddish and cast a reddish hue onto the tooth at the gumline. *With this in mind, do you think it would be more appropriate to try to match the shade of a tooth before or after placing a rubber dam?*

> If the gingiva can influence the appearance of the tooth, then so can the rubber dam. The important factor is that the dam is not natural, so it is necessary to do all shade matching before placing the rubber dam to ensure the most natural reproduction of tooth color.

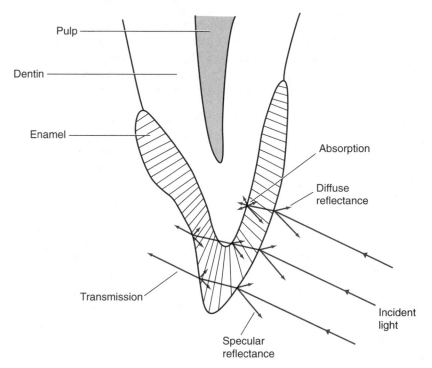

Figure 2–20 Interaction of light with different regions of the tooth.

Today, composites and ceramics can be made with varying degrees of translucency for use in specific portions of a tooth. Opaquing agents, usually metal oxide particles such as titanium oxide, are added to block light penetration. Often these materials are used to cover up a metal structure and make it appear white instead of metallic. Different-colored ceramics or composites can then be added to the opaque layer to make the restoration look more natural.

Many other factors influence color perception, but they are beyond the scope of this chapter. Suffice it to say that this area of dentistry has taken on greater importance in recent years with the increased demand for esthetically pleasing results. Therefore, a basic understanding of color theory is essential for optimizing the appearance of dental restorations.

Corrosion

Tools, automobiles, bridges, dental appliances, and many other everyday objects are made from steels and similar metals. Although these materials are very durable, they can undergo surface and structural deterioration when they are unprotected and left exposed to the environment. The deterioration of a metal by a chemical or electrochemical reaction is termed **corrosion**. Another type of deterioration that involves only the surface and whose end result is usually discoloration is called **tarnish**. Tarnish is responsible for the yearly sale of millions of dollars' worth of products used to clean silver objects in our homes. The difference between corrosion and tarnish is basically one of extent, with corrosion being irreversible and of much greater concern. This was touched on briefly when the solubility of metals was discussed and concerns were raised over the biologic effects of the ions released. Solubility, however, refers to a passive loss of ions, whereas corrosion refers to an active deterioration that produces ions at a faster rate.

With the exception of the noble metals, discussed later, most dental metals corrode in the warm, salty, and acidic oral cavity. The rate is usually very slow, however, and the consequences are minimal. This is true of all implant metals for medical and dental applications. We generally do not find "rust" in the oral cavity. Rust is essentially a brownish iron oxide compound formed when steel or iron (the main element in steel) is exposed to an environment containing two essential ingredients: water and oxygen. Because both of these molecules are present in the oral cavity, we cannot use simple steel or iron appliances. Steel can be made corrosion resistant, however, by the inclusion of chromium. Chromium is responsible for the stainless quality, or corrosion resistance, of stainless steel. When sufficient chromium is added to steel, it forms an oxide "skin," or barrier, on the surface of the object, which keeps it from actively corroding. In other words, the surface has been made passive or has been **passivated**. Most dental metals, with the exception of noble metals and amalgam, are corrosion resistant because of the formation of a passive, protective film on their surface. The film is extremely thin and completely transparent, so it cannot be seen with the naked eye or with any type of microscope. However, certain types of spectrometers that can identify the presence of elements in small concentrations can be used to verify its existence and composition.

The passive film usually can reform quickly if it is broken or disrupted. One impediment to this "healing" process, however, is the presence of chlorine, which inhibits the reformation of the film and accelerates corrosion. Chlorine is also responsible for producing the tarnish discoloration seen on many partial dentures soaked repeatedly in certain denture cleansers. This poses a potential problem for many of our dental metals because chlorine is present in abundance in the oral cavity. The significance of chlorine-enhanced corrosion is reduced by the fact that there are other molecules present in saliva that help protect the metal. Therefore, the composition of the solution in which the corrosion occurs is of primary importance in determining its extent and effects. This solution is called an **electrolyte**, and it is one of four essential components required to establish a corrosion cell.

Electrochemical corrosion involves oxidation-reduction reactions that take place at the surface of objects in an electrolyte. Therefore, two different materials are needed in addition to the solution. The final component of the cell is an electrical connection between the two materials (Fig. 2-21). Because electrical current involves the flow of electrons, there must be a path, or connection, to carry the electrons. The corrosion cell, then, consists of two metals in contact in a solution. When two different metals are connected, a difference in voltage occurs between the two, and a current will flow between them. The greater the difference in voltage, i.e., the more dissimilar the metals in terms of their rate of dissolution, the greater the flow of current will be. Because one metal is more active than the other, it will dissolve or be corroded first. This metal is referred to as the **anode** in the reaction, and it is at this surface that the metal is oxidized and metal ions are generated. The other metal serves as the **cathode**, or the site at which reduction occurs. The two reactions must occur together.

If a patient were to have an amalgam restoration completely across the occlusal surface of a premolar (i.e., a mesial-occlusal-distal or MOD restoration), and the restoration were in contact with a gold crown in an adjacent molar, an active corrosion situation would be established. One would expect the gold crown, the more corrosion-resistant metal, to serve as the cathode and the amalgam to serve as the actively corroding anode (Fig. 2-22). The metallic contact represents the path, and the saliva is the electrolyte. This coupling of two dissimilar metals is called a **galvanic cell** and is similar to a battery. A battery generated in the mouth is cause for concern because there is an accelerated release of ions, which often is

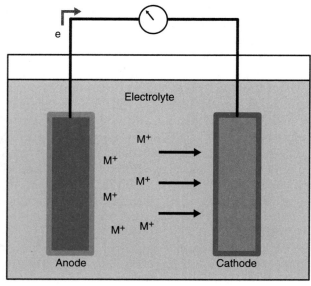

Figure 2–21 An electrochemical corrosion cell.

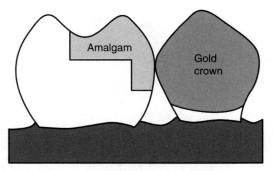

Figure 2–22 A galvanic cell established between an amalgam and gold crown in contact.

sensed as a metallic taste; a more rapid destruction of the less corrosion-resistant metal; and the possibility for pain produced by the flow of electric current. The patient usually does not experience perceptible effects, but it still is desirable to avoid these situations. In addition, although corrosion is accelerated, deterioration to the point where replacement of the amalgam restoration is required would take many years. Usually, this situation may cause slight sensitivity, which subsides with time. In certain cases, however, immediate measures must be taken to alleviate the pain.

An example helps to illustrate this phenomenon. A patient has a new class II amalgam (mesial-occlusal) placed in an upper first molar. Within a month, a full gold crown restoration is placed on the adjacent premolar, in direct contact with the amalgam. The patient returns to the office the following day complaining of a metallic taste and pain in the tooth with the amalgam. The dentist places a wooden wedge between the molar and premolar, separating the teeth, and the patient notes that the pain ceases. Upon removal of the wedge, contact is established between the two teeth, and the patient again complains of pain. The dentist replaces the wedge and paints a layer of dental adhesive bonding resin on the surfaces of the amalgam and gold crown that are in contact. The resin is hardened with a visible light-curing source, and the wedge is removed. The patient's pain is relieved as a result of the insulating effect of the very thin resin layer. In time, movement between the teeth will cause the resin to wear away. The teeth usually do not become sensitive again, however, since the alloy surfaces oxidize to provide natural insulation and the teeth have settled down after the placement of the restorations.

Another type of corrosion common in the oral cavity is called **crevice corrosion**. Whenever a gap, slot, or groove exists next to or on a metal, a crevice is present. A typical example is the margin around an amalgam restoration. Within the crevice, the oxygen concentration is lower than it is on the outside, and the acidity is usually greater. Plaque often collects at these sites, further increasing the acidity. This causes accelerated corrosion within the crevice. The corrosion is somewhat beneficial for the amalgam because the corrosion products, usually metal oxides, fall into and fill up the crevice to seal out bacterial leakage from the saliva. Thus, corrosion may actually improve the longevity of the restoration by reducing the potential for **secondary decay** (i.e., recurrent caries). The metallic ions themselves also may serve as bacteriostatic or bactericidal agents. Conversely, this process probably accelerates the deterioration of the margins (Fig. 2-23). This type of deterioration also can be harmful when it occurs in thin sections of appli-

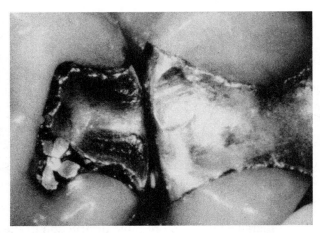

Figure 2–23 An amalgam restoration showing extensive deterioration at the margins.

ances or at solder joints, where the structure can become weakened because of the loss of material to corrosion.

The concept of crevice corrosion implies that it is generally desirable to achieve and maintain smooth, clean metallic surfaces in the oral cavity. This is one reason for polishing amalgam restorations after placement. Even a smooth surface, however, can tarnish and corrode if conditions are right. Note the blackening on amalgam surfaces caused by sulfide tarnishing, especially when the patient does not practice adequate oral hygiene. An understanding of the causes and results of intraoral corrosion may be a powerful tool for the practitioner to motivate the patient toward improved hygiene.

■ *Mechanical Characteristics*

Numerous tests of mechanical properties can be used to characterize a material. Many times, these tests are useful predictors of the likelihood of clinical success for a given material. In most cases, however, they simply provide a relative measure of the suitability of that material for its specified function. The oral environment is complex, and we have only a cursory knowledge of the absolute requirements for each type of restoration. Although we can generate a list of ideal characteristics, they provide only relative guidelines. Most of the information that exists to guide the clinician's selection of materials is based on experience and the evaluation of failures. This does not mean that subjecting a material to a full battery of mechanical testing is a waste of time. These tests provide useful and important information to be used for comparison with other materials that may have succeeded or failed. Such testing also ensures that the material meets some minimal level of quality control and performance, which falls under the purview of the specification program previously discussed. The dental health care provider, however, must be cognizant of the limitations that accompany this information, especially when making a decision about a new product. This section describes many of the mechanical properties that are routinely examined. Where appropriate, their usefulness in predicting clinical success is emphasized. First, some terminology must be introduced with respect to the application of force and its effect on a material.

Types of Forces

There are three basic types of **forces**. A force that tends to pull an object apart is referred to as **tensile** (Fig. 2-24*A*). An object pulled by such a force exists in a state of tension. When the application of force is down on the object, tending to squeeze it together, it is called **compressive**, and an object subjected to this force is said to be in compression (Fig. 2-24*B*). Bending is a combination of these two forces. A beam that is bent, such as a dental bridge spanning the space between two teeth, experiences a compressive force on the top surface under the opposing tooth, whereas the bottom of the bridge, where the pontic is connected to the abutment teeth, is put in tension. The third type of force tends to slide the top of an object over the bottom and is called **shear** (Fig. 2-24*C*). Consider the analogy of placing a deck of cards on a table and pushing on the top card, causing the rest of the cards to slide over one another. Most forces in the oral cavity are complex and are made up of a combination of these forces.

Stress and Strain

Forces of equal magnitude can be applied over two different-sized pieces of the same material and produce different effects. Specifically, the smaller or thinner piece is more prone to be broken or bent because there is less material to support the force. Therefore, it is more appropriate to describe force application in terms that are independent of the size of the object. This is easily accomplished by dividing the force, measured in pounds or kilograms (kg), by the area over which it is applied, measured in inches or meters (m). This force per area is defined as **stress**. The units are pounds/inch^2 (psi) or kg/m^2. Another popular unit is the megapascal (MPa), which can be calculated by dividing the stress value in psi by 145 (i.e., 1 MPa = 145 psi). Whenever an object is exposed to a force, stress is generated within the object to counter the force and keep the object together. Therefore, stress is the material's response to a force. When the stress exceeds the cohesive strength of the object, the object breaks.

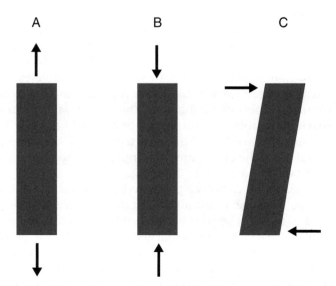

Figure 2–24 The three main types of forces: tensile (**A**), compressive (**B**), and shear (**C**).

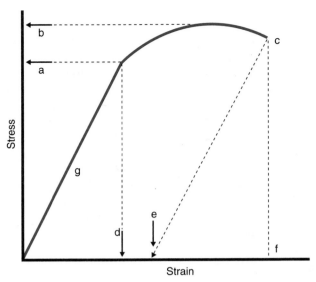

Figure 2–25 A stress-strain diagram identifying elastic limit (*a*), ultimate strength (*b*), fracture stress (*c*), maximum flexibility (*d*), percent elongation (ductility) (*e*), strain at failure (*f*), modulus of elasticity (*g*).

Another result of applying a force to an object is that the object experiences some deformation or change in dimension, called **strain**. This strain is calculated as a change in length divided by an initial length and is measured in the "units" of inches/inches, or m/m (i.e., no units, usually given as a percent). The ability of an object to resist dimensional change under a given stress is related to its stiffness. For any material, it is possible to monitor the change in dimension for a given application of stress and plot a curve (Fig. 2-25). This **stress-strain diagram** provides many useful pieces of information to characterize the mechanical properties of a material.

Stress-Strain Diagram

The example of an orthodontic wire being bent will be used to examine the stress-strain diagram. As the wire is bent to exert stress, it begins to deform slightly. If one were to let go of the wire after this minimal bending, the wire would spring back to its original shape, like a rubber band that is stretched and released. Therefore, the change in dimension, or strain, was completely elastic and recoverable. This region of the stress-strain curve is linear, and the slope of the line is a measure of the stiffness of the material. The proper name for the stiffness of a material is **elastic modulus**, sometimes referred to as Young's modulus. The units of the elastic modulus are MPa/m/m (stress/strain), or MPa, similar to stress. Representative values of the elastic modulus and other properties are compared for several types of dental materials in Table 2-2.

The elastic modulus is a good predictor of a material's ability to resist bending or change in shape and is an important property for dental bridges, orthodontic wires, and many other restorations and appliances. Eventually, as one continues to bend the wire, a point is reached at which letting go of the wire allows it to spring back, but not completely, to its original shape. In other words, enough stress has been generated to exceed the **elastic limit** of the material. The elastic limit is defined as the maximum stress level at which complete recovery of strain occurs on release of the stress. This property also is a useful predictor of the ap-

TABLE 2–2. **Approximate Values for Mechanical Properties of Selective Dental Materials**

Material	Elastic Modulus (GPa)	Tensile Strength (MPa)	Compressive Strength (MPa)	Elastic Limit (MPa)	Knoop Hardness (kg/mm^2)
Tooth					
Dentin	20	10	300	170	70
Enamel	80	40–50	385	350	350
Porcelain	70–95	25–40	150	145	590
Cement	1–14	1–12	5–120	5–120	25–40
Gold	75–100	220–900	—	70–600	75–345
Amalgam	25–35	45–55	300–450	250–400	165
Composite	5–15	45–65	200–300	150–200	40–80
Acrylic	2	20–25	75	50	20

propriateness of a material for structural application in dentistry; it describes the stress necessary to cause a permanent change in dimension. The strain associated with the stress at the elastic limit is called the **maximum flexibility** and is a measure of the maximum elastic strain that can be produced. Impression materials, which often must be severely deformed to be removed from undercuts, must have the capacity to spring back without suffering any permanent change in shape or loss of accuracy.

Through the application of sufficient stress, a small but permanent change in the wire's dimension is produced. This permanent strain is called **plastic deformation**. Despite the fact that the material has been deformed, however, it has not broken. If one were to put greater stress on the wire, eventually a stress level would be reached at which the wire breaks apart. This point is the **ultimate strength**, the maximum stress that can be withstood before breaking. The total plastic deformation that accompanies this stress level is called the **percent elongation**, or **ductility**, and is a measure of the amount of dimensional change that the wire can undergo before breaking. As one might expect on the basis of this discussion, glasses and ceramics cannot undergo plastic deformation without breaking and, therefore, have a low ductility. Materials with low ductility are defined as **brittle**. The ultimate strength of a ceramic is similar to its elastic limit, since any stress above its elastic limit causes it to break.

Other data obtained from the stress-strain curve are **toughness** and **resilience**. These are obtained by calculating the area under the entire curve (toughness) or under the linear portion of the curve (resilience). Toughness is a measure of the amount of energy that the material can absorb without breaking. Resilience is a measure of the amount of elastic energy that a material can absorb and subsequently deliver to another object—for example, to cause movement of teeth in orthodontic applications.

All of these data can be generated by one experiment to provide useful information for characterizing a material. Similar experiments can be performed in compression and in tension. These tests will provide data on the compressive strength and modulus and tensile strength and modulus. Because many applications of dental materials require them to be resistant to bending forces, the flexural test has become popular in recent years. In addition, because most dental materials have higher compressive strengths than tensile strengths and because most restorations that fail mechanically do so because of tensile or flexural forces, the appropriateness of the compressive properties of a material as a predictor of clinical performance is questionable.

Other Properties

There are additional properties useful for comparing materials and tooth structures, which must be determined by other tests.

Hardness

Hardness refers to the ability of a material to resist forces of indentation. Hardness often is equated with being resistant to wear and abrasion, but this is not necessarily true, especially for posterior composites. An evaluation of the hardness of a dental material is appropriate, however, in that some minimal level is required to ensure that a material is not excessively affected by chewing food and toothbrushing. The low hardness of denture-base material correlates with its low toothbrush abrasion resistance, and denture-wearing patients must take care not to be overly aggressive during the cleaning of these prosthetic devices by using brushes with hard bristles. Hardness also is an important property to consider for **model** and **die** materials on which crown and bridge patterns are made, because a soft surface may become scratched or chipped, compromising the accuracy of the final restoration.

Fatigue

Fatigue is common among students, long-distance runners, and certain dental materials. The repeated application of stress to an object causes tiny cracks to be generated within its structure. These tiny cracks do not cause failure initially. With each application of stress, however, the cracks grow until eventually the material breaks. This is analogous to the repeated application of mental stress leading to a climactic nervous breakdown. Fatigue can be avoided through the appropriate design of restorations and selection of materials. Metals, plastics, and ceramics can all fail by fatigue. It is one of the most difficult properties to test but possibly the most important for predicting clinical longevity.

Creep

Creep is defined as the gradual but permanent change in dimension that occurs in an object subjected to a constant load. Most materials undergo creep only at temperatures approaching their melting points, so this is not of concern for ceramics and most metals used in dentistry. Creep can and does occur, however, in dental amalgam and plastic dental materials.

Fracture Toughness

A material's **fracture toughness** is an intrinsic property that describes its ability to resist the propagation, or movement, of an existing crack or flaw. There is some evidence that it may become a useful predictor of the clinical behavior of composites used in situations in which they are subjected to high stress (e.g., class I, II, and IV restorations). In general, high fracture toughness indicates good resistance to cracking.

Wear

Wear is a complex phenomenon that occurs when two surfaces are brought into direct contact (two-body) or into indirect contact with a third body acting between them. A common example of two-body wear is sandpaper directly removing material from a piece of wood or metal. A common example of three-body wear is toothpaste being dragged between the tooth surface and the toothbrush bristles to remove material from the surface of the tooth. Wear depends on many factors, including the hardness, strength, and roughness of the two surfaces and the abrasive third body, the force being applied to the surfaces, and the presence or absence of a lubricant, such as water. Many types of wear can occur in the oral cavity. The two most common are abrasion and attrition. Abrasion usually occurs under low forces and results in the removal of material by the scratching and gouging of one surface by the second surface or the abrasive third body. Attrition usually refers to wear under heavier loads and involves fatigue-like failures, especially in sites of direct contact between two surfaces.

■ *Biologic Characteristics*

Concerns over the biologic effects of dental materials have always existed, but the ability to test for and predict these effects is rudimentary at best. Clearly, the optimum way to ascertain whether the physical and mechanical characteristics of a given material are adequate is through use (i.e., clinical trials). The complicated nature of the host-foreign body response makes this even truer for the biologic characteristics. Specific examples of situations where a risk from the use of a material exists will be identified throughout this text. In general, the incidence of these occurrences is small and most often related to an allergic response or to hypersensitivity. The more common manifestation of a biologic response to dental restorations is the formation of secondary caries and pain associated with postoperative sensitivity. Before considering individual materials, it is appropriate to review briefly some of the factors that influence these two conditions.

The importance of a seal between the restoration and the tooth tissue was alluded to earlier in this chapter. It is generally believed that the largest concern with regard to dental restoratives is not their own toxicity or lack of biocompatibility but their inability to seal margins adequately, thus allowing the leakage of bacteria or their by-products, which cause secondary decay. Several animal studies have shown the presence of bacteria on the pulpal floor or within the dentinal tubules to be associated with inflammatory responses in the pulp of teeth. In other cases where bacteria have been sealed out, the tooth has been stimulated by the dental treatment and the presence of the restorative material or its base. This stimulation results in the production of **secondary** or **reparative dentin**, without any acute or chronic inflammatory response. The type of material seems to be of little importance. Therefore, the key factor in the reduction or elimination of secondary decay, other than the caries susceptibility and oral flora of the patient, is probably the ability to seal completely the margins of the restoration. Amalgams do this by a process of corrosion that fills open margins, whereas composites or cemented restorations rely on the creation of a tight junction with the tooth to eliminate any gaps. Historically, clinicians have been able to adhere materials to the enamel substrate with greater effectiveness than to the dentin substrate. This underlines the difficulty encountered when using certain restorative materials in cavities that extend beyond the dentin-enamel or cementum-enamel junctions. In these cavities, sealing of the margins has posed a great challenge.

Postoperative sensitivity is a common problem for dental clinicians and patients. Its cause is sometimes difficult to ascertain, but there are several explanations. One theory that has gained much support is the **hydrodynamic theory** of pulp pain. The pulp chamber is under a constant physiologic pressure. This pressure tends to force the fluids that surround the odontoblastic processes within the dentinal tubules in a coronal, or outward, direction. Normally, the enamel of the tooth provides a sealing cap for the dentinal tubules, and the fluids do not seep out. Anything that removes the enamel, however, either caries or dental procedures, allows communication of the pulp with the external environment and causes fluid to move out of the tubules. Chemicals and other agents also can diffuse down toward the pulp against this flow.

> In the hydrodynamic theory, it is suggested that tooth pain is a result of the fluid flow around the odontoblastic processes, which causes adjacent nerve fibers to be stimulated.

Consider the patient who presents with a symptomatic tooth caused by a vertical crack. The clinician determines the extent of the crack by blowing air on the tooth. The air causes the fluid in the crack to dry quickly and pulls more fluid up to take its place, thus stimulating the tooth and producing pain. In a similar manner, a deep restoration with an open margin is sensitive because fluid can be drawn out of the space. Normally, this may not be painful, but anything that causes the fluid movement to increase in speed, such as blowing air on the margin, will stimulate the tooth. The consumption of hot and cold foods and beverages produces a similar response. In this case, the thermal change causes rapid expansion or contraction of the fluids in the dentinal tubules. The result is a rapid movement of the fluids past the odontoblastic processes and their accompanying innervation, causing pain. *Is it possible to have tooth pain during chewing but not during the intake of hot or cold beverages?*

Any movement of the fluids in the tubules can provoke tooth pain. If a gap exists between the base of a restoration and the dentin floor of the cavity, a fluid-filled space will be produced below the restoration as the pulpal fluids move out under pressure. If the restoration is sealed, biting on it will cause pain because the space containing the fluid is compressed, driving the fluid down into the tubules and stimulating the nerves. If the restoration were not sealed, biting on the restoration would not cause pain because the fluid could be displaced slowly outward with little stimulating effect on the cellular processes within the tubules.

Although these few examples do not cover all cases of tooth sensitivity, they do serve as a reminder that the sealing of the margins around restorations and the complete bonding of restorations to all areas of tooth structure are two laudable goals for the dental team. As specific materials are discussed in this text, many of these concepts will be reemphasized. In some cases, it will be apparent that the pain can be alleviated without removing the restoration; removal, however, often is the only solution.

Summary

The physical and mechanical properties of dental materials play important roles in determining the clinical success of dental restorations and dental procedures. Ideal materials should have certain characteristics. They should not cause adverse biologic reactions, such as toxicity or allergy. Restorations should not leak salivary fluids, which may promote pulpal sensitivity and further tooth decay. Restorative materials must be strong enough and stiff enough to withstand oral stresses. They should not transmit excessive heat to the tissue. Dental materials must be relatively easy to manipulate and place and, ideally, would be repairable and cleanable. All materials do not meet all requirements. Therefore, knowledge of the properties and limitations of the available materials is fundamental to their correct use and application.

STUDY QUESTIONS AND PROBLEM SOLVING

1. **Which type of bonding in a material is most associated with high electrical and thermal conductivity?**
   a. Ionic
   b. Metallic
   c. Covalent
   d. Van der Waals
2. **Gaps at the margins of composite restorations and teeth may be opened during the ingestion of foods and beverages as a result of:**
   a. Differences in thermal conductivity
   b. The presence of pulpal pressure
   c. Differences in thermal expansion coefficients
   d. Inadequate adhesion
3. **An ideal base for a deep amalgam restoration should be mixed to a heavy consistency and placed to a thickness of approximately:**
   a. 0.5 mm
   b. 2.0 mm
   c. 1.0 mm
   d. 3.0 mm
4. **A significant weight gain in a denture base would be associated with:**
   a. Swelling
   b. Water sorption
   c. Leaching of unreacted molecules
   d. Change in the fit
5. **A pit and fissure sealant is most likely to adhere to enamel if the tooth surface is:**
   a. Low in surface energy
   b. Wettable
   c. Smooth and nonporous
   d. Covered with saliva
6. **The hue of natural teeth is generally:**
   a. 6–8
   b. Yellow
   c. 2–3
   d. White
7. **Replacement of the enamel portion of a tooth is optimally done with a composite having high:**
   a. Opacity
   b. Value
   c. Translucency
   d. Chroma

8. **When an amalgam is in contact with a gold onlay, a galvanic cell is established in which the amalgam:**
   a. Oxidizes
   b. Releases metallic ions
   c. Serves as the anode
   d. Degrades more quickly

9. **Tarnish differs from corrosion in that tarnish:**
   a. Is much more harmful to a metal
   b. Discolors metals and can easily be polished out
   c. Does not cause metal ion release
   d. Involves an electrochemical reaction

10. **The elastic modulus of a material is a measure of its:**
    a. Hardness
    b. Toughness
    c. Percent elongation
    d. Stiffness

11. **In which material is the greatest stress generated when subjected to a force of 100 kg: A, cross-sectional area = 1 cm^2; or B, cross-sectional area = 5 cm^2?**
    a. A
    b. B
    c. The stress is the same

12. **Which property describes the capability of an impression to be removed from around the teeth without permanently deforming?**
    a. Maximum flexibility
    b. Percent elongation
    c. Elastic modulus
    d. Ductility

13. **After drinking cold beverages, a patient experiences severe pain in tooth 21, which has had a PFM crown for several years. A likely cause for this pain is:**
    a. A crack in the tooth below the crown margin
    b. Dissolution of the cement, producing a gap at the margin
    c. A gap between tooth and cement at the interior, away from the margins
    d. An inflammatory response to the cement

SELECTED READINGS

Anusavice KJ. Phillips' Science of Dental Materials. 10th ed. Philadelphia: WB Saunders, 1996.
   A complete text on dental materials, including chapters on the physical and mechanical properties of materials.

Brannstrom M. Dentin and Pulp in Restorative Dentistry. London: Wolfe Medical Publications, 1982.
   This book describes the hydrodynamic theory of pulp pain and the reaction of the pulp to various restorative treatments and materials.

Certosimo AJ, O'Connor RP. Oral electricity. General Dentistry 4:324–326, 1996.
   This case report of a patient experiencing oral galvanism shows a logical approach to diagnosis and treatment of this condition.

Craig RG (ed). Restorative Dental Materials. 9th ed. St. Louis: CV Mosby, 1993.

A very inclusive text on dental materials with separate chapters on the physical, mechanical, and biologic properties of materials, as well as corrosion, adhesion, and the nature of the different classes of materials.

Harper RH, Schnell RJ, Swartz ML, Phillips RW. In vivo measurements of thermal diffusion through restorations of various materials. Journal of Prosthetic Dentistry 43:180–185, 1980.

This article describes an in vivo study in which the temperature at the pulpal floor was determined under amalgam and composites restorations used with or without various cement bases of different thickness. The conclusion was that the choice of base was unimportant but that a thickness of 0.75 to 1.0 mm was optimum.

Hume WR, Gerzina TM. Bioavailability of components of resin-based materials which are applied to teeth. Critical Reviews in Oral Biology and Medicine 7:172–179, 1996.

This article reviews the literature concerning the leaching of components from dental composites and their ability to diffuse into the pulp chamber under a dental restoration. The allergenic potential of these compounds is also discussed.

Knispel G. Factors affecting the process of color matching restorative materials to natural teeth. Quintessence International 22:525–531, 1991.

This article describes the basic concept of color perception in dentistry and modern color measurement systems. Two composite systems are used to explain the concepts.

Mahler DB, Terkla LG. Analysis of stress in dental structures. Dental Clinics of North America 789–798, 1958.

This monograph describes the stresses and strains induced in dental materials used in several clinical applications.

Mair LH, Stolarshi TA, Vowles RW, Lloyd CH. Wear: Mechanisms, manifestations and measurement. Report of a workshop. Journal of Dentistry 24:141–148, 1996.

This article provides a summary of the terminology and mechanisms of wear that occur in the oral cavity, particularly with respect to dental composites.

O'Brien WJ (ed). Dental Materials and Their Selection. Chicago: Quintessence Publishing, 1997.

This inclusive text on dental materials contains an excellent chapter on the properties of materials, including separate chapters on color and adhesion. There is also a chapter comparing the properties of ceramics, metals, and polymers.

Swift EJ Jr. Bonding systems for restorative materials—a comprehensive review. Pediatric Dentistry 20:80–84, 1998.

This article provides a review of the subject of dentin bonding, including its development, current status, and clinical methods suggested to improve the performance of these materials.

Chapter 3

Preventive Materials

Pit and Fissure Sealants
History and Rationale
Materials
Handling and Placement of Resin-Based
  Sealants

Preventive Resin Restorations

Fluoride-Releasing Agents
Gels and Varnishes
Glass Ionomers
Resins

Mouthguards

Summary

Objectives

- Compare and contrast preventive and restorative dental materials.
- Describe the composition and uses of resin-based pit and fissure sealants.
- Discuss the causes of failure and clinical success rates for pit and fissure sealants.
- Describe the preventive resin restoration.
- Describe the composition of fluoride gels and varnishes.
- Describe the general composition of glass ionomers used as preventive materials.
- Compare the clinical results for filled or unfilled resin and glass ionomer pit and fissure sealants.
- Discuss the release of fluoride from glass ionomers and resin-based materials in terms of the quantity and the rate of release.
- Identify the composition and describe the physical characteristics of a mouth-protecting material.
- Describe the procedures involved in the formation of a stock and a custom mouthguard and compare the benefits of each.

Prevention is not a new term or new idea in dentistry. Anyone familiar with G. V. Black's principles for cavity design will recall the phrase "extension for prevention." Unfortunately, such procedures, although effective, were not conservative of existing tooth structure. In fact, extension for prevention is considered radical by many in light of recent developments in cariostatic materials and resin adhesives. These materials have the potential to minimize secondary caries as well as reduce the amount of tooth structure removed for a given restoration. The current concept of prevention has as its goal the complete elimination of caries, both primary and secondary.

It is now universally agreed that the main reason for the significant decline in primary caries in adolescents is fluoridation and the exposure to fluoride-containing products, such as dentifrices, mouth rinses, and oral supplements. These advancements, coupled with a more educated public who understand better than their ancestors the importance of diet and oral hygiene, have proven to be effective preventive therapy for tooth decay. Although fewer teeth in today's youth may require filling, the more elderly population is more likely to retain their teeth, thus shifting the treatment priorities to the geriatric patient in whom root caries is fairly prevalent. Therefore, caries has not been eliminated, and there is no shortage of work for today's dental practitioners.

The dental team's main concern is to minimize discomfort and loss of tooth structure in their patients. The ideal way to achieve this goal is through the prevention of tooth decay in all age groups, and many materials and treatments have been developed to accomplish this. But the development of even more effective preventive treatments remains a high research priority in the global health care field. It is an interesting paradox to consider: The people who are involved in this field are actually working to put themselves out of business.

This chapter discusses many of the materials used as preventive dental materials, including pit and fissure sealants, fluoride-containing resins and glass ionomers, and other fluoridated agents. The fluoridated agents, such as gels and varnishes, are used to prevent caries of smooth surfaces by making them more chemically resistant to microorganisms. Sealants are used to prevent caries of occlusal grooves and fissures by filling them and physically separating them from the caries-producing bacteria. Fluoride-releasing resins, such as sealants and composites, act in both manners. Glass ionomers are used as liners, sealants, and restoratives, primarily to prevent further decay. Finally, mouthguards are used to prevent traumatic tooth injury from external forces or bruxing and to hold topical fluorides next to the teeth. Fluoride is also included in many restoratives, cements, and dentin adhesives, but these will be discussed in later chapters.

■ Pit and Fissure Sealants

History and Rationale

Prevention of caries in the deep grooves and fissures of teeth is more difficult than is prevention of caries on the smooth surfaces. Pits and fissures are difficult to clean and are more likely to trap plaque and bacteria. The acids produced by bacteria can be concentrated within these sites, leading to demineralization of the tooth. Fluoridation is not as effective in these areas as it is on smooth surfaces. Fluorides are provided as gels or liquids, which may not always penetrate deep, narrow crevices. The extent to which this will be a problem is determined by the anatomy of the occlusal grooves.

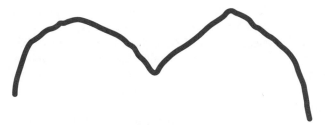

Figure 3–1 A shallow groove in a molar.

When a groove is shallow and smooth, it may be readily cleaned by a brush and dentifrice (Fig. 3-1). Food and debris are unlikely to be trapped. When the groove extends deeper into the tooth, however, forming a pit and fissure as a result of the developmental process, the site is no longer readily cleaned (Fig. 3-2). Food debris and plaque collect here, and if conditions are favorable for opportunistic microorganisms, caries may begin to form.

Several alternatives exist for treating deep pits and fissures. When the bottom of the groove is hard and the explorer does not catch within it, one option is to do nothing but wait and continue to evaluate to see if the condition changes with time. Another option is to instrument the tooth conservatively by running a small bur through the fissure, slightly opening it to provide a more efficient cleaning path. This procedure has been called a "prophylactic odontotomy." Still another option is to cut a somewhat larger groove into the tooth and place a dental amalgam (i.e., silver filling; see Chapter 6). This latter option can be effective, but it is the least conservative. The tooth must be prepared to ensure that the amalgam can be placed with sufficient width and thickness to resist fracture during chewing. A more conservative option is to fill the pit and fissure with a liquid plastic material that hardens to keep food and plaque out of the deep groove. Although filling pits and fissures with chemicals and other materials dates almost to the turn of the 20th century, the development in the 1960s of the **acid-etch technique** for bonding resins to enamel made this alternative treatment option viable.

Normally, enamel surfaces are smooth; however, they can be microscopically roughened by the application of an acid solution. The acid, usually a 37% solution of phosphoric acid in water, is applied to the enamel surface for 15 to 30 seconds. The acid may be in the form of a liquid or a gel, with the latter produced by mixing the liquid with some polymer or silica thickening agent. Laboratory and clinical studies have shown liquid and gel etchants to be equally effective in promoting bonding to teeth.

The time required for the tooth to be exposed to the acid may depend on the age and composition of the tooth. Teeth with a very high fluoride content are more acid resistant and often require longer contact with the acid to produce ad-

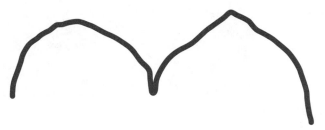

Figure 3–2 A deep pit and fissure in a molar.

equate etching. Altering the time of etch beyond 15 seconds, however, has not had a systematic influence on clinical results.

Enamel is composed of crystalline calcium phosphate materials (i.e., hydroxyapatite), and its surface is partially demineralized by the relatively weak acid. The demineralization of the tooth surface occurs in the outer 10 to 20 μm (the diameter of a human hair is 50 μm). A microscopic roughening takes place as the inner portions or cores of the crystalline enamel rods are etched away, producing a tremendous increase in surface area (Fig. 3-3). The surface changes appearance from smooth and glossy to frosty looking, like a frosted drinking glass. This frosty surface has a very high surface energy and wants to be wetted by anything, including moisture from the breath, biologic molecules from the saliva, or organic molecules from pit and fissure **resin** sealants. The key is to wet the surface with a resin before it can be contaminated by moisture or saliva, which would block the microscopic porosities. When resin monomers are applied to the etched surface, they flow into all of the microscopic roughnesses and porosities, forming resin tags. Once polymerized, these tags lock into the roughness of the etched enamel and bond tenaciously by mechanical forces. There is no true chemical adhesion between the resin and the tooth, but a strong adhesion is created by mechanical interlocking.

The acid-etch technique was developed by Dr. Michael Buonocore in the late 1950s and early 1960s. At that time, the conventional wisdom was against the idea of placing an acid onto sound tooth structure. After all, acids were the cause of the demineralization processes that produced cavities; hence, if not well controlled, they might also cause damage to oral tissues. More than a decade passed before the acid-etch technique became accepted by dental practitioners as a safe and effective way to bond resins and composites to enamel. *Although the technique has been used with great success over the years, it still requires careful consideration of certain variables to enhance success.*

All of the factors that dictate adhesion are at work during the application of pit and fissure sealants to etched enamel. Obviously, the surface must remain uncontaminated to allow intimate contact between the resin monomers and the

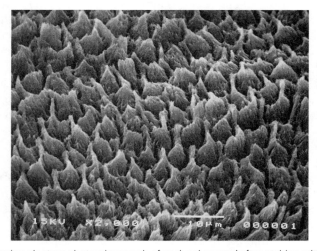

Figure 3–3 Scanning electron photomicrograph of occlusal enamel after etching with phosphoric acid for resin bonding. At this magnification, the diameter of a human hair would be the entire width of the photo.

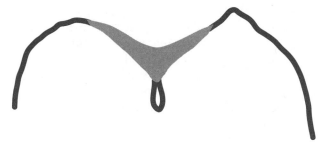

Figure 3–4 A deep pit and fissure that is not completely penetrated by the fluid resin sealant.

rough surface. Therefore, sealants ideally are placed under rubber dam isolation. Certain studies reporting on the long-term clinical success of pit and fissure sealants have shown that excellent results can be achieved with cotton roll isolation, as long as the clinician is careful to maintain a dry field. This is most effectively accomplished with four-handed dental treatment. Another important consideration is the viscosity of the resin. The resin must flow and adapt to the rough surface to cover it and achieve intimate contact. Although the commercial materials are formulated with a low viscosity for this purpose, they may not completely flow into deep pits because the resin cannot always displace the air entrapped within the pit (Fig. 3-4). *What effect might this have on the outcome of the procedure?*

Two things must be considered when the sealant cannot penetrate an entire pit. First, there will be no bonding or adhesion to that part of the fissure. Therefore, there must be a sufficient bonding area above the pit to retain the sealant. Second, the inability to clean the pit before sealant application means that decay may be trapped under the resin after it has hardened in place. Initially, there was concern over the progress of caries left under sealants. Several studies subsequently showed that caries becomes arrested under a pit and fissure sealant and that cultivatable bacteria are virtually nonexistent after sealing. These studies dissipated concerns over the continued development of caries under sealants, as long as the tooth remained sealed to separate the bacteria from their source of nourishment and oxygen. Many clinicians, however, still use a handpiece to perform a conservative widening of the fissure before sealant application to help clean the pit and enhance penetration of the resin for optimal retention and sealing.

Ensuring that the sealant remains in place is an important part of a sealant program. One long-term clinical trial has shown that even in the absence of sealant replacement, only 30% of the teeth were filled or carious at the 15-year recall period, compared with 82% of the control teeth. It was suggested that with recalls at 6-month or 1-year intervals, during which the presence of the sealant can be verified and fresh material reapplied if needed, 100% success may be achievable.

Materials

Several materials have been used as sealants for pits and fissures. The most common is the resin component of dental **composites** (composites are further discussed in Chapter 5). This resin usually is composed of a specific organic **monomer** often abbreviated as bis-GMA (2,2-bis[4(2-hydroxy-3-methacryloyl-oxy-propoxy)phenyl]propane), in addition to other monomers, such as triethylene glycol dimethacrylate. The other monomers are added to dilute the viscous bis-GMA and enhance its flow and mixing characteristics. All of these monomers are based on a chemical structure containing carbon-carbon double bonds ($C=C$) that react by a process called **polymerization**. This process is discussed in detail in Chapter 12, but, simply stated, polymerization refers to the linking together of many compatible molecules to produce a larger molecule, or **polymer**, via a chemical reaction. Polymerization of pit and fissure sealants forms highly cross-linked polymer networks. In many ways, a polymer network resembles a fish net, except that it is not as regularly arranged.

The polymerization reaction can be brought about by mixing equal drops of two liquids containing essential chemical **activators** (amines) and **initiators** (peroxides). The activators and initiators serve to begin the polymerization reaction of the monomers. They are similar to but slightly different from **catalysts**. The resin liquid hardens within 1.5 to 2 minutes, providing ample working time to brush the material onto an etched tooth. A second and more popular method for polymerizing the resin is to use blue-light energy from a handheld light source. The chemical initiator that is required to start the reaction is not activated until it is illuminated by blue light; therefore, no mixing is required and the materials are supplied as one-part, or single-component, systems (Fig. 3-5). One of the advantages of the light-cured systems is a longer **working time**. Because the material will not set until it is illuminated, the operator has a longer period of time to work with and place the material before it begins to harden. Another benefit of the light-cured materials is that they do not need to be mixed and, therefore, have fewer air bubbles than do the two-component, self-curing systems. The light-cured sealants also have a greater surface hardness. The hardening of many plastics is inhibited by the presence of oxygen. Light-cured resins seem to be less affected than self-curing, or mixed, materials. Thus, the surface of a light-cured resin may be slightly harder than a self-curing resin because of less **air inhibition** during polymerization. Despite the differences, however, clinical studies have shown similar retention rates for the self-curing and light-cured materials. This is in agreement with the fact that both have equivalent bond strengths to etched enamel. One study reported that 50 to 60% of the sealants placed were completely retained over a 5-year period.

Polymer resin sealants wear under the occlusal forces of chewing, resulting in the loss of sealant material over time. Studies have measured this loss as 15% of the sealant volume during the first 6 months. Manufacturers have attempted to reduce this loss of material by adding tiny glass filler particles to the monomers to reinforce the sealants. This produces dilute and flowable composites, which are slightly more wear resistant. A side effect of the fillers, however, is that they may act as an abrasive to the opposing dentition when they become exposed on the surface of the sealant. The overall effect of this wear has not been determined. Despite their slightly greater strength and wear resistance, clinical results for filled sealants are similar to those for unfilled sealants.

One additional benefit derived from the incorporation of fillers into the resin is an increase in opacity. The more opaque sealant is easier to visualize in the mouth than a transparent liquid sealant. One study showed that the probability of failing to see a clear sealant on a tooth was approximately 25%, whereas the probability of missing a filled sealant was less than 2%. This becomes increasingly important as the sealant wears and is more difficult to identify. Manufacturers have produced clear tinted sealants to minimize this problem, but they still are not as visible as sealants with filler particles.

Other materials used as pit and fissure sealants include glass ionomer restoratives. The use of these materials as preventive restorative materials is discussed later in this chapter. Their use as sealants, however, was encouraged because they

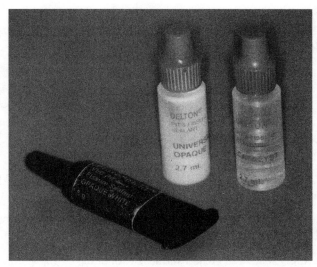

Figure 3–5 Tube of a single-part, light-cured sealant and vials of a two-part, self-curing pit and fissure sealant.

contain fluoride and there was evidence that this fluoride leached out of the material over time. The benefits of a fluoride-releasing sealant are obvious. Glass ionomers have not gained great popularity as sealants, however, because they tend to wear and chip away much faster than do resin-based sealants. Clinical studies have shown a poor retention rate for these materials, with 84% of them being at least partially chipped or worn from the tooth within 3 years. This does not compare favorably with the self-curing sealants of the filled or unfilled variety, of which only 10% have been shown to be partially lost from teeth over 5 years. Evidence shows that even in cases where the glass ionomer appears to be completely lost, however, some glass ionomer almost always remains in the pit, even though it cannot be detected clinically. Although the clinical loss of sealant is alarming, caries reduction for teeth sealed with glass ionomers is the same as or better than that for resins. Therefore, although glass ionomer is lost much more rapidly, it may be equally effective as the completely retained resin for a short time. In the long run, one would expect that the resin-based sealant would show better results because of its greater retention.

In an effort to optimize both retention and fluoride release, filled resin sealants containing fluoride have been developed and used. The fluoride is present either within the fillers or as a sodium fluoride additive. These materials also adhere to enamel as nonfluoridated resins and show similar results clinically. In vitro studies show that they minimize the demineralization of adjacent tooth structure that is exposed to artificial caries environments, in part because the fluoride that they release becomes incorporated into the enamel. The fluoride is released at a fast rate during the first few days after placement but diminishes to a low and constant level thereafter. This behavior is similar to that of the glass ionomers, although the amount of fluoride released from these resins is usually much less than that released from glass ionomers.

Handling and Placement of Resin-Based Sealants

Because retention and clinical success of resin-based sealants depend on mechanical bonding to etched enamel, care must be taken to prepare the tooth correctly

PROCEDURE DISPLAY 3-1

Resin Pit and Fissure Sealant Application

STEP 1
❏ Clean enamel surfaces with pumice in a prophylaxis cup. Wash and dry.

STEP 2
❏ Place moisture isolation (i.e., rubber dam, cotton rolls).

STEP 3
❏ Etch tooth with phosphoric acid for 15–30 seconds. Wash and dry.

STEP 4
❏ Dispense sealant into tray. Mix 10–15 seconds if self-curing variety.

STEP 5
❏ Apply sealant to etched surfaces with brush or applicator.

STEP 6
❏ If light-curing sealant, illuminate for 40 seconds with light source.

STEP 7
❏ Finish by removing "air-inhibited" layer with cotton or gauze.

STEP 8
❏ Check sealant for complete coverage.

for bonding. **Rubber dam** isolation is ideal, but the materials often are used with teeth that are newly erupted, and it is not possible to isolate them with a dam. Careful cotton roll isolation is then appropriate. The ideal time to apply sealants is as soon as possible, but at least within 2 years of eruption. The procedure is summarized in Procedure Display 3-1.

The first step in sealant application is to clean the entire occlusal surface of the tooth or teeth with a pumice slurry on a prophylaxis brush. The area is then thoroughly washed and dried before placing the rubber dam or cotton rolls. The next step is to etch the tooth surface with a 37% solution of phosphoric acid. The acid can be applied as a liquid or a gel for approximately 15 to 30 seconds. The etch time may vary among clinicians, but at least 15 seconds is appropriate to ensure adequate etching with minimal risk of underetching. The surface is then washed with water spray for 10 to 15 seconds to remove all of the acid and etching debris and is thoroughly dried. Resin sealant bonding to enamel is inhibited by moisture, and thus the drying step is critical. The enamel should appear frosty at this point. If the surface is not frosty, the etchant should be reapplied for 30 seconds and then washed and dried.

The next step is to dispense the sealant. If it is a self-curing sealant, equal drops are dispensed into the supplied plastic well and mixed for 10 to 15 seconds with a stick or brush (Fig. 3-6). The fluid resin can then be painted onto the etched enamel, with care taken not to apply pressure to the surface, which would fracture the frail enamel rods and reduce bond strength (Fig. 3-7). The tooth should be sealed within 60 seconds because the working time of this material is only 90 seconds. The resin should be hardened after 2 minutes. Hardening is monitored by probing the sealant with an explorer.

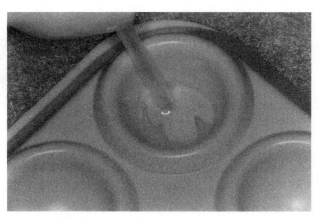

Figure 3–6 Mixing the two liquids of a self-curing sealant.

If a light-cured sealant is used, it can be applied directly to the tooth with a brush (Fig. 3-8) and then exposed to the light source for 40 seconds. It is important to expose the entire surface to the light. A 13-mm light tip that covers the entire occlusal surface is recommended. If a smaller tip is used, it is best to cure the material in two distinct sections instead of waving the light tip over the surface. The light tip should be held as close as possible to the resin to maximize light intensity (Fig. 3-9). A plastic tip can be placed over the source tip to avoid contamination with the resin if it touches the liquid.

Once the sealant is hardened, the surface is finished by wiping it with a cotton pellet or gauze to remove the excess resin that remains uncured because of air (oxygen) inhibition. The sealant is checked to ensure complete coverage and is removed from unetched areas. Defects can be repaired by reetching and reapplying sealant. Finally, the occlusion should be checked and excess sealant removed.

The biocompatibility of sealants has been questioned because of a potential for estrogen-mimicking effects attributed to specific molecular components or contaminants (i.e., BPA or bis-phenol A and bis-phenol A dimethacrylate). Studies have shown that BPA, an epoxy component used in many other industries, can have estrogenic properties. The compound has a very low potency, however, especially when compared with the natural hormone, estradiol. Dental resins do not

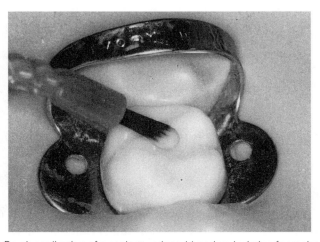

Figure 3–7 Brush application of a sealant under rubber dam isolation for moisture control.

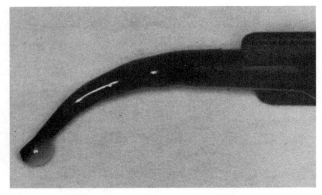

Figure 3–8 Spiral brush for applying a light-cured sealant.

typically contain BPA, though it may be present in trace amounts as a contaminant in some materials. Exposure to BPA or its dimethacrylate from a dental resin has not been shown to cause any adverse condition in humans. Currently, there is no evidence for discontinuing or even questioning the use of resin-based dental sealants because of toxicity concerns. As with all resin-based materials, however, adequate curing and the physical removal of unreacted monomers at the surface by wiping with gauze or cotton is sound practice to minimize exposure to any foreign molecules present in the materials.

■ *Preventive Resin Restorations*

The **preventive resin restoration** (PRR) involves the placement of a dental composite within an **incipient** lesion of the pits or fissures, with minimal excavation of the tooth. Application of composite is followed by sealing the entire occlusal surface of the tooth with a pit and fissure sealant (Fig. 3-10). An alternative is to fill the cavity with glass ionomer and then seal the occlusal surface of the tooth with a sealant. The PRR is typically used on premolars and molars. The restoration is more conservative than a typical amalgam, in which the pits and fissures are prepared and included in the cavity design. One study reported that only

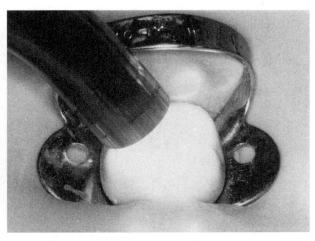

Figure 3–9 Light-curing a sealant on a tooth.

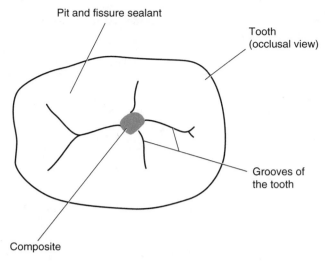

Pit and fissure sealant

Tooth
(occlusal view)

Grooves of
the tooth

Composite

Figure 3–10 Tooth restored with a preventive resin restoration (PRR). The restoration includes minimal tooth preparation restored with a dental composite, followed by etching and surface sealing of the occlusal enamel, including the pits and fissures, with a transparent sealant.

5% of the occlusal surface was involved in preparation for a PRR, compared with 25% for typical amalgam restorations.

Numerous clinical studies have examined the efficacy of PRR, and most have arrived at the same conclusion. The success rate is highly favorable, with the most common causes of failure being loss of the sealant because of wear. As expected, the incidence of caries associated with these restorations increases with time and has been reported to be in the range of 5% over 4 years and 10% after 6 to 7 years.

■ *Fluoride-Releasing Agents*

Several materials are available as fluoride sources for teeth. Some are used in the office, whereas others can be applied by the patient at home, like mouth rinses (Table 3-1). Fluoride is usually present as sodium fluoride, but the dentifrice may contain sodium monofluorophosphate or stannous fluoride. Other materials with fluoride are restorative materials that provide fluoride by a slow, timed-release mechanism. These latter provide a constant source of fluoride, although the level of protection is difficult to determine. Examples of fluoride-containing gels and varnishes, as well as restorative materials such as glass ionomers and composites, are shown in Figure 3-11.

Gels and Varnishes

Fluoride-containing gels and varnishes are used to prevent the formation of caries. The effectiveness of fluorides in preventing decay is well established. The fluoride gel or varnish treatment is an infrequent, in-office adjunct to normal home cleaning with fluoride toothpastes and dietary fluoride supplementation. Home-use rinses are also available for daily treatment.

Fluoride gels usually contain approximately 1.25% fluoride. The fluoride is present in several forms, including sodium fluoride and hydrogen fluoride. The

TABLE 3–1. **Types of Fluoride Sources—Comparison of Dose and Frequency of Use**

Source	Typical Dose (ppm)	Frequency of Use
Fluoride water	1	Continuous
Fluoride supplement (table)	250–1000	Daily
Mouthrinse (home)	200/900	Daily/weekly
Dentifrice	500–1500	2–3 times daily
Gel (in office)	6000–7000	Annually or biannually
Varnish	22,600	2–4 times a year

gels are called **APF**, which stands for "acidulated phosphate fluoride." The gel also contains a small amount of phosphoric acid, plus a thickening agent, coloring, and flavoring. Because of the acidic components, the gels have pH values near 3 to 5. The gels are applied in soft trays like mouthguards and are held in the mouth for several minutes. Existing composite and porcelain-ceramic restorations can become slightly etched and roughened during the application of an APF gel. There are gels with pH closer to neutral (pH 7), however, which may be less harmful to the surfaces of these restoratives. The results of several studies have been reviewed and show a 22 to 26% overall caries-inhibiting effect attributed to the use of fluoride gels.

Varnishes also are available for use by dental personnel. One popular brand contains 5% sodium fluoride (22,600 ppm) in an alcohol solution with natural resins to make it sticky and adherent to the teeth as the alcohol evaporates (Fig. 3-12). Varnishes are applied to the teeth of children (or adults) with a brush several times a year. A typical treatment regimen might be to apply the varnish to the teeth several times over the course of a 1-week period, repeating the procedure at intervals of 6 or 12 months. Numerous studies have been performed, and for one

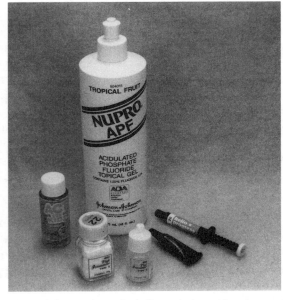

Figure 3–11 Fluoride-containing products, including gel, rinse, glass ionomer, resin pit and fissure sealant, and resin dental composite.

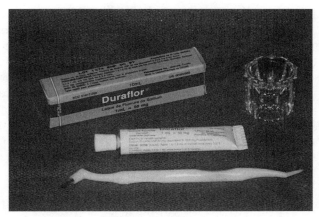

Figure 3–12 Fluoride varnish material, dappen dish for dispensing, and brush for application to the teeth.

specific brand, an average 38% reduction in caries has been shown. At least one study, however, has shown that the caries-preventing effect does not continue once the treatment stops, even though the fluoride content of the teeth has been raised by the application of the fluoride varnish.

Glass Ionomers

Glass ionomers are dental materials used in a variety of applications, including liners, bases, sealants, restoratives, and luting cements. They are composed of an acidic polymer liquid (polyacrylic acid) that is mixed with a silicate glass powder containing calcium, aluminum, and fluorine. When the powder and liquid are mixed, the acidic liquid dissolves some of the powder, releasing metal ions with positive charges. These ions react with the negatively charged groups on the polymer molecules to form a hard matrix that holds the rest of the glass particles together. The hard matrix traps the fluoride ions released from the glass. Over time, these fluoride ions will be slowly dissolved into the saliva or into adjacent tissues in the mouth. A more detailed description of these materials is provided in Chapters 4 and 5.

When used as restorative materials or sealants, glass ionomers are believed to be effective at minimizing the formation of secondary caries. Their physical properties are poor in comparison to dental composites, so their use as restorative materials has been limited. Their use is expanding, however, principally owing to the development of light-cured **resin-modified glass ionomers**, which possess the qualities of both glass ionomers and composites.

As is true with most fluoride-releasing agents, the fluoride in glass ionomers is released in large amounts during the initial period within the oral cavity. Although the rate of release declines rapidly with time, these materials have been shown to continuously release fluoride for periods of 1 year or longer. Furthermore, the fluoride is taken up by adjacent tooth structure. The dilemma, however, is that no one is sure how much fluoride is necessary for caries prevention. Therefore, although the level of fluoride release is low after the first month, it may be sufficient to prevent decay. This quality is one of the major factors contributing to the popularity of these materials.

These materials exhibit another interesting characteristic. In the same manner that they release fluoride (i.e., by diffusion of the ion out of the material), glass ionomers can acquire or take up fluoride. Studies have shown that glass ionomers can be "recharged" with fluoride by exposing the material to a fluoride-containing solution. In this case, the glass ionomer soaks up fluoride, which can then be released later in the mouth. The application of a fluoride gel to a glass ionomer may be one way of achieving this "recharging" during a normal office procedure. The acidic form of the fluoride gel may also dissolve the surface of the glass ionomer, however, so a neutral gel would be more appropriate.

Resins

Various resin pit and fissure sealants, adhesives resins, and dental composites have been formulated with fluoride-containing compounds in the hope of producing cariostatic materials. In general, these materials release fluoride in a manner similar to that of the glass ionomers, in that the release is rapid early but slows dramatically with time. In addition, fluoride is released from resin-based materials such as composites and sealants less readily than from glass ionomers, presumably because the resins are less soluble in oral fluids. A full discussion of composites is presented in Chapter 5; at this point, it suffices to reiterate that dental composites are polymeric materials containing glass-reinforcing fillers. Fluoride is added either to the polymer resin component or to the filler particles. Composites from one manufacturer contain fluoride as a special fluoride-containing filler particle (ytterbium trifluoride). Fluoridated polymers also have been developed but have not been successful commercially. Although both fluoridated polymers and composites release a significant amount of fluoride, only limited data are available to prove that these materials have any therapeutic effect.

■ *Mouthguards*

Mouthguards are used by participants in sporting activities to protect the dentition from direct or indirect trauma. Although mouthguards usually are associated with football, they are routinely worn in all full-contact or semi-contact sports, especially by the young. Some estimates show that tens of thousands of dental injuries may be prevented each year by the wearing of suitable mouthguards. The mouth protector resides between the teeth and absorbs the energy of a blow to the head or mouth that would otherwise cause the maxillary and mandibular teeth to impact on one another; the result is fewer cases of chipped or broken teeth.

Mouthguards generally are made from semirigid but soft plastics; a common material is a polymer of polyvinylacetate and polyethylene. The material generally comes in thin sheets less than ⅛-inch thick that can be custom fitted to the dentition by heating and forming within the mouth. The materials possess the characteristic of being **thermoplastic**, which means that they become softened and moldable on heating but become rigid enough to hold their shape when cooled. The materials have only minimal strength and resistance to tearing. Therefore, their service life depends on the activities of the user. A person who bites or chews on the mouthguard or a person who clenches and grinds during wearing will eventually bite through the guard and require a new one.

Stock mouthguards can be purchased and formed at home. The material is similar to that used to carry fluoride gels to the patient during in-office fluoride treatments; however, these guards can be customized relatively easily. The clear or colored plastic can be softened by heating in boiling water (100°C) for a minute or so. The guard is then allowed to cool to a temperature that can be tolerated by the tissues before being placed into the mouth and having the person bite down on it gently. Biting too hard causes tearing, but biting too passively produces an ill-fitting device. After several minutes, the material will have cooled sufficiently to maintain its shape on removal from the mouth (Fig. 3-13). At this point, the edges can be trimmed with a knife or scissors to remove distal extensions and reduce the chances of irritating soft tissues. As expected, a stock mouthguard is serviceable and reasonably priced, but a custom-made guard is preferable.

A custom-made maxillary mouth protector can be made in a dental office from the same material used for stock guards; however, the procedure is more complicated and expensive. First, an impression is made of the arch. Then, a **stone** model is produced from the impression. Dental stone is similar to **plaster** (i.e., plaster of Paris), except that it is harder and stronger. These materials, along with other **gypsum** products, are described fully in Chapter 9. The thermoplastic guard material is then formed on the stone model by using a vacuum technique. Finally, the guard is trimmed and finished for maximum comfort and protection. A full description of the procedure follows.

After the stone model of the maxillary arch is produced, a line is drawn in pencil around the teeth at approximately the point of the attached gingiva and the oral mucosa. The guard will later be trimmed to this line. Thus, for maximum comfort, the guard will not have a palatal component. The model is then soaked in water for a brief period to minimize the potential for the guard material to stick to it during forming. The model is then centered on a suitable vacuum-forming unit (Fig. 3-14). A sheet of the guard material is then placed within the heating portion of the vacuum unit, and the unit is heated to soften the plastic. When the heated plastic material sags, it is placed over the model by lowering the heating unit, and light pressure is applied. Excessive pressure will cause the plastic to become too thin in the cuspal areas. The vacuum pulls the softened plastic down onto the model, producing an intimate contact between the two. The machine is then cooled for several minutes while pressure and vacuum are maintained. The model and the guard material may then be removed and placed into cool water. When the guard is sufficiently cool, it is removed from the model and trimmed with a blade, sharp knife, or scissors to remove the palate and any sharp edges. The edges of the guard can be heated in an alcohol flame and then smoothed by hand to produce the final product.

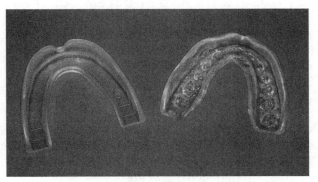

Figure 3–13 Stock mouthguard before and after being formed to the dentition.

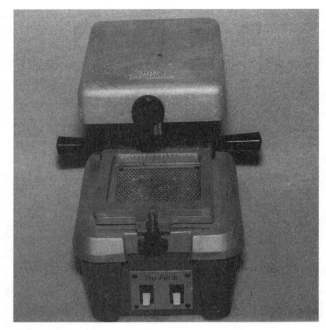

Figure 3–14 Vacuum-forming device for producing a custom mouthguard.

Summary

Preventive materials are used to eliminate dental caries and tooth damage before they can occur. Polymeric pit and fissure sealants, small resin composite restorations, fluoride-releasing gels and varnishes, glass ionomer restoratives, and plastic mouthguards are examples. The materials are produced in a variety of formulations for different applications. Some (i.e., glass ionomers and certain varnishes) help to prevent tooth decay by providing an intraoral source of an anticaries agent, such as fluoride. Others, such as composites and resin sealants, serve to seal the tooth from bacteria and their acidic by-products. Custom-made mouthguards serve to cushion the teeth from potentially damaging intraoral and extraoral forces. The conservation of hard and soft oral tissues is a primary goal for dentistry, and the development of preventive materials for this purpose continues to be an important area of study.

STUDY QUESTIONS AND PROBLEM SOLVING

1. Which of the following is (are) *not* a common component(s) of resin-based pit and fissure sealants?
   a. Plaster
   b. Small glass filler particles
   c. bis-GMA monomers
   d. Phosphoric acid
2. Which of the following is (are) true of light-cured pit and fissure sealants as compared with self-curing sealants?
   a. They contain fewer porosities
   b. Their strength is twice as great
   c. They require only half the time to place
   d. They have greater surface hardness

3. **A patient who received occlusal sealants on all molars 5 years ago returns with occlusal decay on several previously sealed teeth. Possible reasons for the lack of success include:**
    a. Poor oral hygiene practices
    b. Excess loss of sealant as a result of wear
    c. Poor initial bonding of the sealant
    d. The sealant did not contain fluoride

4. **A preventive resin restoration might be indicated for a patient with:**
    a. Extensive caries of both lower first molars
    b. An incipient lesion in an upper premolar
    c. A deep groove in a caries-free second molar
    d. Recurrent decay around an existing amalgam in a first molar

5. **Compared with any of the resin-based sealants, glass ionomers:**
    a. Have been shown to have greater retention rates in clinical studies
    b. Release fluoride at a greater rate and to a greater extent
    c. Have similar short-term preventive capabilities
    d. Are more resistant to chipping

6. **Which of the following is (are) *not* a recommended use(s) for a glass ionomer?**
    a. Luting cement for a gold crown
    b. Thermal insulating base under an amalgam
    c. Restoration of a first molar with a fractured cusp
    d. Veneering anterior teeth

7. **The preparation and placement of a resin-based pit and fissure sealant may include which of the following steps?**
    a. Mixing two resin components by kneading them together in gloved hands
    b. Applying an acidic solution to the enamel surface of the tooth
    c. Washing the tooth as the final step just before applying the sealant
    d. Removing an unreacted resin layer with a gauze as the final step

8. **Fluoride gels differ from fluoride varnishes in that:**
    a. Gels are for home use only
    b. Varnishes are more acidic and more dangerous
    c. Varnishes can cause surface deterioration of restorations
    d. Gels are held in the mouth in trays

9. **Mouth protectors are commonly made:**
    a. From hard plastics formed on metal frameworks for reinforcement
    b. By softening a plastic in boiling water and then forming on the teeth
    c. By a custom technique to improve fit and comfort
    d. From polyacrylic acid liquid and glass particles

SELECTED READINGS

Beltran-Aguilar ED, Goldstein JW, Lockwood SA. Fluoride varnishes. A review of their clinical use, cariostatic mechanism, efficacy and safety. Journal of the American Dental Association 131:589–596, 2000.

This article summarizes the in vitro and in vivo studies on the use and efficacy of fluoride varnishes. The authors conclude that semiannual applications of the varnish is the most proven treatment regimen and that these materials are safe and easy to use.

Ellwood RP, Blinkhorn AS, Davies RM. Fluoride: How to maximize the benefits and minimize the risks. Dental Update 25:365–372, 1998.

This article reviews current thoughts on the various fluoride delivery systems and their safety and efficacy in preventing dental caries.

Feigal RJ. Sealants and preventive restorations: Review of effectiveness and clinical changes for improvement. Pediatric Dentistry 20:85–92, 1998.

This article describes the literature supporting the use of sealants and preventive resin restorations.

Gilpin JL. Pit and fissure sealants: A review of the literature. Journal of Dental Hygiene 71:150–158, 1997.

This article reviews the scientific literature regarding pit and fissure sealants, including their use, efficacy, and acceptance in dental practice.

Helfenstein U, Steiner M. Fluoride varnishes (Duraphat): A meta-analysis. Community Dentistry and Oral Epidemiology 22:1–5, 1994.

This article uses a statistical technique called meta-analysis to review the clinical studies of fluoride varnishes. The study concludes that fluoride varnishes are effective and that the caries reduction is inversely correlated with study duration when these materials are used.

Mejare I, Mjor IA. Glass ionomer and resin-based fissure sealants: A clinical study. Scandinavian Journal of Dental Research 98:345–350, 1990.

This article reports a study comparing glass ionomer to two resin-based sealants over a 5-year period. The study shows the resin sealants to be well retained over the period, whereas nearly all of the glass ionomers were lost. Caries was recorded in 5% of the resin-based sealants, but there were no cases reported for the glass ionomer-sealed teeth, demonstrating the effectiveness of fluoride release from these materials.

Mertz-Fairhurst EJ, Curtis JW Jr, Ergle JW, Rueggeberg FA, Adair SM. Ultraconservative and cariostatic sealed restorations: Results at year 10. Journal of the American Dental Association 129:55–66, 1998.

Ultraconservative sealed composite restorations are compared with ultraconservative sealed amalgam restorations over a 10-year period in class I lesions. The study showed that caries was arrested in the sealed amalgam and composite restorations and that sealant was retained at a similar rate over composite and amalgam.

Ripa LW, Wolff MS. Preventive resin restorations: Indications, technique, and success. Quintessence International 5:307–315, 1992.

This review article discusses the diagnostic criteria for pit and fissure occlusal caries and treatment planning. A technique for placing a preventive resin restoration with a glass ionomer liner is presented. The literature concerning success rates for these types of restorations is highlighted.

Simonsen RJ. Retention and effectiveness of dental sealant after 15 years. Journal of the American Dental Association 122:34–42, 1991.

This article reports on the success of a filled pit and fissure sealant applied under cotton roll isolation and followed over a 15-year period without reapplication.

Stookey GK. Caries prevention. Journal of Dental Education 62:803–811, 1998.

This comprehensive article discusses the use of fluoride in water fluoridation programs, professional gel treatments, home-use dentifrices and mouth rinses, and varnishes. The efficacy of the various methods of delivery is presented.

Waggoner WF, Siegal M. Pit and fissure sealant application: Updating the technique. Journal of the American Dental Association 127:351–361, 1996.

In this article, the authors discuss available options for sealant materials and discuss important factors in their placement.

Williams B. Fissure sealants: A review. Journal of the International Association of Dentistry for Children 20(2):35–41, 1990.

This article provides a review of the history and development of pit and fissure sealants. It contains over 125 references to support the conclusion that the use of these materials is effective from the standpoint of cost and caries reduction.

Chapter 4

Intermediary Materials and Cements

Objectives

- Explain the difference in intent when placing a liner rather than a base.

- Describe the composition and uses of varnishes in dentistry.

- Compare the different forms of calcium hydroxide materials used as liners.

- Describe the application of calcium hydroxide and the benefits expected from its use.

- Describe the procedure for dispensing and mixing lining materials.

- Explain why glass ionomer is considered to be an excellent lining or basing material.

- Describe the mixing of zinc phosphate cements, and explain why the technique differs from that used to mix glass ionomer.

- Explain how the working time of zinc phosphate cement can be prolonged.

- Compare the composition and properties of the materials used as luting cements in dentistry.

- Compare the clinical performance of glass ionomer and zinc phosphate as luting cements for crowns and bridges.

■ *Definition of Terms*

The concept of preventive dental materials was introduced in Chapter 3. To a certain extent, the main focus of this chapter is similar to that of Chapter 3, i.e., prevention. The difference lies in the fact that most of the materials discussed in this chapter are used after caries or tooth erosion has already occurred. The role of these materials is to minimize the occurrence of secondary caries or postoperative sensitivity, thus helping to prevent further problems. These materials generally are used in combination with another restorative material. Some of them have therapeutic value, and all are used for specific purposes. They are often called **intermediary materials** because they occupy the intermediary space between the tooth and a restorative.

The terms "liner" and "base" are used synonymously by some practitioners, but others clearly distinguish between them. For our purposes, we will abide by the following broad definitions. A **liner** is applied in a thin layer to seal the dentin on the floor and walls of the cavity from the influx of bacteria or irritants from restorative procedures. This sealing is necessary because the pulp may be in open communication with the oral cavity through dentin tubules that may have been opened by caries or the preparation of the cavity. The placement of glass ionomer liner to seal the dentin under a composite restoration is a typical example (Fig. 4-1*A*). **Varnish**, by this definition, is also classified as a lining material when it is coated onto the walls and floor of a cavity preparation before an amalgam is placed (Fig. 4-1*B*). Resin adhesives are also used for this purpose. In contrast, **bases** are applied in thicker layers to provide thermal or electrical protection to the pulp. Bases must be strong enough to support a restorative material. This does not imply that the base is used to strengthen the restorative but simply that the base must have sufficient structural integrity to withstand forces from the restorative material during its placement and function. A common example is the use of a glass ionomer or zinc phosphate cement base under a deep amalgam restoration. Note that glass ionomer can be used as either a base or a liner, depending on the intent. The materials used as varnishes, liners, and bases, the manner in which they are mixed and placed, and their physical and clinical characteristics are addressed in the pages that follow. Because many of these materials are also used to lute, or attach restorations to teeth, the chapter ends with a discussion of dental cements.

■ *Varnishes*

Uses of Varnishes

Much in the same way that varnishes are painted onto coffee tables and boat parts to seal wood surfaces from the damaging effects of moisture, several types of varnishes are used in dentistry. The most common use of a varnish is as a sealer of the dentinal tubules of an amalgam cavity preparation (Fig. 4-1*B*). As is discussed in Chapter 6, amalgam undergoes a slight contraction during hardening. This shrinkage leads to the formation of openings around the margins of new restorations. With time, corrosion will fill in the gaps and eliminate **marginal leakage**. During the first few months, however, it is desirable to seal opened dentinal tubules that may be present under the amalgam. Varnish has been used for this purpose, although its benefits are somewhat controversial. In addition to sealing the dentin from the migration of agents into the tooth, the varnish also may pre-

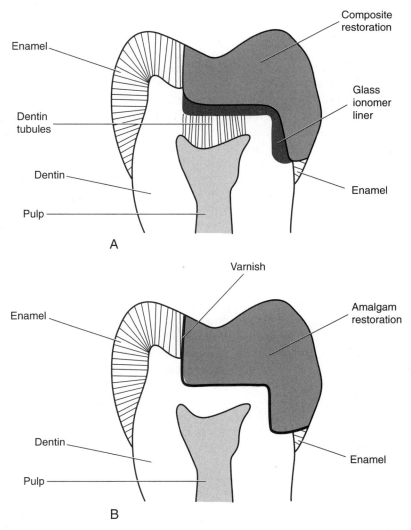

Figure 4–1 A. A glass ionomer liner placed under a composite to seal the dentin. **B.** A varnish or resin adhesive coating the walls and floor of a cavity under an amalgam restoration.

vent the outward migration of metallic ions from the amalgam to the tooth. This phenomenon is responsible for the esthetically undesirable darkening of tooth structure adjacent to amalgams. Varnishes help to minimize this problem, although its occurrence has diminished markedly since the introduction of modern amalgams, which are more corrosion resistant than were their predecessors.

Types of Varnishes

Varnishes are liquids composed of resins or polymers suspended in a solvent. Varnishes that seal the tooth under amalgams contain either the natural copal resin or cellulose. Another type contains calcium hydroxide, but this is discussed later in the section on liners. Other liners can be used to seal the dentin under composites; they are made of polyurethane polymers, which are also suspended in a solvent. The solvent is a volatile organic liquid, such as acetone, chloroform, or ether.

Handling and Placement of Varnishes

Varnishes are supplied in bottles (Fig. 4-2). They are applied to the cavity or, in the case of a glass ionomer varnish, to the restoration with a thin brush or small cotton balls (i.e., pledgets). The solvent within the fluid acts as a "vehicle" that carries the resin or polymer to the tooth site and then evaporates, leaving behind a resin or polymer film to coat and seal the tooth. The films are porous, so the material usually is applied twice (within 20 to 30 seconds) to provide a more uniform coating. The final thickness of the varnish layer will usually be on the order of 5 to 10 μm (a human hair has a diameter of about 50 μm), although some of the polymer coatings may be thicker. Because loss of solvent will cause the material to become viscous and difficult to collect and brush onto the tooth, the cap should be replaced on the bottle immediately after dispensing the varnish into a suitable container. Should the varnish become thick, additional solvent can be added to "thin" the varnish and improve its flow.

Characteristics of Varnishes

Resin-based cavity varnishes are insoluble in water. They are, therefore, fairly resistant to oral fluids and should remain on the tooth or restorative surface for a long time. Because they are applied in such thin layers, however, they can be easily scratched or worn from surfaces. They adhere physically, not chemically, to a surface. Certain varnishes are used to coat fresh glass ionomer restorations to prevent moisture loss. Varnishes can be easily abraded. Because these varnishes need to be present only for the first 24 to 48 hours while the glass ionomer fully hardens, however, later abrasion and removal is of little consequence.

The benefits associated with the use of varnishes in amalgam therapy are questionable. Its presence does not guarantee that postoperative sensitivity will be eliminated; the converse is also true. The use of varnish is the clinician's personal choice and may have little effect on the success of the restoration. No harm is associated with its use, however. Some in vitro studies show that leakage around amalgam restorations is reduced when varnishes are used; other studies show that varnished dentin is less permeable to acid than is unvarnished dentin. Therefore, before placing an acidic zinc phosphate cement base under an amalgam restoration, varnish can be applied to the tooth to protect the pulp. Similarly, many clin-

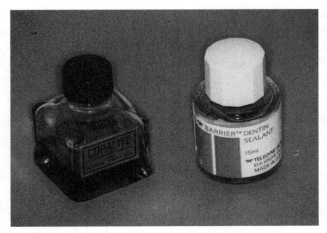

Figure 4–2 Bottles of cavity varnish and dentin sealer.

icians coat the exposed dentin of crown preparations with varnish before cementing crowns with zinc phosphate cement. The decision to use a varnish, or even a liner, is in part determined by the depth of the cavity. Deep cavities may be classified as those extending to within 0.5 to 1.0 mm of the pulp. This means that 1 mm or less of dentin remains to insulate and protect the pulp. Although it is difficult to gauge clinically, this **remaining dentin thickness (RDT)** is an important parameter. Studies suggest that restorative procedures and materials generally do not irritate the pulp when the RDT exceeds 0.5 to 1.0 mm.

Varnishes should not be used with composite or resin restoratives. The components of the varnish inhibit the curing of the resin materials and eliminate the chance for resin adhesives to bond to tooth structure. *Considering the adhesive characteristics of glass ionomers, would a cavity varnish be indicated to seal the dentin under one of these restorations?*

■ *Liners*

Uses of Liners

Lining materials are used to seal tooth structure against the leakage of irritants present in saliva or restorative materials. They also are used to provide a protective cap or covering to the pulp in deep cavities. A liner is placed as a direct **pulp cap** when there is a pulpal exposure and the liner is placed directly on the pulp. An **indirect pulp cap** refers to a situation in which there is a suspected exposure and the capping agent is placed over a small amount of remaining caries but not in direct contact with the pulp.

Types of Liners

Three types of materials are commonly used in dentistry as cavity liners, although they are not used interchangeably. The three materials are calcium hydroxide, glass ionomer, and **zinc oxide eugenol (ZOE)** cement.

Calcium Hydroxide

Calcium hydroxide is a basic compound with an approximate pH of 11. As such, it is mildly irritating to the vital pulp tissue. It also has **bacteriostatic** properties, which means it keeps bacteria from actively spreading. Both of these qualities make it a good lining material for restorations in close proximity to the pulp. It was long believed that calcium hydroxide was necessary to promote the formation of the secondary dentin that served to "wall off" and protect the pulp from external insults. Recent studies, however, have shown that the calcium hydroxide itself is not necessary for secondary dentin formation; what is needed is a mild irritant in conjunction with a sealed cavity (i.e., salivary bacteria must be excluded). Although calcium hydroxide does not bond to dentin, it does have antibacterial properties. It continues to have a high pH after setting because the material dissolves readily in aqueous solutions, liberating hydroxyl ions. This high pH provides a stimulus for the tooth to repair itself in the absence of bacterial infection. Thus, calcium hydroxide is not the only material that can serve this purpose, but it has a long history of clinical success to recommend it.

Calcium hydroxide is supplied in several forms. It may be sold as a liquid containing the compound calcium hydroxide suspended in a solvent; it also is supplied as a paste, in which the calcium hydroxide is suspended in methylcellulose. In these

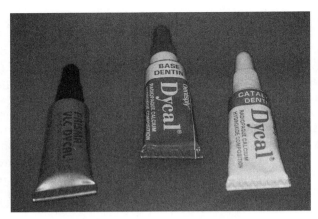

Figure 4–3 Tubes of a visible light-cured calcium hydroxide liner and of the base and catalyst pastes of a self-curing calcium hydroxide liner.

first two forms, the material is used like a varnish. In its third common form, calcium hydroxide is supplied as a two-paste system in tubes marked "catalyst" and "base" (Fig. 4-3). The calcium hydroxide is mixed with several other ingredients, such as zinc oxide and calcium phosphate. A catalyst is present to cause the calcium hydroxide to react and form a hard, amorphous compound within a matter of minutes under oral conditions. Finally, a fourth calcium hydroxide paste formulation contains a polymer resin (i.e., urethane dimethacrylate, similar to the resin in some composites) that can be hardened by illumination from a handheld blue light source (Fig. 4-3). *What benefits would be derived from a light-cured calcium hydroxide?*

Light-cured calcium hydroxide has a rapid setting reaction and a lower solubility in water. Therefore, it is more stable and does not dissolve as readily as the conventional material. Studies also show that it is not harmful to the pulp.

Glass Ionomers

For the same reason that glass ionomers are attractive as restorative materials, they are attractive as liners. Their adhesive characteristics make them ideal for sealing dentin under many types of restorations. They also release fluoride, which may give them anticarious properties.

Glass ionomer liners are supplied in two forms (Fig. 4-4). The earliest versions of these materials were conventional glass ionomers supplied as powder and liquid systems. The powder contained silicate glass particles, and the liquid contained a polyacrylic acid copolymer in water. Several manufacturers supply the powder and liquid components in predosed capsules, like amalgams. The capsules are **triturated**, or mixed at high speed, in an amalgamator (see Fig. 6-3) for 10 to 15 seconds, and then the cement is ejected from the capsule with a special gun cartridge.

Another version of glass ionomer is supplied as a powder and liquid system, but the liquid has been modified to include a light-curable resin component. This resin may simply be added to the liquid or, more effectively, chemically attached to the polyacrylic acid copolymer. Because both components have light-sensitive ingredients, the liquid and powder are supplied in brown bottles (Fig. 4-4). These resin-modified glass ionomer liners are popular because they can be hardened quickly in the cavity, like the light-cured calcium hydroxide materials. As mentioned earlier, they are stronger and less moisture sensitive than are the original forms. Further details about the composition and packaging of glass ionomers are discussed in Chapter 5.

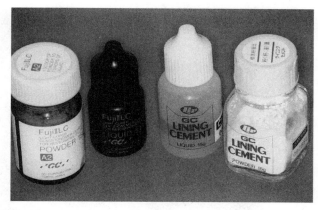

Figure 4–4 Liquid and powder for visible light-cured and self-curing glass ionomer liners.

Zinc Oxide Eugenol

This liner material has the same formulation as the ZOE used as a temporary cement or restorative material (see Chapter 10). The material is supplied in two tubes of paste labeled "catalyst" and "base." One paste contains zinc oxide and an accelerator in a resin; the second contains eugenol with an inert filler to make a paste. Other components also are added. Setting takes place by the reaction between zinc oxide and eugenol to form a crystalline compound called zinc eugenolate. Other oils beside eugenol can be used to make eugenol-free pastes, which are appropriate for patients allergic to eugenol. ZOE also is supplied in powder and liquid form, with both components packaged in bottles (Fig. 4-5).

ZOE has a near-neutral pH, so it usually is not irritating to the pulp. Also, eugenol has a sedative (obtundent) effect on the pulp, making ZOE useful as a liner for placement over calcium hydroxide in cases of near-pulp exposure. Eugenol can be toxic, however, when presented to tissue in high concentrations, and thus the ZOE should not be placed directly on an exposed, vital pulp.

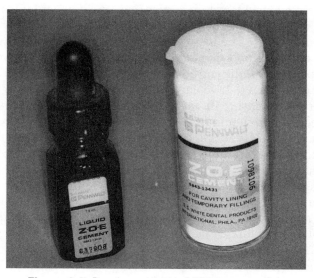

Figure 4–5 Powder and liquid of ZOE base material.

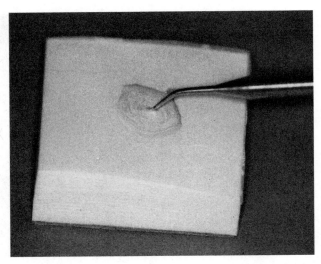

Figure 4–6 A two-paste, self-curing calcium hydroxide formulation being mixed on a pad with an applicator.

Handling and Placement of Liners

Liners supplied as two pastes are mixed with a steel spatula or other suitable mixing instrument on an oil-impervious paper pad supplied by the manufacturer. The coating on the pad keeps the liquid of the liner from soaking into the paper, which would change the powder-to-liquid ratio and affect the handling and properties of the material. Equal lengths of base and catalyst pastes are dispensed on the pad and quickly mixed together for about 20 seconds, until the paste is homogenous in color (Fig. 4-6). The liner is then applied to the dentin in a thin layer with a special applicator. The light-cured calcium hydroxide materials are hardened with a 20-second exposure from a handheld visible light-curing unit immediately after placement (Procedure Display 4-1).

Glass ionomers or ZOE liners that are supplied as powder and liquid systems are mixed on glass slabs or coated paper pads. Disposable paper pads are often preferable because glass ionomers adhere well to glass and can be difficult to remove if allowed to set on a glass slab. The powder jar is first fluffed or shaken to loosen the powder, and then the supplied scoop is lightly filled and emptied onto the mixing pad. The manufacturer's directions should always be consulted to ensure correct proportions of powder and liquid. The powder is then divided into two parts. Next, the correct number of drops of liquid are dispensed onto the pad, with care taken to hold either the dropper or the dropper bottle vertical to ensure accurate dispensing of each full drop (Fig. 4-7). The first half of the powder is mixed into the liquid for 15 seconds to produce a creamy consistency, and then the second half is added. Glass ionomers have a working time of 1.5 to 2 minutes, which is 1 to 2 minutes shorter than the working time of ZOE. The material can be placed into the tooth in the same manner as calcium hydroxide; a thickness of approximately 1 mm is recommended. Setting time for the ionomer is about 4 minutes. Although ZOE will take longer to set on the pad in the operatory, moisture and heat will hasten its set; it also will harden within 4 to 5 minutes in the mouth (Procedure Display 4-2).

The resin-modified glass ionomer is treated in a manner similar to the conventional glass ionomer, except that the entire quantity of powder is mixed into the liquid all at once within 15 seconds. Because these materials harden by the

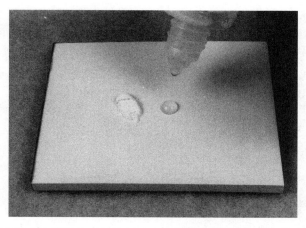

Figure 4–7 One scoop of a glass ionomer powder on a pad, with the liquid being dispensed from the bottle in preparation for mixing a liner.

same mechanism as conventional glass ionomers (see Chapter 5), even without the application of visible light, the working time is still limited to approximately 2 minutes. The material is placed in a thickness of approximately 1 mm and light-. cured for 30 seconds with a handheld visible light-curing unit.

Characteristics of Liners

The three liner materials have different characteristics. ZOE is a weak material, having a compressive strength of only 5 to 6 MPa. Similarly, calcium hydroxide is

PROCEDURE DISPLAY 4-1

Mixing a Calcium Hydroxide Liner

Equipment checklist
❑ Tubes of calcium hydroxide "catalyst" and "base"
❑ Oil-impervious pad
❑ Stainless steel cement spatula
❑ Timer or watch with second hand

STEP 1: **Proportioning**
❑ Dispense equal lengths of "catalyst" and "base" near each other on pad

STEP 2: **Mixing**
❑ Quickly mix pastes together for 20 seconds—first with tip of spatula and then scrape mix from pad and swipe across surface to blend
❑ Identify complete mix by homogenous color (no streaks)

STEP 3: **Applying liner**
❑ The mixed liner is picked up on the tip of an applicator, transferred to the cavity preparation, and dabbed into place

STEP 4: **Cleanup**
❑ Remove unset cement from instrument and spatula under running water
❑ Throw away top sheet of pad

PROCEDURE DISPLAY 4-2

Mixing Glass Ionomer Cement

Equipment checklist

❏ Glass ionomer cement powder (with scoop) and liquid
❏ Paper pad or glass slab (can be chilled in the refrigerator or under cold water for 5 minutes and then meticulously dried)
❏ Stainless steel cement spatula
❏ Timer or watch with second hand

STEP 1: **Proportioning**

❏ Shake and "fluff" jar to loosen powder
❏ Load scoop level with powder and dispense onto slab
❏ Form flat square of powder with spatula
❏ Divide square into halves
❏ Dispense liquid from dropper bottle near powder (remember to keep bottle vertical for accurate dispensing)

STEP 2: **Mixing**

❏ Draw one powder increment into liquid, smearing over large region of slab for 15 seconds to produce a creamy mix
❏ Draw second increment into mix, continuing to mix as above for another 10 to 15 seconds
❏ Determine consistency by pulling 0.5- to 0.75-inch-long ribbons of creamy cement from the mix with the spatula

STEP 3: **Lining and Cementations**

❏ For lining: Follow Step 3 in Procedure Display 4-1
❏ For cementation: Restoration is usually coated or filled with a thin layer of cement with the spatula

STEP 4: **Cleanup**

❏ Remove unset cement from slab and spatula under running water
❏ If cement is allowed to harden, remove from slab and spatula by soaking in warm water and then scrubbing with baking soda

weak, with a strength of 8.5 MPa, although the light-cured types are stronger. In contrast, conventional glass ionomer liners have compressive strengths of 50 to 100 MPa, with the light-cured versions being even stronger.

Calcium hydroxide is soluble in water and will dissolve in time under a leaking restoration. *What problems does this create, and how might it influence the placement and use of this material?*

If the liner were initially used to line the floor of the cavity completely, but subsequently dissolved and disappeared over time, the net result would be an unsupported restoration. This lack of support could make the restoration more prone to fracture during chewing. This is the main reason why calcium hydroxide should not be used to line the entire dentin surface under a composite or an amalgam restoration. At one time this was a common procedure, but glass ionomers have now supplanted calcium hydroxide for this purpose. Because of the incorporation of a light-cured resin component, the light-cured calcium hydroxide liners are much less soluble than were the original materials. Because they have no adhesive capacity with regard to the tooth surfaces, however, it still is not recommended that they be placed over all exposed dentin. Calcium hydroxide materials are optimally used for only the deepest portions of a cavity preparation in small quantities in "spot" applications and as a pulp-capping agent (Fig. 4-8). Studies also have shown that they are well tolerated by the pulp and, therefore, are ideal for this purpose.

ZOE, like calcium hydroxide, is more soluble in water than is glass ionomer. In addition, eugenol inhibits the hardening (polymerization) of resins and does not adhere to tooth structure. Therefore, ZOE is not recommended as a lining material under dental composites.

Both conventional and resin-modified glass ionomers are popular lining materials, although they have slightly different characteristics. Both appear to have similar biocompatibility when tested in animal studies and human clinical trials. Some of their physical characteristics differ, however, as a result of the incorporation of the resin component into the liquid of the light-cured types. The polymerization reaction increases the strength of the resin-modified version of the glass ionomer. As a further consequence of the increase in strength, the adhesive bond to dentin also is increased (from approximately 4 to 5 MPa to 8 to 10 MPa). Perhaps the most important dividend of the resin addition is the reduced moisture sensitivity of the light-cured version. When placed in thin layers and allowed to dry, this material is not prone to cracking like the conventional glass ionomer. This beneficial characteristic helps to minimize leakage and sensitivity problems when the material is used as a liner. The purpose of a liner is to seal the dentin. The dentin cannot be sealed, however, if the liner contains cracks that provide paths for fluids to penetrate. Therefore, the resin-modified glass ionomer often is preferred over the conventional material for such applications.

To function optimally for many years, a liner must have sufficient strength and resistance to solubility. The same is true for a base. The liner also must be fluid enough to be uniformly distributed over all of the exposed dentin to ensure complete protection. Strength and solubility resistance are optimized by maximizing the powder-to-liquid ratio, simply because the powder portion is the strongest and least soluble part of the cement. These cements should always be mixed with the highest powder-to-liquid ratio possible. The limiting factor is the viscosity of the

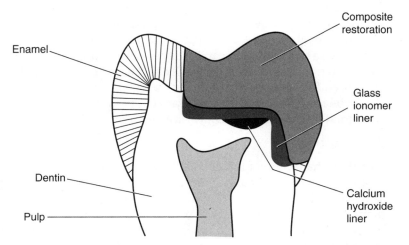

Figure 4-8 Placement of calcium hydroxide under a glass ionomer liner and composite restoration. The calcium hydroxide is limited only to the deepest portions of a cavity preparation because of its low strength and high solubility.

material. As the powder-to-liquid ratio is increased, so is the viscosity of the mix, which makes it more difficult for the liner to flow over all of the exposed dentin. At the same time, the working time is reduced when a thick mix is produced. Therefore, the ideal mix is produced by delaying mixing until the clinician is ready and then mixing deliberately at the powder-to-liquid ratio recommended by the manufacturer to optimize properties and fluidity. The temperature of the operatory can also have a significant effect. Therefore, under warm conditions, acceptable mixes are best achieved by mixing on a chilled glass slab to extend the working time and maximize the amount of powder that can be incorporated into the liquid.

■ *Bases*

Uses of Bases

As previously defined, bases are placed in relatively thick layers (at least 0.75 to 1.0 mm) to provide thermal insulation under deep (less than 1 mm of dentin remaining) metallic restorations. Bases can also seal the dentin at the same time, especially if they are made from glass ionomers or resin-modified glass ionomers.

Types of Bases

Essentially any dental cement can be used as a base. All have similar insulating capabilities, and all have thermal conductivity values similar to those of the natural dentition. The conventional and light-cured glass ionomers already discussed are commonly used as bases. In addition, a reinforced version of ZOE can be used as a base material under amalgam restorations.

Zinc Oxide Eugenol

There are two types of reinforced ZOE, one containing a polymer and the other aluminum oxide particles with the chemical ethoxybenzoic acid (EBA). Both are powder and liquid systems. The polymer-reinforced version contains 20% acrylic polymer in the form of small spheres, which is added to the zinc oxide powder. The liquid is the normal eugenol formulation. The second type is called EBA. The powder is a zinc oxide formulation with aluminum oxide reinforcement particles. The liquid contains EBA and eugenol in approximately a 2:1 ratio. The EBA helps to produce a stronger matrix to hold the particles together, thus creating a stronger base or temporary restorative material. These reinforced ZOE bases often have been used for patients with sensitive teeth. The rationale has been that the pulp would be less affected by the neutral ZOE than it might be by the acidity of other common base materials, such as glass ionomer or zinc phosphate cement.

Zinc Phosphate

Zinc phosphate cement mixed to a thick, viscous consistency is commonly used as a base to provide thermal and mechanical protection under amalgam restorations. The material is packaged as a powder and liquid system. The powder is composed mainly of zinc oxide particles to which magnesium oxide is added. The acidic liquid contains phosphoric acid in water (approximately a 33% acid concentration). A small amount of aluminum phosphate is added to enhance the setting reaction. When the powder is mixed with the liquid, the acid begins to dissolve the outside of the zinc oxide particles, releasing zinc ions into the phosphoric acid liquid. The

DISPLAY 4-1

> ### Factors Accelerating the Setting Rate of Most Cements
>
> Use of small particles in the cement powder
> Use of a high powder-to-liquid ratio
> Mixing at elevated temperatures
> Overmixing (i.e., mixing longer than necessary)
> Mixing zinc phosphate rapidly in few steps

negatively charged phosphoric ions react with the positively charged aluminum and zinc ions to form a zinc phosphate compound, which serves as a matrix to hold the original particles together. Several factors influence the rate of the reaction, including the size of the zinc oxide particles, the powder-to-liquid ratio, the mixing technique, and the mixing temperature. In general, smaller-sized particles, faster mixing, higher mixing temperatures, and the use of more powder all hasten the setting rate (Display 4-1). Of these, all except particle size are under the control of the clinical staff and should be considered when these materials are mixed. Therefore, it is important to keep several factors in mind during the mixing and manipulation of bases. These are the same factors that affect the setting rate of liners and were addressed previously.

Handling and Placement of Bases

The mixing of glass ionomer as a liner has already been discussed. Usually, the only difference between mixing a cement as a base or as a liner is the consistency. Bases usually are mixed to a higher powder-to-liquid ratio for maximum strength. Because a clinician may exert more than 5 to 6 pounds of force during the condensation of amalgam, the base that is placed must be strong enough to withstand the condensation forces, even though it has just been placed itself. Therefore, it also must have a rapid setting rate, and this is enhanced by the higher powder-to-liquid ratio. A base of insufficient strength may be displaced or fractured during condensation of the amalgam, reducing its efficiency.

Glass ionomer and ZOE cements are mixed rapidly in a single increment or, at most, in two separate increments of powder. The mixing of zinc phosphate cement is very different. Zinc phosphate must be mixed slowly, in stages, to avoid heat buildup within the material. As zinc oxide and phosphoric acid react, heat is released. This heat hastens the setting rate and severely shortens the working time. The detailed procedure for the proper mixing of zinc phosphate is outlined in the next section, on cements; however, the same principles apply for mixing bases. The difference is that the base is mixed to a much thicker consistency to form a putty-like material that can be applied to the floor of the cavity with an amalgam condenser (Fig. 4-9). When mixed at ambient temperatures, the setting time for the base is approximately 5 to 6 minutes.

Characteristics of Bases

The characteristics of ZOE and glass ionomers were discussed in the section on liners; therefore, this section concentrates mainly on zinc phosphate. Zinc phosphate

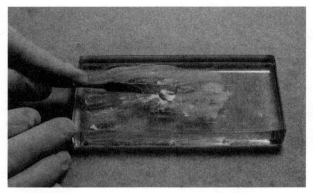

Figure 4–9 A zinc phosphate cement after being mixed on a glass slab to a putty-like consistency for use as a base.

is an acidic cement. This characteristic may be cause for concern when zinc phosphate is placed near the pulp, and partially explains why zinc phosphate usually is used in conjunction with calcium hydroxide liners in deep cavities. The pH of the setting material is low (approximately 2 to 3) and remains low for many hours after the initial hardening has occurred. Figure 4-10 shows the rise in pH with time for a zinc phosphate mixed to a base consistency. Note that the neutralization of the acid to move the pH closer to 7 occurs slowly, similar to the way the material acquires strength with time. Therefore, although the base reaches a clinically useful hardness and strength within minutes after mixing, the setting reaction continues for hours and days, further improving all of the properties of the material. The behavior of glass ionomer is similar to that of zinc phosphate, although it experiences a slightly more rapid rise in pH during setting.

The compressive strength of a zinc phosphate base at 24 hours is similar to that of a glass ionomer (nearly 100 MPa), and both are superior to any of the ZOE formulations (Table 4-1). The material has a very low solubility in water, lower than that of glass ionomer, although its solubility in the mouth is slightly greater than that of glass ionomer (this apparent contradiction will be discussed later). Zinc

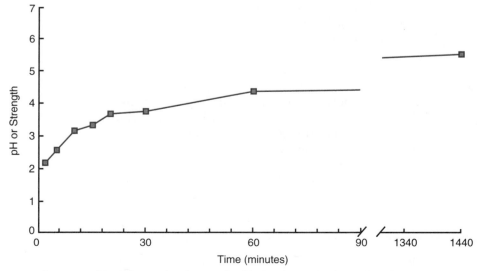

Figure 4–10 Rise in both pH and strength with time for a mix of zinc phosphate cement.

TABLE 4–1. Approximate Physical and Mechanical Properties of Several Dental Cements

	Compressive Strength (MPa)	Tensile Strength (MPa)	Elastic Modulus (GPa)	Water Solubility (%)	Oral Solubility	Pulp Response
ZOP	70–100	5.5	13.5	0.06	Medium	Moderate
ZOE	6–30	—	—	0.04	High	Mild
ZOE/EBA	55	4.1	5.0	0.05	Medium	Mild
ZOE/resin	48	4.1	2.5	0.08	Medium	Mild
PC	55	6.2	5.1	0.06	Medium	Mild
GIC	85	6.2	7.3	1.25	Low	Mild-moderate
RMGIC	130–170	12–14	3–4	1.00	Low	Mild-moderate
Resin	70–170	30	3–5	0.01	None	Moderate

ZOP, zinc phosphate; ZOE, zinc oxide eugenol; ZOE/EBA, zinc oxide eugenol/ethoxybenzoic acid; PC, polycarboxylate; GIC, glass ionomer cement; RMGIC, resin-modified glass ionomer cement.

phosphate provides a stiffer base than glass ionomer, but it does not form a chemical bond to the tooth surface. Despite its lack of chemical adhesion to teeth, zinc phosphate has a long history of successful use in dentistry and continues to be an acceptable material and the choice of many clinicians.

■ *Cements*

Uses of Cements

Cements are used for a variety of applications in dentistry. The most obvious use is for permanently retaining metal inlays, onlays, crowns, and bridges to tooth structure. Cements used in this manner are called **luting** agents because they *lute*, or adhere, one surface to another. Other uses of conventional types of cements include the bonding of orthodontic bands to molars and cementing pins and posts to teeth to retain restorations. The use of conventional cements to bond porcelain or ceramic veneers, inlays, crowns, and bridges has been superseded by the use of resin cements with formulations similar to those of composites. Resin cements are also used to attach the wings of certain types of metal "resin-bonded bridges" to teeth (Fig. 4-11), to bond metal or ceramic brackets to enamel for orthodontic applications, and to cement composite or ceramic inlays, onlays, crowns, bridges, or

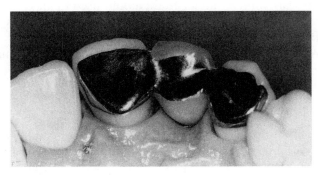

Figure 4–11 Lingual view of a resin-bonded bridge replacing a lateral incisor.

veneers to teeth. The requirements for the cements used in the different applications vary, but many of the formulations are interchangeable. Although there are certain reasons for choosing a specific formulation for a certain application, many clinicians achieve good results using only one or two types of cements for all clinical applications.

Types of Cements

Several types of luting cements are used in dentistry; many of them have already been discussed in relation to their use as base materials. The common cements are zinc phosphate, zinc polycarboxylate, glass ionomer, ZOE, and resins (actually composites). Another type of cement, silicophosphate, was used in the past but essentially has been replaced by glass ionomers. Although called a cement, another type of material, silicate cement, was used in the past as a restorative material but has since been replaced by composites and glass ionomers.

The cements have different handling and physical characteristics but can be used almost interchangeably. Although it has been suggested that certain cements should not be used in certain applications, there are few clinical data, except for ZOE, to support the restricted use of any cement. ZOE usually is considered a temporary cement because it has limited strength and durability. The use of this material as a temporary restorative is fully discussed in Chapter 10.

Zinc Phosphate

Zinc phosphate cement is manufactured in two forms. The type I form is used for luting castings, and the type II form is used for all other applications. The only difference between the two is the size of the zinc oxide particles. The type I cement has smaller particles that enable the cement to flow out into thin (less than 25 μm) layers between a casting and the tooth. The type II form contains larger particles and can routinely achieve a film thickness of 40 μm. The zinc phosphate cements used for bases have the same composition as those used for luting agents, with the only difference being the consistency to which they are mixed.

Zinc Polycarboxylate

Zinc polycarboxylate was the first cement to produce true chemical adhesion to tooth structure. It is composed of a powder much like that of the zinc phosphate cement. Some stannous fluoride often is added to the powder to improve handling characteristics and properties, but it does not seem to provide a beneficial anticarious effect. The major difference between phosphate and carboxylate cements is in the liquid portion. The liquid of the polycarboxylate is a polyacrylic acid copolymer in water and is similar to the liquid used in glass ionomer cements. The liquid can be freeze-dried and added to the powder, which is then simply mixed with water containing a small amount of an additive.

A carboxylate cement adheres to tooth structure through an ionic interaction between negatively charged molecules in the cement with positively charged atoms, such as calcium, in the tooth structure.

Glass Ionomers

The composition of glass ionomers has already been fully described in Chapter 3. Briefly, the powder contains a calcium-aluminum silicate glass that is soluble in acid. The liquid is a copolymer of polyacrylic acid and either itaconic or maleic acid. A small amount of tartaric acid is added to the liquid to provide a reasonable working time, which is then followed by a rapid set. Originally, polyacrylic acid was used alone in glass ionomers, but the polymer had a tendency to dry out and increase in viscosity during storage. The copolymers are less apt to thicken and thus have greater stability. The restorative, base, liner, and luting agent have essentially the same chemical composition. The potential beneficial effects of the fluoride release from these cements make them desirable materials. In addition, they achieve true chemical adhesion to tooth structure in the same manner as the polycarboxylates.

The similarities between the compositions of the cements should be obvious. It should be apparent that a mixing and matching of powders and liquids has taken place to produce the many different types of dental luting cements. The chart in Table 4-2 should help to clarify cement compositions.

Resin-Modified Glass Ionomer

Resin-modified glass ionomer cements have a composition similar to the resin-modified glass ionomer liner and/or base material discussed earlier in this chapter. The difference is that these cements may be used to lute metallic restorations and, therefore, cannot be light-cured. Instead, the materials are formulated to have two self-curing reactions, one for the glass ionomer and one for the added resin. This is further explained in Chapter 5. The resin-modified glass ionomer cements are stronger, more water insoluble, and more adherent to tooth structure than is the conventional glass ionomer cement.

Resin Cements

Resin cements are basically fluid composites. The fluidity is achieved by reducing the amount of filler particles added to the composite. The resins may be bis-GMA (2,2-bis[4(2-hydroxy-3-methacryloyloxy-propoxy)phenyl]propane) or urethane dimethacrylates with the appropriate diluents. The fillers usually are barium glasses, although some resin cements are filled with microscopic silica particles. The filler may make up 30 to 60% by weight of the cement, although there is a trend to produce materials that are more heavily filled for better strength and wear resistance. Because these cements do not adhere to tooth structure, they usually are used in conjunction with an etching treatment. A resin adhesive can also be used when dentin is present. Although some resin cements are only self-curing cements, many are dual-cured formulations, containing chemicals for both a self-curing and a light-cured reaction. Dual-cured cements (Fig. 4-12) commonly are used to cement composite or porcelain inlays, onlays, crowns, and veneers because these restorations will partially transmit light; however, it is not possible to illuminate the cement through a metal casting or bridge. The concept behind dual

TABLE 4–2. **Simplifying the Composition of Dental Cements**

| | Powders | |
Liquids	Silicate Glass	Zinc Oxide
Phosphoric acid	Silicate cement	Zinc phosphate
Polyacrylic acid	Glass ionomer	Polycarboxylate
Eugenol	—	Zinc oxide eugenol
Dimethacrylate monomers	Resin	—

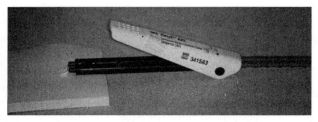

Figure 4–12 Dual-cure resin cement supplied in a convenient two-barrel dispenser.

curing is that the areas that are not exposed to the light source eventually (i.e., within 10 to 15 minutes) will harden on their own from the self-curing reaction. Nevertheless, the properties of dual-cured cements are optimized when they are light cured.

Compomer

Compomers are a class of materials also referred to as **polyacid-modified resins**. They are essentially resin composites that contain additional acidic monomers similar to glass ionomers. These materials, like composites and unlike resin-modified glass ionomers, do not contain water in their formulation, however. They are anhydrous. Therefore, compomers are more similar to composites than to glass ionomers. They initially harden by a polymerization of the resin monomers. After absorbing water from the oral cavity, they have the potential for a delayed acid-base reaction (like glass ionomers). In addition, they release fluoride, though typically to a lesser extent than do glass ionomers. They are formulated in light-cured or self-cured versions to be used as cements for all types of dental restorations, and they have properties similar to resin cements. These materials will be more fully explained in Chapter 5.

Handling and Placement of Cements

The mixing of cements for luting applications is addressed using the specific example of zinc phosphate. Although mixing techniques vary between materials, most of the procedures have already been discussed for the other cements. The procedure for zinc phosphate is the most complicated and must be understood to maximize the desirable physical characteristics and clinical success of the material.

Hardening of most dental cements takes place when the powder and liquid are mixed together to produce a chemical reaction between their components. Usually, the particles in the powder are partially dissolved by the acidic liquid, releasing ions that react with the negative charges of the molecules in the liquid. This reaction forms a matrix that rigidly binds the original particles together. The rate of the reactions depends on several variables, including the powder-to-liquid ratio, temperature, water concentration in the mix, and mixing time. The operator has control over each one of these variables and must manipulate them to produce ideal mixes.

This detailed procedure for mixing zinc phosphate is essential to provide the operator with ample working time. The reaction is exothermic, meaning it gives off heat. When enough powder becomes dissolved in the acidic liquid, the acid becomes neutralized and gives off heat. Because the heat accelerates the setting rate, it is important to slow the interaction between the powder and liquid. This is accomplished by several means. *Can you predict what these might be?*

First, the mixing can be done on a chilled glass slab. Because heat accelerates the chemical reaction, the chilled slab will slow the setting rate by reducing the mixing temperature. The glass slab can be chilled by placing it into a refrigerator or under cold water for 5 minutes. In either case, before proceeding, the slab needs to be completely dried because moisture on the slab will cause the cement to set faster. If the slab is cooled to a temperature below the dew point, it will "sweat" when exposed to room humidity, condensing water onto its surface. The water will become incorporated into the mix, speeding the chemical reaction that forms the cement matrix by hastening the rate at which the acid becomes neutralized. Another benefit from the use of a chilled slab is that the slower reaction rate keeps the viscosity low. When the viscosity of the mixture is low, more powder can be mixed into a given amount of liquid while adequate flow characteristics are main-

PROCEDURE DISPLAY 4-3

Mixing Zinc Phosphate Cement

Equipment checklist
- ❑ Zinc phosphate cement powder (with scoop) and liquid
- ❑ Glass slab (chilled in the refrigerator or under cold water for 5 minutes and then meticulously dried)
- ❑ Stainless steel cement spatula
- ❑ Timer or watch with second hand

STEP 1: **Proportioning**
- ❑ Load scoop level with powder and dispense onto slab
- ❑ Form flat square of powder with spatula
- ❑ Divide square into quarters
- ❑ Divide one quarter into two one-eighth portions
- ❑ Divide one one-eighth portion into two one-sixteenth portions for a total of six increments
- ❑ Dispense liquid from dropper bottle near powder

STEP 2: **Mixing**
- ❑ Draw first one-sixteenth increment into liquid, smearing over large region of slab for 10 seconds
- ❑ Draw second one-sixteenth increment into mix, continuing to mix as above for another 10 seconds
- ❑ Draw a one-eighth increment into the mix and continue mixing as above for 10 to 15 seconds
- ❑ Draw a one-quarter increment in and mix for 10 to 15 seconds
- ❑ Draw a second one-quarter increment in and mix for 10 to 15 seconds
- ❑ Draw the final one-quarter increment in and mix for 10 to 15 seconds
- ❑ Determine consistency by pulling 0.5- to 0.75-inch-long ribbons of creamy cement from the mix with the spatula

STEP 3: **Loading restoration with cement**
- ❑ Restoration is usually coated or filled with a thin layer of cement with the spatula

STEP 4: **Cleanup**
- ❑ Remove unset cement from slab and spatula under running water
- ❑ If cement is allowed to harden, remove from slab and spatula by soaking in warm water and then scrubbing with baking soda

tained. Because cements with higher powder-to-liquid ratios are the strongest, it is desirable to maximize the powder-to-liquid ratio. The use of a chilled slab allows this to be done without sacrificing handling characteristics.

The second important point is that zinc phosphate should be mixed by incorporating small increments of powder into the liquid over a relatively long period of time. This slow mixing of powder and liquid also controls the rate at which the acid becomes neutralized, thus slowing the setting rate and lengthening the working time. It also is beneficial to mix over a large area of the slab to allow heat to dissipate from the mix, thus keeping the overall temperature lower and prolonging the working time.

One of several common methods for mixing zinc phosphate is described in Procedure Display 4-3. The appropriate amount of powder is dispensed onto a glass slab and then divided into six portions with a long, thin cement spatula (Fig. 4-13). The liquid is then dispensed from the dropper bottle adjacent to the powder. The liquid should not be dispensed first because water may begin to evaporate from it during the time that the powder is dispensed, altering the working time.

The first small increment is drawn into the liquid with the spatula and mixed for 10 seconds with a smearing motion over a large portion of the slab (Fig. 4-14). A large surface area allows the heat created by the neutralization of the acid to dissipate, thus keeping the mix cool. The same is done for the second small increment, making sure to scrape the mix from the slab periodically to avoid leaving any of the powder unwetted by the liquid. This process continues until the cement has reached the desired consistency. Often this is determined by touching the spatula to the mix and pulling up: A ribbon of creamy cement should flow from the spatula blade. When the ribbon becomes 0.5 to 0.75 of an inch long, it should slide off the spatula and flow back into the mix on the slab, blending with the rest of the mix (Fig. 4-15). If the cement immediately drips off of the spatula as it is raised, it may be too fluid. If it is too stiff to be drawn out into a thin ribbon, it may be too viscous. The total mixing time should take 1 to 1.5 minutes, providing a cement with a working time of several minutes. Once mixed, the cement is coated onto the dental appliance, and the appliance is seated in the patient.

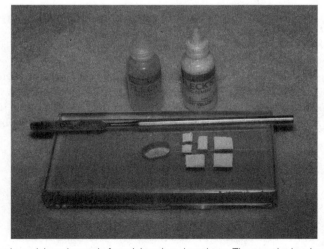

Figure 4–13 A glass slab and spatula for mixing zinc phosphate. The powder has been dispensed and divided on the slab, and the liquid has been dispensed from a dropper bottle near the powder.

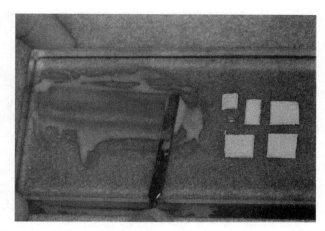

Figure 4–14 First increments of zinc phosphate powder being mixed into the liquid, with a sweeping motion over a large area of the slab used to minimize heat buildup.

The slab and spatula are easiest to clean when they are washed off before the cement has set. The cement is water soluble and is easily removed at that point. Set cement can be removed from a slab or spatula by soaking in warm water. Baking soda also can be used to aid in removing set cement.

As previously mentioned, glass ionomers are also packaged in an encapsulated form for use as a dental cement. The capsule, similar to that used for dental amalgam, is mixed in a triturator, or dental amalgamator, for 10 seconds typically at a speed of 3000 to 4000 rpm (Fig. 4-16). The cement is usually dispensed from the capsule directly into the restoration to be luted with a special handheld dispenser.

Characteristics of Cements

All dental cements are brittle materials. They have relatively high compressive strengths but are fairly weak in tension (Table 4-1). The resin cements are the strongest of the cements. They have the highest tensile strength, and their compressive strength is similar to that of zinc phosphate and glass ionomer. The strength of the polycarboxylate cements is intermediate. The ZOE cements are the weakest of the group; the low strength of ZOE cements limits their use to tempo-

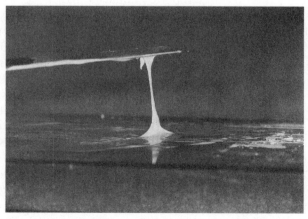

Figure 4–15 Cement ribbons being pulled from the zinc phosphate mix, showing a correct consistency for luting.

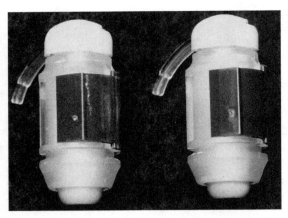

Figure 4–16 Glass ionomer in capsules similar to those used for dental amalgam.

rary applications. Resin-modified glass ionomers and compomers are intermediate to glass ionomers and composites. The elastic modulus of the zinc phosphate cement is the highest, being nearly double that of glass ionomer. For this reason, some clinicians have advocated the use of zinc phosphate when cementing long-span bridges, because they question whether glass ionomer could sufficiently resist the bending forces imposed. Given the similar clinical results with each of these cements, there is little evidence that only zinc phosphate should be used for these applications.

The solubility of the cements is a major concern. A primary cause of failure of dental castings is related to the "washout" or dissolution of the cement at the margins of a restoration. This cement loss contributes to leakage, secondary decay, and loosening of the restoration. The solubility of the cements in water does not reflect their solubility in the oral cavity, however, with one exception. The resin-containing cements are the most insoluble of all of the cements, either in water or in the oral fluids (Table 4-1). The other cements also appear relatively insoluble in water, with the exception of the glass ionomers. Note that even ZOE seems to be more stable in water than are glass ionomer cements. In the often acidic, salty environment of the oral cavity, however, glass ionomers have been shown to be the least soluble of the nonresin cements, followed by zinc phosphate and polycarboxylate. The ZOE cements are the most soluble in the oral cavity, another factor that limits their use to temporary applications.

All of the cements will absorb water in the oral cavity. This has not presented a problem for most dental restorations requiring cementation because the restorations have traditionally been made of metal. With the expanding use of all-ceramic restorations, however, water sorption posed a problem for one specific type of resin-modified glass ionomer cement. During the mid-1990s, a higher-than-acceptable incidence of ceramic crown fractures was noted for one brand of these materials. It was believed that the high water sorption in conjunction with the high stiffness of this particular cement produced excessive forces on the crowns, leading to fracture. For this reason, resin-modified glass ionomer cements are not recommended for all ceramic restorations.

The biocompatibility of the various cements is obviously a serious concern. Given that many of the cements are acidic, one would expect differences between the different types. The zinc phosphate cement is the most acidic. Although glass ionomer, resin-modified glass ionomer, and polycarboxylate cements have a similar pH when applied to the tooth (pH 2 to 3), they undergo a more rapid rise in pH during setting than does zinc phosphate (Fig. 4-10). Therefore, the acidic nature of zinc phosphate is enduring, with the pH remaining below 5.5 until nearly 24 hours after mixing. As might be expected, mixing with a lower powder-to-liquid ratio increases the acidity of the zinc phosphate cement, another reason for mixing cements with a high powder-to-liquid ratio. The incidence of postoperative sensitivity and pulpal damage is slightly higher with zinc phosphate cement than it is with the other cements, possibly because of the slower neutralization of the acidity. Zinc phosphate is routinely used without any adverse effects, however, suggesting that at least some of the biologic concerns can be alleviated through the appropriate mixing and handling of the material. The polycarboxylate cement undergoes the most rapid rise in pH, reaching a value of 5 within 30 minutes of mixing. Perhaps this explains why it is considered by many clinicians to be the most biocompatible of the acidic cements. The pH of the glass ionomer cements rises somewhat more slowly than does that of polycarboxylate, placing them between zinc phosphate and polycarboxylate in terms of tissue compatibility. ZOE has a neutral pH and, therefore, is the most benign of the cements. Resin cements and compomers also are neutral, but postoperative sensitivity and pulpal inflammation can be related to their setting shrinkage, which can contribute to marginal leakage. More will be said about this in the next chapter.

The cements all have a satisfactory working time, although zinc phosphate might be considered to be superior to the rest (with the exception of the dual-cure resin cements). The rapid set of the glass ionomers creates problems during the simultaneous cementation of several units, especially because the time available for cleanup of the excess cement in the mouth is greatly reduced. Some clinicians prefer a zinc phosphate cement for inlays and onlays in which a significant amount of marginal cleaning will take place. The use of preencapsulated glass ionomer and polycarboxylate formulations provides increased working time because mixing is accomplished mechanically within 10 to 15 seconds. Although these systems are more costly, the convenience and the more reproducible consistency from mix to mix would appear to outweigh the cost factor.

Summary

Intermediary materials occupy space between dental restoratives and tooth structure to seal (liners) or insulate (bases) the tooth or to protect it from the restorative material or oral environment. Cements are used to attach restorations temporarily or permanently. Resin, polymer, and ceramic-type materials are used to produce varnishes, calcium hydroxide for liners, zinc phosphate for bases and cements, ZOE for bases and temporary cements, polycarboxylate for cements, and glass ionomers for liners, bases, and cements. The materials have different characteristics. The poorer strength and solubility resistance of ZOE preclude its use as a permanent cement. Glass ionomers have properties similar to those of zinc phosphate cements but also adhere to teeth and release fluoride. Therefore, ionomers have become popular permanent cements, as have insulators and sealers under amalgam and composite restorations. Most materials, with the exception of liquid varnishes, are provided in a form that requires mixing of two components to produce a paste that is applied and then dries or hardens within the tooth. Powder and liquid systems can be mixed to different consistencies for different applications. For example, strong bases for providing thermal and mechanical protection under amalgams require viscous mixes with high powder-to-liquid ratios. In contrast, cements must be mixed at lower viscosities to enable them to flow out from between the restoration and tooth during placement. Generally, thicker mixes made by adding more powder provide greater strength, stiffness, solubility resistance, and faster rates of hardening than do thinner mixes.

STUDY QUESTIONS AND PROBLEM SOLVING

1. **A base is placed on the floor of a deep cavity under a gold restoration to:**
   a. Provide thermal protection for the pulp
   b. Seal the dentin from toxic gold particles
   c. Prevent gold atoms from penetrating into the tooth
   d. Improve the stiffness of the restoration

2. **During the warm part of the year, the office air-conditioning system experiences problems, causing the operatory temperature to be noticeably warmer than usual. How will this affect the way you mix zinc phosphate cement for a bridge?**
   a. Mix the powder into the liquid faster to leave enough working time
   b. Chill the slab in the refrigerator before mixing to prolong the working time
   c. Mix only one half of the recommended powder to slow setting
   d. Dispense the liquid first to allow time for water to evaporate to slow setting

3. **A patient complains that tooth 3, which contains a crown, is sensitive to hot and cold, and the dentist notices that there has been a substantial loss of cement at the margins and suspects that it is leaking. Which of the following characteristics of the cement best explains the reason for the cement loss?**
   a. Low compressive strength
   b. Solubility in oral fluids
   c. High thermal conductivity
   d. Low elastic limit

4. **Which of the following materials is most often placed into a deep cavity with the intent of protecting the pulp and promoting reparative dentin formation?**
   a. Zinc oxide eugenol
   b. Glass ionomer
   c. Calcium hydroxide
   d. Zinc phosphate

5. **What would be the rationale for placing a liner of glass ionomer under a large and deep composite restoration in a molar?**
   a. Provide thermal insulation for the tooth
   b. Seal the dentinal surfaces under the composite
   c. Improve the strength of the restoration
   d. Minimize chances for postoperative sensitivity

6. **Glass ionomers are considered by some to be the material of choice for applying a base under an amalgam restoration because they:**
   a. Chemically adhere to dentin and enamel
   b. Are twice as strong as all other bases
   c. Are completely insoluble in oral fluids
   d. Provide fluoride protection under leaky fillings

7. **A patient with a history of very sensitive teeth requires an amalgam restoration of a maxillary molar. Which base material may be the best choice for this patient, and why?**
   a. Glass ionomer, because it will never dissolve
   b. Zinc phosphate, because it is very stiff
   c. Zinc oxide eugenol, because it has a neutral pH
   d. Light-cured calcium hydroxide, because it is so strong

8. **Which of the following is least likely to have a significant effect on the setting rate of zinc phosphate cement?**
   a. Powder-to-liquid ratio
   b. Size of the powder particles
   c. Stiffness of the mixing spatula
   d. Size of the mixing area

9. **Which of the following is *not* present in glass ionomer cements?**
   a. Eugenol
   b. Polyacrylic acid
   c. Silicate glass
   d. Tartaric acid

10. **Compomer cements differ from resin-modified glass ionomer cements in that compomers:**
   a. Initially harden by an acid-base reaction
   b. Are stronger and more wear resistant
   c. Have monomers for a polymerization reaction
   d. Release fluoride into the saliva

SELECTED READINGS

Hilton TJ. Cavity sealers, liners, and bases: Current philosophies and indications for use. Operative Dentistry 21:134–146, 1996.
   A comprehensive and scientific review of the evidence for the use of the various types of materials available as bases and liners in restorative dentistry.

Knibbs PJ, Walls AWG. A laboratory and clinical evaluation of three dental luting cements. Journal of Oral Rehabilitation 16:467–473, 1989.
   This article shows that the in vitro erosion in water of glass ionomer cements is less than that of polycarboxylate and zinc phosphate cements. In addition, a clinical study was conducted to evaluate the marginal integrity of 250 restorations cemented with these materials over a 3.5-year period. Zinc phosphate gave the best clinical performance.

McComb D. Adhesive luting cements—classes, criteria, and usage. Compendium of Continuing Education in Dentistry 17:759–762, 764, 1996.
   This article describes glass ionomers, resin-modified glass ionomers, and resin cements and provides a comparison of their biologic and physical properties, their indications, and their limitations. The article also makes recommendations for their clinical usage.

Milosevic A. Calcium hydroxide in restorative dentistry. Journal of Dentistry 19:3–13, 1991.
   The composition and properties of a variety of calcium hydroxide materials are summarized. The antibacterial effects and tissue reactions also are reviewed. It is concluded that the mechanism of hard tissue repair in association with calcium hydroxide preparations is not clear, nor is its antibacterial nature. These uncertainties contribute to the unpredictable outcomes that are often associated with calcium hydroxide materials.

Mitchem JC, Gronas DG. Clinical evaluation of cement solubility. Journal of Prosthetic Dentistry 40:453–457, 1978.
   This study shows that the in vivo solubility of dental cements is different from the in vitro solubility, casting some doubt on the results of simple water storage as a means of predicting the solubility of dental cements.

Mount GJ. Polyacrylic cements in dentistry. American Journal of Dentistry 3(2):79–84, 1990.
   This review article describes the development, composition, and properties of polycarboxylate and glass ionomer cements. The differences in composition of glass ionomers used as luting agents, liners, and restora-

tives are presented. It concludes that both are excellent permanent cements but that the popularity of glass ionomers has superseded that of the polycarboxylates. Clinical procedures for the use of glass ionomers for luting, lining, and restoring are provided.

Nicholson JW, Crool TW. Glass-ionomer cements in restorative dentistry. Quintessence International 28:705–714, 1997.

A review of the composition, chemistry, properties, and use of conventional and resin-modified glass ionomer cements. Specific clinical examples of the use of these cements are highlighted and presented.

Smith DC, Ruse DN, Zuccolin D. Some characteristics of glass ionomer cement lining materials. Journal of the Canadian Dental Association 54:903–908, 1988.

The pH, bond strength to dentin and composite, and radiopacity were evaluated for several glass ionomer liners. The best bond to dentin was shown to be in the range of 5 to 6 MPa, and all of the liners were more radiopaque than dentin, enhancing clinical diagnosis for secondary decay.

Tam LE, McComb D, Pulver F. Physical properties of proprietary light-cured lining materials. Operative Dentistry 16:210–217, 1991.

The physical properties, such as strength, fluoride and calcium release, and pH were evaluated in this study of four different light-cured lining materials. The results showed that the more composite-like the liner was, the stronger it was but the less fluoride or calcium it released.

Direct Esthetic Anterior Restoratives

Objectives

- List and explain the function of the three main components of dental composites.

- Compare the composition, properties, and appearance of the different types of composites.

- Discuss the procedure of placing and curing a light-activated dental composite to optimize the properties and marginal seal of the restoration.

- Select a type of composite for a specific clinical application, based on the demands of the situation.

- Compare the properties of composites, compomers, and glass ionomers and describe how specific differences may influence clinical performance.

- Compare the composition and properties of the different types of glass ionomer restoratives.

- Describe the proper technique for mixing a conventional glass ionomer restorative.

- Explain the importance of maintaining a moist, but not wet, environment during the placement of a glass ionomer restorative.

- Compare the composition and properties of compomers to composites and resin-modified glass ionomer restoratives.

- Describe the basic components of dentin adhesives and briefly explain how they achieve adhesion to tooth structure.

There is a movement in dentistry toward **esthetic** restorations. The choice between a metallic tooth replacement and one that mimics the appearance of natural teeth is an obvious one. Nowhere is this more important than in the anterior region of the mouth. The ability to lighten dark or stained teeth, to close conservatively a large gap between two central incisors, or to increase the bulk and reshape a tooth may mean the difference between a person who smiles and one who is embarrassed to open his or her mouth to speak. Esthetic dentistry may, at times, cross the line between reparative and cosmetic dentistry in that often there is no symptomatology associated with the treatment.

The esthetic dentistry movement may have begun when the **acid-etch technique** was finally incorporated into everyday dentistry. Nearly a decade separates the discovery and the routine use of this procedure because the application of an acidic solution to vital tooth structure was not readily accepted. Once the procedure gained a foothold in the profession through its successful use with dental composites, however, the esthetic possibilities for dentistry in the anterior as well as the posterior regions of the mouth were greatly expanded. Some of the beneficial qualities of composites are their adequate strength, excellent esthetics, and moderate cost.

■ *Historical Perspective*

Before the development of dental composites, the conservative repair of anterior teeth was a difficult task for the clinician. The materials that were available included the **silicate cements** (actually a restorative, not a cement) and the **unfilled acrylics** (similar to those used to make dentures). The formulation of these materials is described in other chapters (silicates, Chapter 4; unfilled acrylics, Chapter 12). Although either of these materials could produce acceptable restorations, their longevity and esthetic qualities were not ideal. One of the biggest problems related to their use was marginal staining, a consequence of the lack of adhesion between the restoration and the tooth (Fig. 5-1) that allowed leakage of salivary components and the collection of stains at this interface. Such leakage often was associated with secondary decay, especially for the unfilled acrylic. Secondary decay was less of a problem for the silicates because they released fluoride.

Even after composites became accepted, the silicate cements were used still in pediatrics because of the beneficial effects of the fluoride. Today, glass ionomers and compomers have replaced silicates as the anterior restorative for patients requiring the additional protection of a fluoride-releasing agent. In actuality, there is a strong similarity between the glass powders used in the silicate cements and the glass ionomers.

In addition to the leakage and esthetic shortcomings of silicates and unfilled acrylics, both materials suffered from limited strength and abrasion resistance when exposed to biting stresses. Although the acrylics, like the silicates, were not soluble in saliva, they were plastics and had a very high coefficient of thermal expansion, which was considered to be another factor contributing to marginal leak-

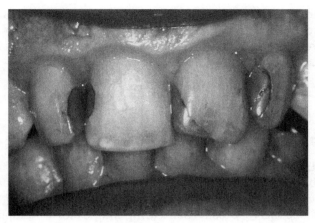

Figure 5–1 Staining around the margins of class III and class IV unfilled acrylic resin restorations because of a lack of adhesion. Note also the general surface discoloration.

age. Clinicians needed a material with mechanical and thermal stability, better adhesion, and enhanced esthetics to perform longer-lasting and more reliable esthetic dentistry. This call was answered by the development of the dental composite and the acid-etch technique in the late 1950s to early 1960s. The two men most responsible for these discoveries were Dr. Rafael Bowen and Dr. Michael Buonocore, respectively. Some 10 years later, the glass ionomers were introduced as material that could be used as a luting agent for cast metal restorations or as restorative materials themselves. A unique feature of these glass ionomers was their ability to react chemically with tooth structure to produce adhesion without the necessity for acid etching.

More recently, new restoratives having characteristics intermediate to composites and glass ionomers have been developed. Resin-modified glass ionomers have most of the same qualities as conventional glass ionomers, but they are stronger and less moisture sensitive. Compomers are similar to composites, but they have greater fluoride release, and some clinicians find them easier to use.

■ *Uses of Composites, Glass Ionomers, and Compomers*

Dental composite, glass ionomer, and compomer restoratives are used in many applications for anterior teeth. Composites are used in class III (interproximal cavities in incisors and premolars that do not involve the incisal angle), class IV (interproximal cavities in incisors and premolars that involve the incisal angle), and class V (cavities on the gingival third of the teeth) cavities; as veneers that cover teeth stained by drugs or chemicals, such as fluoride; to fill in spaces (or **diastema**) between teeth; and to enhance the size or contour of small or misshapen teeth. Because of their limited strength, the composite still requires some tooth structure for support, and in cases in which there is little tooth remaining, a ceramic or porcelain bonded to a metal crown may be indicated instead. Glass ionomer restoratives are used mainly in class V cavities or erosion-abrasion lesions, where their ability to adhere to enamel, dentin, and cementum is a great advantage. The glass ionomers are not indicated for restorations on which heavy stress is generated and, therefore, are not acceptable for replacing incisal edges (class IV); composites are the material of choice for these restorations. Compomers are indicated for the same applications as glass ionomers, predominantly class III and class V restorations. Other potential uses for these materials, especially composites, include buildups or **cores** for cast crowns and as esthetic repair materials for fractured or chipped porcelain restorations.

■ Dental Composites

Types and Packaging

Dental composites are manufactured in two different forms: **self-curing** (or auto-curing) composites and **light-curing** composites. The original composites were self-curing, but because of the popularity of light-curing composites, only a few are made this way today. Self-curing composites are supplied as pastes in two containers to keep the catalysts separated until the material is mixed (Fig. 5-2). Equal amounts of material are dispensed from both containers and mixed on a paper pad with a plastic spatula. A limitation of this system is the fixed working time; the material will harden within several minutes whether the operator is ready or not.

In the early 1970s, composites containing different catalysts were developed. These single-paste systems were hardened by exposure to the light from a hand-held ultraviolet (UV) lamp. The benefit to the clinician lay in the ability to place the material without time constraints, because it would not harden until directly exposed to the light source. The system was popular, but concerns over the health hazards of exposure to high-intensity UV radiation and problems in achieving complete curing of deep restorations limited its acceptance. Later in the 1970s, new composites were developed that contained a different catalyst system sensitive to blue light instead of ultraviolet. Although the visible light traveled more deeply into the composite than did the UV light, concern still existed that the bottoms of the restorations would not be exposed to adequate light intensity to harden completely. Therefore, the restoration should be built up in a succession of thin layers to ensure adequate hardening. And although the light is in the visible range, concern remains about the potential for retinal damage if one looks directly at the intense blue light for long periods. Special orange-tinted glasses and filters thus are recommended during light operation.

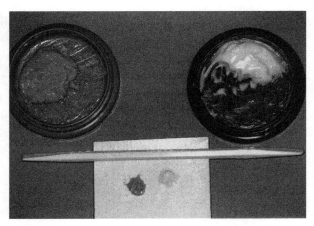

Figure 5–2 A self-curing composite and equal portions of base and catalyst dispensed onto a pad in preparation for mixing.

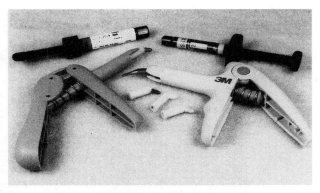

Figure 5–3 Packaging of light-cured composite, showing two individual syringes, two intraoral direct application syringes, and several compules with color-coded caps to denote different shades of composite.

The visible light-curing systems have become the choice for modern composites. The material is supplied either in syringes from which the paste is extruded or in small disposable compules that are placed into a dispensing syringe for direct injection into the tooth (Fig. 5-3).

Composition

As defined previously, a composite is a mixture of two different classes of materials. Dental composites are mixtures of polymers (often called resins) and glass particles (or fillers). They also contain chemicals to begin the hardening reaction and pigments to produce the different shades to match a variety of teeth. Finally, the filler particles are always coated with a coupling agent, called a **silane**, which is used to enhance the bonding between the filler particles and the surrounding polymer matrix (Fig. 5-4). The particles are surrounded and separated from each other by a small amount of polymer resin. The properties of these materials depend on many factors, including the amount of filler and resin, the size and properties of the filler particles, the properties of the polymer matrix, and the adhesion between the polymer and filler particles. Many types of composites are available; the most efficient way to classify them is according to their filler characteristics.

Composites originally were made with ground quartz (crystalline silicon dioxide) because it produced good translucency and tooth-like esthetics when mixed with the resin. Chunks of quartz were ground into irregularly shaped particles with an average size of 20 to 40 μm. The largest particles, however, were 50 to 100 μm, or approximately equal to one to two times the diameter of a human hair (Fig. 5-5). The particles were added to the liquid resin, which was made up of organic monomers, to produce a paste that was approximately 75% by weight filler and 25% by weight resin. The set composite was strong and hard but difficult to polish because of the presence of the large particles, which always left the surface somewhat rough. Enamel is very smooth and is characterized by a surface luster, so even a microscopically rough surface on a restoration will look and feel different from a natural tooth. *The size of the large particles was a significant drawback. Can you suggest a reasonable solution to improve the polishability of composites?*

To enhance the polishability and ultimately the esthetics of these anterior restoratives, smaller reinforcing fillers were needed.

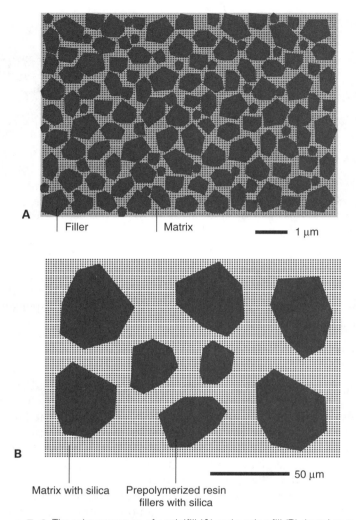

A | Filler | Matrix   ▬▬ 1 μm

B

Matrix with silica   Prepolymerized resin fillers with silica   ▬▬ 50 μm

Figure 5–4 The microstructure of a minifill (**A**) and a microfill (**B**) dental composite.

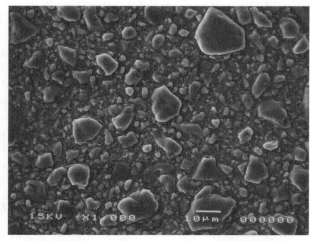

Figure 5–5 Scanning electron photomicrograph of the polished surface of a conventional dental composite.

The answer came in the use of small silica particles, also called fumed or pyrolytic silica. The particles, called microfillers, are produced by a chemical process that includes heating in a flame to produce spheres with diameters around 0.04 μm, or one tenth of the wavelength of visible light. Because of their small size and high surface area, these particles are ideal thickeners for paints and other liquids. Because they are such good thickeners, however, it is difficult to mix a lot of them into a resin to produce a composite with good handling characteristics. Therefore, there is a severe limit on the number of small fillers that can be added to a composite. This limitation has a detrimental effect on the strength of the composite, which depends on the quantity of fillers. Composite manufacturers have used a special technique to maximize the amount of microfiller particles and improve their strength and stiffness. Although the details are beyond the scope of this text, the main idea is that small, "minicomposite" pieces called **prepolymerized resin fillers** are added to the paste (Fig. 5-4*B*). These prepolymerized resin fillers are made by adding large amounts of microfiller particles to a dilute resin and hardening it by heating the paste in an oven. This increases the overall filler concentration and strengthens the composite while maintaining good handling characteristics. Many different types of **microfill** composites are available, although almost all still have less filler than do composites with larger particles (Table 5-1). Because of their small particle size, however, these microfill composites can be polished to a very smooth and shiny surface and thus have excellent esthetic qualities (Fig. 5-6).

The ideal combination of esthetics and durability in a dental composite is achieved with the materials referred to as **hybrids** (Fig. 5-7). Hybrid composites contain a mixture of small and microscopic particles, which make up 70 to 80% of the total weight of the composite (Table 5-1). The most common are the minifills. Their largest particles are either 1 to 2 μm (small, fine particle hybrids). Hybrids with larger fillers are called midifills, and they contain particles with an average size of 3 to 8 μm (midsized hybrids). Generally, the materials that have larger particles have greater amounts of fillers and, consequently, higher strength. The particles can be made of quartz, but a variety of other glasses containing barium, aluminum, strontium, zinc, zirconium, etc. are used to produce composites that are **radiopaque** (impenetrable by x-rays), thus enhancing their visibility on

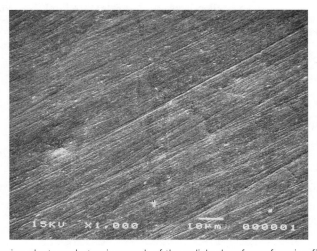

Figure 5–6 Scanning electron photomicrograph of the polished surface of a microfill dental composite.

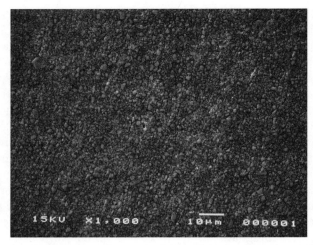

Figure 5–7 Scanning electron photomicrograph of the polished surface of a minifill dental composite.

a radiographic film. This is important for diagnostic purposes, especially when composites are used in posterior teeth. Table 5-1 shows the different composite types and their characteristics.

Composites with altered viscosity and handling characteristics have been produced for use in specific applications. Flowable composites are, typically, diluted minifill composites made more fluid by reducing the overall filler content to less than 45 vol%. They are easily dispensed from a very small gauge needle directly into a cavity preparation. In contrast, packable composites have a very thick and heavy consistency and are designed for posterior teeth. These composites have similar filler volume as normal minifill and midifill composites, but the heavy con-

TABLE 5–1. Classification of Dental Composites

Composite Class	Filler Type	Filler Size (μm)	Filler Volume (%)	Examples
Conventional	Quartz or glass[a]	Average = 20 Range = 1–100	50–60	Adaptic Concise Profile
Microfill	Fumed silica (SiO_2) PPRF	Average = 0.04 Range = 10–50	30–55	Silar/Silux Durafill Helioprogress
Small hybrid	Quartz or glass	Average = 0.5–1.0 Range = 0.1–3	50–60	Herculite XR Charisma Z100, Z250
	Fumed silica	Average = 0.04		Tetric Ceram
Midsized hybrid	Quartz or glass	Average = 1.0–3.0 Range = 0.1–10.0	65–70	Bisfil-P Occlusin Clearfil
	Fumed silica	Average = 0.04		P-50

PPRF, prepolymerized resin fillers.
[a]Silicate glasses with barium, strontium, zirconium, zinc, aluminum, or other additives.

sistency is produced by using modified fillers or by altering the distribution of particle sizes to include more smaller fillers.

The composite's resin component is the binder that holds the filler particles together. Over time, the resin has undergone less commercial development than the filler. The resins of most dental composites contain monomers, organic molecules with molecular weights between 100 and 1000 g/mole. The monomers are liquid at room temperature. Hardening is achieved by a chemical reaction that converts the individual monomers into long, chain-like structures, with each monomer serving as an individual link in the chain. The giant organic molecules formed from the reaction are called polymers, and they possess a very high molecular weight. As discussed in Chapter 3, the chemical reaction that produces polymers from monomers is called polymerization. A full description of the process is provided in Chapter 12.

The monomers used in dental composites are called dimethacrylates. The two that are used most often are bis-GMA (2,2-bis[4(2-hydroxy-3-methacryloyloxy-propoxy)phenyl]propane), the molecule developed by Dr. Rafael Bowen in the late 1950s, and the urethane dimethacrylates. These are the same resins used in resin cements. Because the resins are somewhat viscous (bis-GMA is as thick at room temperature as refrigerated molasses), they are usually diluted with another low-viscosity dimethacrylate, TEGDMA (triethylene glycol dimethacrylate), to produce a fluid resin that can be maximally filled with glass particles. The monomers then polymerize by a chemical reaction, producing a **cross-linked** structure. Cross-linked polymers are discussed further in Chapter 12 but can be envisioned as spider webs, with each ring of the web being the individual polymer chains and the cross-links being the short segments that hold the rings (i.e., the polymer chains) together.

In addition to the resin and filler, the composites contain chemicals to promote the hardening, or polymerization, reaction. For light-cured composites, an initiator (camphoroquinone) is added along with an another compound (an amine) to accelerate the reaction. For the self-curing systems, an initiator (benzoyl peroxide) is added to one paste and an activator (an amine) to the other. In the light-cured material, the visible light causes the camphoroquinone to become reactive, whereas in the self-curing system, the amine causes the peroxide to become reactive (Display 5-1). Either type can prematurely harden. Heat can pro-

DISPLAY 5-1

Simplified Explanation of the Curing of Self-Curing and Light-Curing Resins

Self-Curing		Light-Curing
Paste A	**Paste B**	**Paste**
Monomers	Monomers	Monomers
Initiator	Activator	Initiator
		Accelerator

Mixing A and B, or light-curing the paste, causes the following:

Initiator + activator (or accelerator) → reactive initiator

Reactive initiator + monomers → reactive monomers

Reactive monomers + monomers → polymers

mote the reaction of the peroxide, so the self-curing materials should always be stored in the refrigerator. Their **shelf life** can be 2 years or longer when stored correctly. Heat or exposure to the operatory lights can cause the camphoroquinone to react, so the light-cured composites should be refrigerated (although this is not as important as for the self-curing materials) and never exposed to the operatory lights for more than several seconds (i.e., secure the cap on the tube or syringe when not dispensing). Light-cured composites that are refrigerated can have a shelf life of several years, although it is advisable to use them within 2 years for optimum results.

The polymerization of the self-curing material is brought on by mixing the two paste components. Mixing brings the initiator and activator together to start the polymerization reaction. If the reaction were to begin immediately after mixing, the assistant and clinician would not have sufficient working time to place the material. Therefore, manufacturers add some **inhibitor** molecules to each paste to delay the polymerization and provide ample working time; this inhibitor also ensures that the pastes do not prematurely harden during storage. Inhibitors also are added to light-cured composites to improve storage stability and to help keep the material from prematurely hardening under the operatory lights.

Handling and Mixing

The mixing of a self-curing composite is reasonably simple. Equal quantities (determined by eye) of the pastes in each container are removed with a plastic spatula (Fig. 5-2). Care is taken to use different ends of the spatula for each container to avoid cross-contamination of the jars, which would prematurely harden the pastes. The pastes are dispensed onto the supplied paper pad and are folded into one another with the plastic spatula for 15 to 20 seconds to ensure adequate mixing of the components. A plastic spatula usually is supplied because some of the fillers are abrasive to steel spatulas, causing metal particles to be incorporated into the mix and producing a gray composite.

The working time generally lasts 1.5 to 2 minutes after mixing is complete. Setting takes place within 4 minutes from the start of mixing but is quicker in the mouth. *Is it obvious why setting would be hastened in the mouth, where the temperature is higher than it is in the office?*

> The material should not be disturbed after the working time has ended and the initial setting period has begun. Such activity produces voids and disrupts the polymerization, thereby reducing strength and esthetics. Therefore, the self-curing restorative must be held in place until it becomes rigid. In contrast, the light-cured material becomes rigid immediately after it is illuminated by the light source. An added benefit is that the light-cured material can be manipulated without concern for the working time, which is essentially "unlimited." Once the clinician is satisfied with the placement of the restoration, he or she illuminates the composite to cause hardening. In actuality, the operatory lights are sufficiently intense and of the appropriate energy to cause premature hardening of the material, so the practical working time is limited to 5 to 10 minutes.

The high-intensity halogen bulbs in the light units generate light that is passed through a blue filter to maximize the light energy at the appropriate wavelength

(470 nm). Many of the original units had fiberoptic bundles in a long cord through which the light was transmitted to a tip that could be used intraorally. Breakage of the fibers led to a loss in light transmission over time, however, and a new design was created. Most current light-curing units have the light source and the intraoral tip together and are held by a gun-type device with a trigger (Fig. 5-8). The power source is a separate unit attached to the gun by an electrical cord. Portable, battery-operated units are also available. The tips, which also contain glass fibers in a rigid tube, can be sterilized between patients by wiping them with appropriate disinfectant solutions. Some solutions can degrade the end of the fibers, which diminishes the intensity of the emitted light; thus soaking the light tips in disinfectants is not recommended. A large amount of heat is generated from the light bulbs during operation. When the bulb overheats, the unit will shut down and be inoperable until the bulb cools sufficiently. Therefore, a fan usually is mounted within the gun to help cool the light source.

Many of the current halogen-lamp curing lights provide for variable intensity and exposure time selections. Because there is currently no consensus as to the optimal curing method, the new lights allow the clinician a wide variety of choices for different types of restorations. Alternate light-curing systems have been developed to reduce light activation times from 40 to 60 seconds down to 10 seconds or less. These systems use higher-intensity lights (plasma arc lamp, PAC) or lasers and generally are several times more expensive than traditional halogen bulb units. The curing reaction proceeds in the same way, but because of differences in composition, all composites cannot be polymerized as efficiently with certain types of PAC lights.

Many of the original self-curing composites contained filler particles that were abrasive to metals and required mixing and placement with plastic instruments. Most modern materials, however, can be placed with metallic instruments, with the type and shape being dictated by the cavity preparation. Because of its more fluid consistency, the material is not easily condensed, like an amalgam is; some of the packable composites with modified filler formulations, however, can be "packed" rather than simply "wiped" into place. The clinician must take care not to introduce air bubbles and voids during placement. Once the restoration has been placed in an anterior tooth, it usually is desirable to place a plastic matrix strip (i.e., Mylar strip) onto its surface before light activation. ***What purpose might the matrix serve during the curing of the material?***

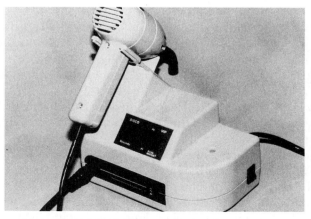

Figure 5–8 A light-curing unit for dental composites.

> The matrix serves two purposes. First, oxygen inhibits the polymerization reaction; thus covering the surface with a nonporous strip keeps oxygen away and allows for maximum hardening. Second, the matrix produces a very smooth, regularly contoured surface. This may minimize the amount of finishing required.

In contrast to the metal matrices used with amalgam, the composite matrix must be clear to transmit the light. The unset composite will stick to the matrix, so the strip, once placed, should not be moved or it will pull the composite away from the tooth.

Setting Reaction

Hardening of composite takes place through a rapid, free-radical polymerization reaction that is further described in Chapter 12. Once the reaction begins, the monomers in the composite paste are transformed into a cross-linked polymer matrix within 15 to 30 seconds. This rapid hardening is often referred to as a "snap-set"; this means that the consistency (handling characteristics) of the material remains the same throughout the working time but that the viscosity increases quickly once hardening begins. The working time for a self-curing composite is usually about 2 minutes after mixing has begun. The total reaction is not complete for several hours, but the material is sufficiently hardened within minutes to be **finished** and **polished**. The reaction is the same for the self-curing and light-cured forms, although it proceeds to completion faster in the light-cured material. *Based on the mode of activation for the setting of self-curing versus light-cured composites, one might suspect that there are certain considerations during placement and curing procedures that may affect their clinical outcomes.* These considerations relate to two of the important limitations, or clinical problems, accompanying these materials.

One problem with composites is the shrinkage that accompanies the polymerization (or curing) reaction. Another problem is the extent of the curing reaction and the factors that limit it. To understand these problems, one must have some knowledge of the manner in which composites harden.

For the monomer molecules to react with one another and form chemical bonds, they must get closer together than they are in the uncured paste. The result is that the overall volume of the composite lessens as it polymerizes; in other words, the composite shrinks. Shrinkage is greatest where the polymerization is happening at the fastest rate. For the self-curing composite, the reaction happens fastest in the center because it is insulated and builds up heat, which accelerates the chemical reaction. Therefore, the shrinkage is directed toward the center of the restoration and away from the cavity walls. This directional shrinkage highlights one of the problems with composites and emphasizes why bonding to the tooth is so important in terms of sealing the cavity.

The reaction for the light-cured material is similar, except that it should start and proceed fastest in the region closest to the activator (i.e., the blue light source). Therefore, it has been argued that shrinkage is directed toward the light. If the light is shone from the occlusal surface, the composite would be expected to pull up and away from the walls of the cavity. For this reason, researchers have suggested that it may be possible to direct the contraction partially toward instead of away from the tooth by curing the composite from the facial and lingual surfaces. This poses a problem because the light also will be absorbed by the tooth, thus reducing the intensity available to cure the composite when there is a thick layer of intervening enamel or dentin. Although the direction of shrinkage is currently a matter of debate, most evidence now suggests that the composite will shrink and be pulled toward all bonded surfaces. Because there are usually bonded surfaces in direct opposition to one another, such as the occlusal and gingival margins of a class V composite, the shrinkage results in forces that tend to pull the material away from the tooth surface, thus compromising marginal integrity.

Another important factor affecting the amount of polymerization reaction that takes place is the quantity of light shone on the material. A short exposure time produces less hardening than does a long exposure time. In addition, the light becomes absorbed by the material as it attempts to penetrate. Therefore, if the cavity is deep, the light may not penetrate to the deepest portion when shone from the occlusal surface. These two factors, duration of exposure and composite depth, must be controlled to optimize the properties of the restoration. ***How can this be accomplished efficiently in the clinical setting?***

The exposure time can be controlled simply by regulating the amount of time the light is held over the restoration. It is generally accepted that a minimal exposure time for composites is 40 seconds, though 60 seconds is often used. Exposure times exceeding 1 minute, however, will not significantly improve the polymerization and simply will generate additional heat within the tooth.

The drawbacks associated with prolonged exposures are increased heat build-up at the site (the light interaction with the tooth and restoration generates some heat) and the reduced lifetime of the bulb in the curing unit (overheating of the bulb causes it to burn out faster). The drawbacks are probably of minor significance, compared with the potential problems created by "undercuring."

The second factor that must be controlled during placement of light-cured composites is the depth of material to be cured. It is logical to build up the restoration in thin increments, curing each one independently instead of placing one large increment (i.e., "bulk filling") and trying to cure the entire restoration with one light exposure.

A general rule of thumb is that each increment should be at most 1.5 to 2.0 mm thick. This will help to ensure complete penetration of the light and maximum curing of the composite at the bottommost portion of the cavity preparation.

These factors are important in all restorations but are obviously more so in posterior teeth, where greater bulks of material are used. Because the intensity of the light source is important (a minimum of 400 mW/cm^2 is required), it is recommended that the tip be placed as close to the surface to be cured as is physically possible (i.e., within 1 to 2 mm). The intensity of the light is inversely related to its distance from the source.

Incremental placement of composites also is important with regard to controlling polymerization shrinkage stress. As the composite hardens, it builds up stresses within itself. These stresses result because the material is constrained by the cavity walls from shrinking freely. When bonding is good, the stresses are transferred to the bonded interface. If the bond is not strong enough, a marginal gap may open. A smaller volume of composite will undergo less overall contraction and should produce less overall shrinkage stress than would larger volumes. Therefore, curing several increments in sequence is expected to generate less overall stress than curing one large increment at once. Theoretically, this places less stress on the bond between the composite and the tooth surface and helps maintain the seal between the two.

Many researchers believe that internal stress is reduced when composites cure more slowly. Evidence to support this is the lower stress generated in the self-cure composites, which have a slower polymerization rate than light-cured composites, while having the same extent of polymerization. For this reason, manufacturers have developed light-curing units that can be operated at a lower intensity to reduce the polymerization rate. Note that this is the exact opposite of the effect achieved by the newer higher-intensity PAC lights and lasers mentioned previously, whose main benefit is a more rapid cure. This controversial issue is currently being intensely studied by scientists around the world. Will it be possible for us to have our cake and eat it too?

One final factor that is important in determining the extent of curing is the shade of the composite. Although there is variation between brands, generally it is best to use the thinnest increments and the longest exposure times for the darker shades of composite. The dark pigments in the darker shades absorb light more efficiently, thus transmitting less light than would the lighter shades.

Finishing

Contouring and polishing of dental composites can be accomplished within a few minutes after the restoration has hardened. Finishing or contouring is accomplished with carbide burs, diamonds, or sandpaper disks and either the slow- or high-speed handpiece. The initial contouring should be done with water spray to avoid heat buildup and damage to the surface of the restoration; clinicians often perform the final finishing dry, however, to improve their view of the margins. Then, strips with abrasive bonded to one side are usually used to finish the interproximal spaces. Final polishing is achieved through the use of aluminum oxide or diamond pastes containing particles as small as 1 μm in diameter.

Characteristics and Properties

Dental composites have many of the characteristics of natural teeth, although they are not an ideal substitute. In this section, various properties and characteristics of composites are discussed in relation to their formulation and the manner in which they are handled. Each of the properties has a certain significance for the clinical success or failure of a composite restoration. When one considers the disparity in the properties of enamel and dentin, the two natural materials that restoratives replace (Table 5-2), the difficulty in using a single material to simulate tooth substance is readily apparent. This is why different types of composites often are combined in a single restoration to achieve this goal more ideally.

The physical properties of composites generally are adequate for use as anterior restoratives (Table 5-2). They have low thermal conductivities and in this respect mimic tooth structure well. Note that there is little difference between the types of composites. Conversely, the thermal expansion coefficient, which describes the extent to which the material expands when heated and contracts when cooled, is higher for composites than for tooth structure. The filler component of composite is inorganic and has a coefficient of thermal expansion that is similar to that of enamel or dentin (see Table 2-1). The resin component, however, has a high coefficient of thermal expansion. Therefore, the more resin there is in the composite, the higher its coefficient of thermal expansion. The clinical significance of this mismatch, which is greatest for microfills because of the higher resin con-

TABLE 5–2. **Values for Various Properties of Dental Composites and Glass Ionomers**

| | Composites | | Glass Ionomers | |
	Microfill	Hybrids	Conventional	Resin-Modified
Setting contraction (vol%)	2 −4	1.5–4	3–4	3–4
Thermal expansion coefficient (α; $10^{-6}/°C$)	50–60	20–40	10–15	30–35
Thermal conductivity (cal · cm/cm² · sec · °C)	1–2	2–3	1.5–2.5	
Tensile strength (MPa)	40–50	50–70	7–15	30–40
Flexural strength (MPa)	75–100	100–160	10–14	55–60
Flexural modulus (GPa)	5–7	8–14	6–7	3–5
Compressive strength (MPa)	400–475	375–475	125–175	200–220
Fracture toughness (MPa · $m^{1/2}$)	0.9–1.1	1.2–1.7	0.4–0.6	0.9–1.1

tent, is not completely known. It is generally believed, however, that a large mismatch in thermal expansion between a restorative and a tooth causes stress to be placed on their interfacial bond because of the different extents of expansion and contraction between the two materials. As long as the bond is strong and durable, there should be no problem. If the bond becomes weakened and breaks, however, the different expansions will lead to the creation of larger interface gaps through which microleakage may occur. The leakage may allow bacterial infiltration, leading to further decay processes. Therefore, the thermal expansion characteristics of composites are not ideal, and the materials have been improved by increasing the filler volume fraction with this thought in mind.

There is another important aspect to the dimensional change of composites. As stated previously, the reaction of most monomers to form polymers is accompanied by a reduction in volume. This **polymerization shrinkage** causes the composite to contract and pull away from the cavity wall. The reduction in volume is substantial, on the order of 2 to 4% (Table 5-2). The amount of contraction depends on the amount of polymerizing monomers. This characteristic provides another rationale for maximizing the amount of filler in the composite. Unfortunately, all composites shrink too much. The dimensional change is sufficient to create gaps along the margins when the restorations are not adequately bonded to the cavity walls. Even when bonding is achieved, the tendency of the composite to contract and pull away from the cavity causes the interface to be in a state of tensile stress. This stress may ultimately cause the bond to fail, thus providing a leakage space. This problem is of primary importance for dental composites. *Is there a way to negate this problem?*

The ideal dental composite would be a material that undergoes negligible dimensional change during curing—in other words, a nonshrinking or nonshrinkage stress composite. Such resin systems exist, but other problems have precluded their use in dentistry. This is an area of intense research interest, and better candidate materials are expected to be made available each year.

One factor that helps to offset the polymerization contraction of composites is water sorption. Polymers absorb water. When the polymer takes up water, it swells. This swelling results in an expansion of the composite, although it is not usually sufficient to completely close the gaps created by polymerization shrinkage. Water also causes some deterioration of the composite, which ultimately results in a slight reduction in physical and mechanical properties.

Color stability is another important physical characteristic of composites. Rougher surfaces have a natural tendency to pick up stain faster than do smoother surfaces. Thus, microfill composites should be more color stable than hybrid composites with larger particles. Color change, however, can be caused by internal changes as well as surface staining. Self-curing composites had a tendency to discolor because of an instability in the amine activator. Improvements were made by incorporating more color-stable activators. Visible light-activated composites have some tendency to yellow with time because they also contain an amine accelerator. The concentration is so small, however, that although a color change may occur, it usually is not significant enough to require replacement. A significant potential problem with color-matching composites is the difficulty in initially achieving the same shade as the surrounding tooth structure. Failure to do so causes the composite to look unnatural from the start. It also is possible that the composite may eventually look lighter than the natural teeth, because the teeth tend to darken with age. Overall, however, clinical problems with color mismatch produced over time have been relatively minor.

Because the stresses generally are low, esthetics is more important than strength for most anterior restorations. For example, aside from toothbrush abrasion, there is little stress imposed on a class III (anterior interproximal) filling. Similarly, most class V (near the gingiva) lesions experience little stress during service. Therefore, the microfill composites are the materials of choice for these restorations. Their esthetic results are unequaled, and their mechanical properties and abrasion resistance are adequate for long-term success. The superb esthetic results of the microfill composites are a function of the small particle size used in their fillers. When the particles are very small, polishing produces smooth, mirror-like surfaces that remain smooth over the years. They mimic enamel well in this respect. Although hybrids approximate microfills in the size of their particles and their ability to take a smooth polish, they remain slightly rougher (Fig. 5-7). Improvements in the strength and polishability of the minifills, however, have led many to consider them as a composite restorative material suitable for all anterior and posterior applications.

In general, dental composites have adequate strength for most restorative applications. Recently, their use has been expanded to include crown and bridge prosthodontics. In situations that require stronger mechanical properties, however, selection becomes most important. Composites generally have tensile strength similar to that of amalgam, although they have lower compressive and flexural strengths (Table 5-2). In the anterior portion of the mouth, this creates a problem only when the materials are used to rebuild incisal edges or when they replace most of the existing tooth structure. Stresses from biting and clenching are high on incisal edges, as are wear rates. A simple examination of the incisal edges of your own teeth should convince you that wear of these surfaces occurs. Also, chipping of front teeth is not an uncommon occurrence, especially in response to some type of trauma. These situations require a material with the highest possible fracture resistance. Generally, fracture resistance is related to the level of filler loading in the composite—the composites that have the most filler also have the highest fracture resistance. Therefore, hybrids may be more appropriate choices than microfills for replacing class IV cavities (i.e., incisal edges).

Clinical Performance

Composites used in the restoration of anterior teeth have enjoyed a high level of success when evaluated in controlled clinical trials. Some studies of private practitioners, however, have reported relatively short lifetimes of only 3 to 4 years for the average restoration. The major reasons for failure usually are secondary caries and marginal discoloration. Both of these problems are related to inadequate marginal adhesion, which should be attainable with the acid-etch technique. Therefore, operator variability probably is most responsible for the difference between the controlled clinical trials and the private practice experience. Under ideal conditions, anterior composites likely will last for 10 years or longer, although this depends on the type of cavity.

The restoration of class III cavities with modern composites is a successful procedure, especially when the margins of the preparation reside entirely in enamel. The color change for modern materials is minimal, and if proper bonding to the margins is achieved, marginal staining and secondary caries are less likely to occur.

The restoration of class IV cavities (incisal edge failures) is more problematic. Often, incisal edges experience a significant amount of force during clenching or biting. This varies from patient to patient because of individual differences in occlusion, but the longevity of class IV restorations in general would be expected to be less because of the greater stress and increased chance for fracture or chipping of the restoration. In this light, one clinical study has shown that composites with greater strength and fracture resistance, such as midsized hybrids, experienced less failure than microfills over a 3-year period in these sites. A layered class IV restoration also is common. A stronger composite, such as a minifill or midifill, is used as a dentin replacement to provide support, whereas a microfill is overlaid on the hybrid to produce optimum surface smoothness and esthetic results. Again, the full enamel margin enhances the chance for complete sealing.

The restoration of class V lesions or erosions is perhaps the most difficult and least successful composite restoration. Failures usually result from incomplete sealing because of the presence of cementum and dentin at the gingival margins. There are several opinions regarding selection of a composite for these cavities. One is that during chewing, stress is produced within the class V restoration, which usually resides at the region of the tooth where flexure is greatest. This stress may contribute to debonding of the weakest margin. For this reason, a less stiff composite (i.e., one with a lower elastic modulus) may "flex" more with the tooth, thereby imposing less stress on the bonded interface. In contrast, the stiffer hybrid composite "flexes" less and stresses the bond more. Therefore, the microfill, with the better polishability and the possibility for reduced stress, may be the optimal choice for this restoration. When the class V preparation involves an incisal margin in enamel and a gingival margin in cementum, the restoration must rely on dentin bonding for retention and sealing. Results with the initial dentin bonding agents were poor because the contraction of the composite produced sufficient stress to pull the composite away from the gingival margin. Clinical studies showed that most of these restorations fell out within 6 months to 1 year after placement. Current dentin adhesives have improved the prognosis of class V composites, as discussed later in this chapter. Perhaps the most successful restoration, to date, for class V lesions, however, has been the glass ionomer.

■ Glass Ionomers

Types and Packaging

Glass ionomers come in several different forms. The material is marketed as a liner, luting cement, or restorative; the latter is the focus of this discussion. Basi-

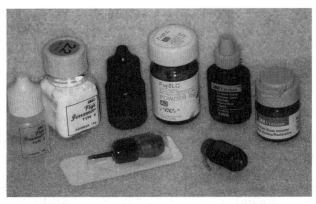

Figure 5–9 Packaging of a glass ionomer restorative material, showing the conventional and resin-modified varieties, in addition to the preencapsulated materials.

cally, glass ionomers are powder-liquid systems that must be dispensed in the correct proportions and subsequently mixed on a pad with a metal or plastic spatula (see detailed instructions in Chapter 4).

Manufacturers also supply the material in a preencapsulated form, similar to dental amalgam (Fig. 5-9). The capsules are mixed in a triturator and dispensed by a "caulking"-type gun, in a way similar to many impression materials. The liquid portion of many of the glass ionomers is viscous and difficult to dispense accurately from a dropper bottle. Therefore, a major benefit of the encapsulated system is a more reproducible proportioning and mixing system. It also is more convenient and aseptic than the hand-mixed systems.

The newest type of glass ionomer material is a light-cured, resin-modified version, which has been marketed as a liner, cement, and restorative. This material also is supplied as a powder and liquid system. It is packaged in dark-colored (black or amber) vials to avoid premature reaction from light exposure. Some brands also come preencapsulated.

Composition

The term "glass ionomer" refers to a mixture of an inorganic glass-reinforcing agent and an organic, ionic polymer. The glass particles are composed of a silicate (calcium aluminofluorosilicate) glass, similar to that used in the original silicate cement restoratives. The inclusion of fluoride in the glass is considered to be a major therapeutic feature of these materials. The glass particles are 40 μm or less in diameter for the restorative material and less than 25 μm for the luting material. *Why should there be a difference between the two?*

The smaller particles allow for thinner films of cement to be formed during the seating of restorations. Thicker mixes can be produced with the larger particles, however, thus producing stronger glass ionomers for restorations. The liquid contains the ionic polymers suspended in water to which a small amount of tartaric acid is added to regulate the working time and setting rate. Metallic oxide pigments are also added to produce the different shades.

The original glass ionomer products had the glass particles and pigments in the powder and the polymer, water, and tartaric acid in the liquid. The viscous liquid is somewhat difficult to dispense accurately from a dropper bottle and becomes thicker with age as the water evaporates when the bottle cap is left off. One manufacturer invented a different packaging system to address these problems. The liquid was freeze-dried to make a polymer powder, and this powder was subsequently added to the glass particles. Without water, the mixture will not react and remains stable. The liquid component, then, was simply distilled water to which a small amount of tartaric acid was added. The presence of tartaric acid in the water for these formulations is noteworthy: An empty liquid vial should never be refilled with tap or distilled water alone because without the tartaric acid, the working and setting time may be inappropriate, leading to a poor mix.

In the early 1980s, a new type of reinforced glass ionomer was produced. This material was made by mixing either amalgam alloy particles or silver or gold particles coated with a glass into the normal powder used for the glass ionomer. Popular brands have been called "The Miracle Mix" and "Ketac-silver." These products have been shown to have slightly greater strength and wear resistance compared with conventional glass ionomer restoratives. They also are highly radiopaque. Their gray color provides a striking contrast to the tooth, which is a desirable feature in a core buildup material because it enhances the clinician's ability to define the margins of the buildup and avoid overcutting the tooth. In this respect they are similar to amalgam, the most popular buildup material, although amalgam is more difficult to cut. Composites, another buildup option, are tooth colored and often have a dye, pigment, or filler (such as titanium) added to improve their contrast as core materials.

The other version of glass ionomers comprises the resin-modified formulations. These are different from the conventional, self-curing formulations, in that the liquid portion is modified by the addition of polymerizing monomer, such as hydroxyethyl methacrylate (HEMA). The molecules may simply be added to the liquid or actually attached to the ionic polymers through a chemical reaction. In any case, a small amount of light-sensitive catalyst is included, similar to that found in composites, to cause a polymerization reaction when the material is exposed to the blue light source. The liquid must be packaged in dark-colored vials for this reason. In some cases, the light-sensitive catalyst is also added to the powder component, which is packaged in an amber vial. The caps should never be left off of these vials because the catalyst may become activated and ruin the product. Some of these products also contain self-curing polymerization promoters to allow them to undergo this part of the reaction even in the absence of light activation. Although initially developed as liners and bases, many formulations are marketed as restorative materials or as core materials for the buildup of a tooth in preparation for a crown. The latter usually are mixed in higher powder-to-liquid ratios to improve mechanical properties and decrease fluidity. This newest version of "packable" glass ionomer has been recommended for occlusal surfaces on primary teeth.

Mixing

Glass ionomers that must be mixed are referred to as conventional or self-curing and are supplied as powder-liquid systems. The liquid is dispensed via a dropper bottle, and the powder is dispensed with an appropriate scoop to ensure optimum handling and mechanical properties (Fig. 5-10). For lining applications where fluidity is necessary, powder-to-liquid ratios of 1.8:1.0 or 2.0:1.0 are usually used. Restorative mixes are made at powder-to-liquid ratios approaching 4.0:1.0. Full details of the mixing procedure at low powder-to-liquid ratios are presented in Chapter 4.

When mixing at a low powder-to-liquid ratio, the pad is sufficient and a plastic spatula, similar to that used for self-curing composites, can be used to mix the two

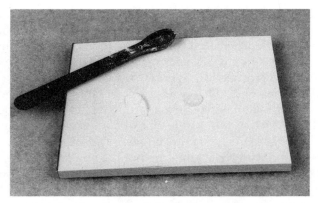

Figure 5–10 A self-curing glass ionomer dispensed onto a mixing pad.

components. Because of the heavy consistency of the restorative material, however, it is often helpful to mix it with a stiff spatula on a glass slab. One half of the powder is mixed into the liquid for approximately 10 to 15 seconds. The second half is then quickly added, with the material folded in on itself until all of the powder is wetted by the liquid and it has a shiny, putty-like consistency. The entire mixing time should not exceed 30 to 40 seconds to allow ample working time (Fig. 5-11). These materials set rapidly, leaving a working time of approximately 2.5 minutes. When the mix no longer appears shiny, it has reached the end of the working time. Glass ionomers can be mixed on a chilled glass slab to prolong the working time when desired. The mixing of the resin-modified glass ionomers is similar. In either case, the manufacturer's directions for each specific material should be followed.

The preencapsulated glass ionomers require the use of a common amalgam triturator set to the correct speed and time (usually about 10 seconds). The capsule must be activated by pressing in the ends to break the internal diaphragm and allow the powder and liquid to mix during trituration. Working time is enhanced because there is less mixing time; however, the greater energy supplied during trituration causes the setting to be somewhat accelerated, so overall working time is approximately 2 to 3 minutes from the time trituration has stopped. These materials generally are injected into the cavity with a special gun but can also be dispensed onto a pad and inserted with appropriate instruments.

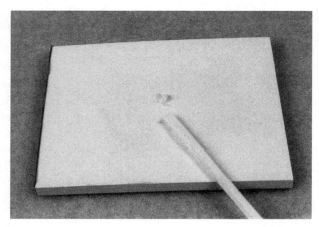

Figure 5–11 A self-curing glass ionomer mixed to a restorative consistency (i.e., like putty).

Handling

One benefit of the glass ionomer material that makes it attractive as a liner or restorative is its ability to adhere to tooth structure by virtue of ionic interactions between the ionic polymer and the calcium in the tooth. The polymer must remain free to form these interactions. As the material begins to react, the polymer becomes tied up and no longer is in a liquid state; thus the surface loses its shiny appearance, and viscosity increases quickly. The material then becomes much less adhesive toward the tooth. In addition, the adhesion depends on the presence of moisture on the tooth. Adhesion is poorer when the bonding surface is completely desiccated. A significant amount of tooth sensitivity has been reported after the use of glass ionomers applied to tooth surfaces that were aggressively dried with air blasts. Therefore, the surface of the tooth should remain moist, but not soaked, to achieve optimum adhesion with glass ionomers. Drying with cotton pellets rather than forced air has been recommended.

After it is mixed, the glass ionomer is placed into the cavity by wiping it into place with a steel or plastic instrument or by injecting it with a syringe. Like composites, it is not thick enough to be condensed like amalgam. Cavities usually are slightly overfilled (i.e., an excess of material is placed above the margins) and then contoured with the instrument to remove the excess. The restoration can be covered with a plastic or metal matrix during setting. Glass ionomers are very sensitive to early moisture contamination, which disrupts setting and causes them to become chalky in appearance (Fig. 5-12). The matrix tends to isolate them from gross moisture until they have hardened. Once the glass ionomer hardens, it is sensitive to becoming dried out. Drying immediately after setting causes the surface and interior to crack (Fig. 5-12). One method used to avoid this drying-out is to coat the glass ionomer with the supplied varnish immediately after the initial hardening has taken place. A more permanent alternative is to place a layer of unfilled bonding resin over the surface and to cure it with a visible light source to produce a resin coating that inhibits moisture exchange.

A major advantage of the new light-cured materials is that because of the resin addition, they are not as moisture sensitive and therefore have less tendency to desiccate or crack. After placement, they are exposed to the visible light source for 30 seconds to cause the initial setting. Because these materials contain resins, the top surface will not cure because of air inhibition. Therefore, the materials should be slightly overfilled and covered with a matrix during light exposure.

Finishing should be delayed for 24 hours because of the moisture sensitivity of conventional glass ionomers. Some manufacturers suggest that finishing can be accomplished within 10 to 15 minutes. Care should be taken to avoid drying,

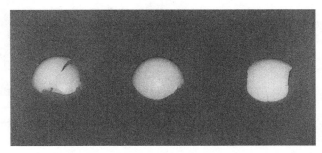

Figure 5–12 Self-cured glass ionomer surfaces showing the effects of desiccation (*left*) and early moisture contamination (*right*), compared with a glass ionomer that was coated with a varnish (*center*).

however, by first coating the surface with Vaseline before finishing with stones, carbides, or diamonds. For finishing, the resin-modified versions can be treated like dental composites.

Setting Reaction

As the liquid of a conventional glass ionomer is mixed with the powder, the acidic polymer liquid attacks the outer surfaces of the glass powder, causing them to dissolve partially. In doing so, positively charged metallic ions, such as aluminum and calcium, are released. These ions chemically interact with the negatively charged groups on the polymer. The polymers become cross-linked by this acid-base reaction, forming an amorphous network that holds the reinforcing fillers in place (Fig. 5-13*A*). Fluoride ions released from the glass particles also become incorporated into the matrix. When the glass ionomer comes into contact with saliva, this fluoride is slowly released, providing a potential anticariogenic effect. Laboratory studies have verified that glass ionomers of all types continue to release fluoride for more than 1 year after setting, although the release is greatest during the first few days or weeks.

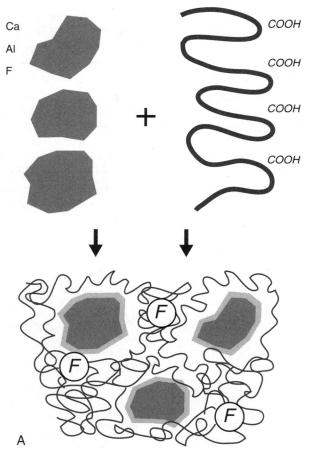

Figure 5–13 The setting reactions for a self-curing (**A**) and a light-cured (**B**) glass ionomer. The *solid dashes* in **B** represent polymerized resin groups that cross-link the polymers.

The setting time for the conventional materials is 4 to 5 minutes, although the material continues to increase in strength for at least 24 hours. The setting is accompanied by a 3 to 4% volumetric shrinkage. The shrinkage of a glass ionomer restorative is less detrimental to bonding than is shrinkage of a composite, possibly because of the slower overall setting rate of the glass ionomer materials.

The resin-modified glass ionomers undergo a two- or three-stage setting reaction (Fig. 5-13*B*). First, light activation causes the polymerizable groups to react and essentially cross-link or "gel" the material in a way similar to composites. This reaction is rapid, taking place more quickly than the slower acid-base reaction found in conventional glass ionomers. There is evidence, however, that the conventional glass ionomer reaction also occurs within 10 minutes or so of the initial set and greatly improves the properties of the material. The materials will also cure in the absence of light exposure because of the third stage of the setting reaction, a self-curing of the polymerizable groups. The properties of these materials are optimal when they are light-cured first, however. Table 5-3 provides a comparison of the different types of glass ionomers and their curing reactions.

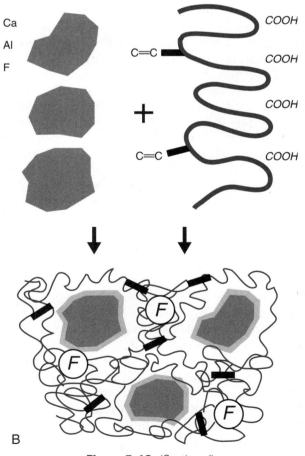

Figure 5–13 *(Continued)*

TABLE 5–3. Glass Ionomers—Types and Setting Reactions

Type	Acid-Base Reaction	Light-Activated Polymerization	Self-Curing Polymerization
Conventional	Yes	No	No
Resin-modified			
• Self-cured	Yes	No	Yes
• Light-cured	Yes	Yes	No
• Dual-cured	Yes	Yes	Yes

Characteristics and Properties

Glass ionomers, like composites, have many characteristics similar to those of natural teeth, although ionomers generally are weaker. Their thermal properties are nearly ideal, and perhaps this contributes to the fact that marginal sealing of glass ionomer restorations is very good. Because water is a part of their formulation, they are slightly soluble in water. Compared with composites they are far more soluble, although this does not seem to be a significant clinical problem for the materials when they are used as restoratives.

The greatest weaknesses of the conventional glass ionomers lie in their mechanical properties; they are much weaker than other restorative materials (Table 5-2). Their low tensile strength and fracture resistance prohibits them from being used in stress-bearing restorations, such as class I, II, or IV cavities. Clinical studies in deciduous teeth indicate that they cannot stand up to the rigors of masticatory stresses, and they are quickly worn down and become unacceptable as permanent restoratives. Similarly, many in the field have expressed concern over the use of glass ionomers as core buildups. They are certainly indicated where sufficient tooth structure (i.e., one half to two thirds of the tooth) remains but have been shown to fail in in vitro tests at lower stresses than composites or amalgams when serving as the sole support for a crown. In class III and V cavities, however, the strength of the glass ionomers is of little concern. The most recent resin-modified glass ionomers were developed for non–stress-bearing applications, as well as for use as a core buildup material when adequate tooth structure remains. Their properties and adhesion may be slightly improved over those of conventional glass ionomers, but they are not considered suitable for use in high-stress regions.

Clinical Performance

Because of their fluoride release, glass ionomers have been used predominantly as anterior restoratives for patients with a high caries rate. As they do not offer a significant improvement over composites for the restoration of class III or class IV cavities for the general population, they do not currently enjoy as much use in these applications. The glass ionomer surface cannot be polished to the same smoothness as composite, nor is the material as translucent. Therefore, glass ionomers do not offer the same esthetic potential as microfill composites. These materials also have very low fracture resistance, which eliminates them from consideration for class IV restorations. There have been clinical trials with glass ionomers in posterior teeth, predominantly for deciduous molars. In general, conventional, metal-reinforced, or resin-modified glass ionomers suffer from a higher incidence of fracture and wear on occlusal surfaces than do composites or amalgam. They should, therefore, be used only with caution in such instances.

From this discussion, it is obvious that the structural integrity of the glass ionomer restoration is a primary concern that limits its use to non–stress-bearing sites. The adhesive nature of the material and the expected beneficial effects of the fluoride release, however, continue to make it attractive for more extensive applications. The development of light-cured glass ionomers was a significant step in this direction. Although the original materials were intended only for use as bases, reinforced versions with enhanced mechanical properties have become available and have extended their usefulness.

At present, the glass ionomers have a niche in restorative dentistry in the restoration of class V lesions or erosions. Although their esthetic qualities and polishability are not the equivalent of those of microfill composites, excellent restorations are still achievable. Numerous clinical studies have evaluated the new dentin adhesives for composites. In most of these studies, glass ionomer is used as a reference material and in virtually all cases has been the material with the greatest success rate. Few if any glass ionomer restorations are lost from class V cavities over 3- to 5-year periods. Newer adhesives for dentin are being developed continually for composite restorations with a comparable level of success.

■ *Compomers*

Compomer is a contraction of "composite" and "ionomer," suggesting a material with intermediate characteristics and properties. Compomers are packaged and handled much like composites. They are single-paste systems that are applied and hardened by light activation, like composites are. These materials have essentially the same composition as composites with one exception. Compomers contain an additional molecule with carboxylic acid groups, similar to the molecules in conventional and resin-modified glass ionomers. This implies that compomers can also undergo an acid-base setting reaction like glass ionomers. Compomers, however, do not contain water (i.e., they are anhydrous). After they have been placed, hardened, and finished, the water in saliva is absorbed by the material, and an acid-base reaction occurs over time. The water causes the carboxylic acid groups to hydrolyze, and the acidity produces an etching of the adjacent glass with the subsequent release of metallic ions. These ions then cross-link the acid groups. The fact that this reaction does not contribute to the initial hardening, as it does for resin-modified glass ionomers, is important to understand.

Compomers have properties that are intermediate to those of composites and resin-modified glass ionomers but are closest to composites. They have generally been shown to have less fluoride release than glass ionomers, although some of the newer versions have been improved in this regard. Compomers are most effective when they are bonded to the cavity walls with dentin/enamel adhesives, similar to composites. Like composites also, they have excellent esthetics. Compomers are very popular in some parts of Europe, and many studies report good clinical success with compomers when they are used in anterior teeth. Earlier formulations demonstrated excessive wear when used on occlusal surfaces in children, however, and this application is not recommended for permanent teeth.

◼ *Enamel and Dentin Adhesives*

The importance of achieving and maintaining adhesion between dental restoratives and tooth structure cannot be overstated. Although bonding to enamel is a well-established procedure, many cavity outlines extend into dentin or cementum and must be treated differently. The adhesive technologies that have been aggressively pursued to bond resins to enamel and dentin are reviewed in this section.

Enamel Adhesives

Unfilled resins have been used for many years for the purpose of enhancing the adaptation and bond of composites to etched enamel surfaces. Initially, these "enamel bond" resins were of the self-curing variety. As light-curing became the technique of choice for most clinicians, light-cured enamel adhesives were produced. These materials are essentially unfilled composites or pit and fissure sealants that are applied to the enamel surfaces with a brush. Their excellent flow properties allow them to coat and fill in the small irregularities of the acid-etched enamel surface in a manner that is superior to that of the thicker, more viscous composites. These resins, like the composite itself, possess no chemical adhesiveness toward the enamel surface and rely solely on mechanical interlocking of the enamel rods for adhesion. As such, they have no beneficial effect when used alone to bond to dentin. Their use has been limited to the enamel portions of preparations.

Enamel bond resins also are routinely used for the intraoral repair of fractured composite restorations. The chipped or fractured composite restoration can be repaired with fresh composite. First, the surface of the fractured restoration is roughened with a diamond or abraded with an intraoral sandblaster (air abrasion) to remove contaminants and create additional sites for mechanical bonding. The surface is then cleaned with phosphoric acid to remove cutting debris and subsequently rinsed and dried. Next, a coating of the unfilled resin is applied to the rough surface and light activated. Its purpose is to enhance the adaptation of the new composite to the old composite. Finally, the new composite is added and light activated. Bond strengths between new and old composites, with an unfilled resin used as an intermediate step, may be 60 to 90% of the strength of the original composite.

Dentin Adhesives

Because of the significant curing contraction that compromised the adhesion of composites to tooth surfaces, it was obvious that some mechanism was required to provide a bond between the composite and dentin or cementum. The first attempt to enhance this bond followed the lead of enamel acid etching. Acid etching of dentin produces a surface far different from that produced on enamel, however, and the initial results were poor.

Etched dentin contains many open dentinal tubules, the number of which depends on the location in the tooth. For example, only 4% of the dentin surface near the dentin-enamel junction may contain tubules, whereas near the pulp, where the tubules are packed much closer together, 30% of the surface area of the dentin may contain tubules (Fig. 5-14). In addition, whereas enamel is composed almost entirely of inorganic mineral, nearly 50% of the volume of dentin is made up of water and organic material, mainly collagen protein. Thus, the composition

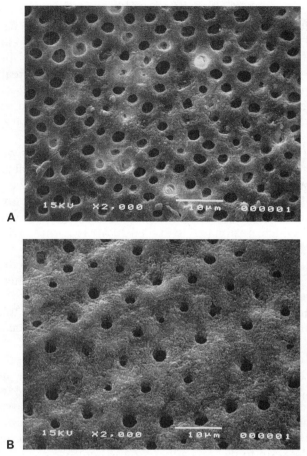

Figure 5–14 Scanning electron photomicrographs of dentin. **A.** High density of tubules near the pulp. **B.** Lower density of tubules near the dentin-enamel junction.

of dentin is much different than that of enamel, and one would expect it to behave differently when etched with acid. The presence of water and organic components lowered the surface energy of the dentin and made bonding with existing resins essentially impossible.

In the 1970s and early 1980s, a tremendous effort was made to identify ways to form chemical bonds between resin adhesives and dentin. This search actually began many years before, but significant commercial advances were not apparent until the 1980s. Researchers produced dentin adhesives whose mechanism of action included the proposed formation of chemical bonds to the hydroxyapatite, or mineral portion of dentin, as well as to the collagen, or organic portion. Although improvements in the bond strengths to dry dentin substrates were achieved, these could not be duplicated under moist conditions, and the results of clinical trials were poor. Although disappointing, these materials still were an improvement over unfilled "enamel-bond" resins, and they paved the way for further developments.

At the time there was great resistance to the placement of phosphoric or other types of acids onto the dentin for fear of harming the pulp. Although there were much conflicting data, some early studies had shown pulpal damage in the teeth of experimental animals that was caused by the application of acids to dentin.

Based on the results of these studies, calcium hydroxide liners were always placed onto dentin surfaces before acid etching of enamel to safeguard the dentin and pulp. These concerns caused many dentin adhesive developers to avoid the use of strong acids as dentin treatments for their adhesives because these chemicals would remove the protective covering of the tubules created by the instrumentation process.

When the dentin is cut by a dental instrument, a layer of loosely adhered debris is left covering the dentinal tubules. Because of its appearance, this layer, which contains the components of the ground dentin, is referred to as the **smear layer** (Fig. 5-15). Many of the earlier dentin adhesives were designed to bond directly to this layer by reacting with the collagen or calcium within it; however, bond strengths of only 2 to 6 MPa (300 to 900 psi) were achieved because the smear layer itself was not bonded well to the dentin below. These bond strengths were not great enough to resist the contraction stress generated by shrinking composites, which is estimated to exceed 20 MPa in some cavities. Therefore, these adhesives were unsuccessful.

Further developments produced bond strengths to dry dentin that measured in the range of 10 to 12 MPa (1500 to 1800 psi). These bond strengths were achieved by first applying a conditioner to the dentin to remove the smear layer. In some cases, the primer, which was acidic, would completely remove the smear layer and leave the tubules open, whereas in others, the acid was milder and removed the smear layer but left the tubules plugged with debris (Fig. 5-16). In any case, the bond strengths of these adhesives to dentin were improved by this treatment. Marginal leakage was not eliminated, however, and clinical success rates still were not acceptable, especially in light of the excellent success of glass ionomers. Much of the reason for the failure can be explained by the effect of moisture within the dentinal tubules. Because the resins were essentially **hydrophobic** (*hydro* = water; *phobic* = hating), moisture effectively limited the ability of the resin to wet and adhere to the dentin.

The most recent additions to the dentin bonding materials are designed to be more **hydrophilic** (i.e., "water loving"). These adhesives are supplied as either one-component or multicomponent systems (Fig. 5-17). Multicomponent systems usually contain three separate components: etchant, primer, and adhesive

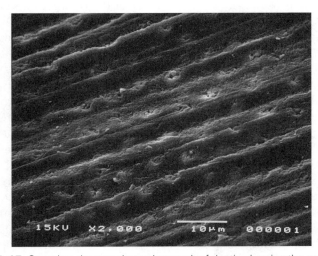

Figure 5–15 Scanning electron photomicrograph of dentin showing the smear layer.

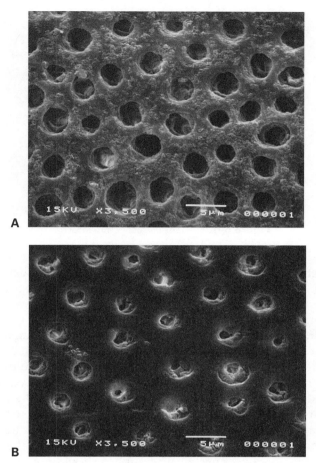

Figure 5–16 Scanning electron photomicrographs of dentin. **A.** Total removal of the smear layer by etching with phosphoric acid. **B.** Milder effect created by less aggressive acids.

resin. The etchant is usually a phosphoric acid gel. The primer is usually a hydrophilic monomer that serves as an agent to wet and penetrate the etched dentin, preparing it to receive the adhesive. One-component systems have a combined etchant and primer (so-called "self-etching primer") or a combined primer and adhesive. In the latter, an acid etch is usually used as the first step, and the primer/adhesive is applied after the etch has been washed off. Therefore, some one-component systems actually require two steps. There is intensive research into these new, simplified adhesives. Currently, it appears that one-component and multicomponent systems produce similar adhesion to dentin and enamel and have similar costs. The procedure for the use of a typical three-component system is described, although not all adhesives are used in exactly the same manner.

Step one involves the application of an acid *etchant*, whose function is either to remove totally or at least to alter the smear layer by demineralizing the hydroxyapatite. This process exposes the underlying dentin or at least makes the smear layer more permeable for the next step. In addition, a significantly roughened surface is produced. Although the surface is not as rough as etched enamel, it is more permeable than normal dentin or a normal smear layer. The acid etchant may be phosphoric acid (either diluted to 10% or at the full strength of 37%), nitric acid, or some other organic acid such as maleic acid or EDTA (ethylenedi-

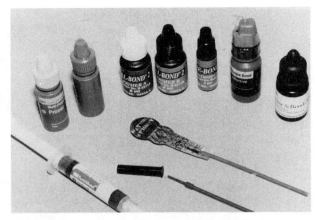

Figure 5–17 Several current commercial dentin adhesive systems.

aminetetraacetic acid). The etchant is applied to the dentin and enamel with a brush, allowed to stand for 15 seconds, and then washed with a copious water spray. The surface is then dried, either by lightly blowing air or by blotting with cotton. For nearly all materials, it is important not to overdry the tooth because bonding is enhanced when some moisture remains in the tubules. This has been referred to as "wet bonding."

Step two involves the application of a separate *primer* to the dentin. The primer contains monomers and hydrophilic molecules (such as HEMA) that serve as wetting agents to improve the penetration of the monomers into the permeable dentin surface. Because much of the mineral has been removed by the acid in the top few micrometers of the surface, the primer penetrates into a mostly organic material composed of collagen fibrils sticking up from the sound dentin to which they are strongly connected. This surface should not be allowed to dry after the etch process. Upon drying, the collagen fibrils collapse and effectively "seal off" the surface from the primer and adhesive. The resins do not penetrate, therefore, and adhesion is reduced. It is very important to follow closely the manufacturer's instructions to avoid this problem. The primer is then applied with a brush. It is not washed off, nor is it dried excessively.

The third and final step is to apply the *adhesive* material. The adhesive is essentially an unfilled or lightly filled resin, similar in composition to the resin in composites except that hydrophilic molecules have been added. The adhesive is brushed onto the prepared dentin surface and is thinned to a uniform layer with the brush; it coats as well as partially penetrates the dentin surface. The adhesive is then light-cured for approximately 10 seconds. The adhesive bonds to the dentin, mostly by surrounding the exposed collagen fibrils and mechanically locking into the rough dentin surface once the adhesive monomers become polymerized. This interface region has been shown to be more resistant to demineralization by acids, suggesting that a zone of resin-reinforced dentin forms to link the resin to the tooth structure. This zone has been called the "hybrid layer" (Fig. 5-18).

Because the adhesive is a resin-like composite, it forms an air-inhibited layer on its surface when it is light cured. This layer polymerizes when the overlying composite restoration is placed, and the two become joined.

The application procedure for the one-component systems varies from brand to brand. Because they employ fewer steps, the application time may be slightly

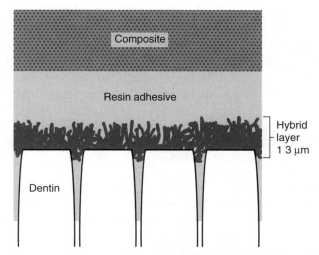

Figure 5-18 Schematic drawing of the hybrid layer formed between a dentin adhesive and the dentin surface, showing penetration within and through the collagen fibrils.

shorter than it is for some multicomponent systems. For example, after etching, washing, and lightly drying, the combined primer/adhesive is applied to the surface with a brush. For some materials, improved adhesion occurs when the primer is lightly scrubbed into the surface with the brush. The surface is then dried with the air syringe. This procedure is critical because these systems all contain a solvent in the primer/adhesive, either acetone or ethanol, that must be eliminated before light-curing for 10 seconds. Because of the presence of the solvent, some researchers suggest that these new adhesives are more sensitive to application technique variables than are many of the multicomponent systems. Therefore, it is imperative to follow the manufacturer's directions.

Bond strengths to dentin with the new adhesives often exceed 20 MPa (3000 psi) and may be equivalent to those on enamel. Although many in vitro studies show that they still do not completely eliminate microleakage at the dentin margins, early results from clinical trials show them to be significantly improved over previous formulations, and they eventually may perform in a manner comparable to glass ionomers in class V lesions. These adhesives also appear to be better able to bond in moist environments, although isolation still is important during the procedure to avoid gross contamination of the cavity preparation with saliva and/or blood.

An additional application of adhesives is in the bonding of amalgam restorations. The application of a dentin adhesive before placing amalgam (see Chapter 6) has been advocated to seal the dentin to reduce the incidence of postoperative sensitivity and to reinforce the tooth and the amalgam at the cavity margin. This technique has grown significantly in popularity. All of the same considerations concerning the use of adhesives for composite are applicable for bonding amalgams.

Summary

Direct esthetic anterior restorations are used to repair missing or decayed tooth structure or to improve the appearance of teeth in the front of the mouth. Composites used in conjunction with resin adhesives and glass ionomers are the materials of choice. The popularity of glass ionomers is increasing because of the potential therapeutic effect of the fluoride they release. They are excellent restorations for gingival areas, where stresses are low. Light-cured glass ionomers have been developed with improved strength and esthetic qualities, compared with the conventional self-curing materials, and can be used in more extensive restorations. These materials are used much like light-cured composites but may adhere to the tooth without the need for the resin dentin adhesives or acid etching of enamel required for successful composites. Composites generally are stronger, more polishable, and more esthetically satisfactory than glass ionomers.

Compomers were developed as a class of materials joining the best qualities of both composites and glass ionomers. In actuality, however, there is little evidence to suggest they offer a significant improvement in clinical performance. Proper attention to light-curing procedures—such as the use of sufficient illumination time and curing restorations in increments to ensure adequate depth of cure and minimize shrinkage forces—is essential for the successful use of composites and compomers.

STUDY QUESTIONS AND PROBLEM SOLVING

1. **Which of the following is *not* a true statement about dental composites?**
   a. They contain monomers that chemically react to transform a paste into a rigid restorative
   b. Glass particles are coated with coupling agents to enhance bonding to polymers
   c. They contain spherical fillers that are generally 100 to 200 μm in diameter
   d. Their strength depends on how much filler they contain
2. **Which type of composite would be expected to have the shiniest surface after polishing with prophylaxis paste?**
   a. Small-sized hybrid
   b. Microfill
   c. Midsized hybrid
   d. All would be the same
3. **Which of the following is *not* recommended in the technique for curing light-cured composites?**
   a. Holding the light tip 1 cm from the tooth
   b. Wearing special glasses with orange filters
   c. Using an exposure duration of 40 to 60 seconds
   d. Placing the composite in increments of 1 to 2 mm
4. **An image-conscious patient returns with a fractured class IV composite restoration that must be replaced. The chart shows the original restoration was a microfill composite placed 6 months ago. What treatment might be suggested to replace the restoration?**
   a. Glass ionomer to prevent further decay
   b. A midsized hybrid because of its greater strength
   c. A microfill composite to maintain maximum esthetics
   d. A small-sized hybrid combining strength and esthetics

5. **When comparing light-cured and self-curing composites, which of the following statements is true for light-cured composites only?**
   a. They contain resin, filler, and initiator molecules
   b. One must wait at least 24 hours to polish them
   c. They shrink when they harden in the mouth
   d. The clinician can take 10 minutes to place them

6. **Light-cured glass ionomers differ from self-curing (conventional) glass ionomers in that light-cured versions:**
   a. Demonstrate greater fluoride release in the mouth
   b. Have greater strength and stiffness
   c. Can be hardened within a shorter period of time
   d. Will not form surface cracks during drying

7. **Glass ionomers should be mixed for approximately 30 to 40 seconds because:**
   a. Longer mixing times delay the setting reaction
   b. Shorter mixing times do not allow the powder to be entirely dissolved
   c. Longer mixing times shorten the working time
   d. Shorter mixing times can compromise the material's strength

8. **A glass ionomer would be most likely to adhere to a dentin surface when it is:**
   a. Isolated by a rubber dam and dried with an air blast for 30 seconds
   b. Isolated from saliva by cotton rolls and dried with an air blast for 30 seconds
   c. Isolated from saliva by cotton rolls and lightly dried with cotton
   d. Isolated by a rubber dam and lightly dried with cotton

9. **Compomers differ from resin-modified glass ionomers in that compomers:**
   a. Do not contain water
   b. Have a delayed acid-base reaction
   c. Have properties similar to composites
   d. Handle like composites

10. **Which of the following is *not* one of the three basic components in most dentin-bonding agents?**
    a. Antimicrobial agent
    b. Surface etchant
    c. Wetting primer
    d. Resin adhesive

11. **Compared with multicomponent adhesives, one-component adhesives:**
    a. Can be applied in only a fraction of the time
    b. Have higher bond strengths to dentin
    c. Require fewer steps
    d. Are much less expensive

SELECTED READINGS

Asmussen E. Clinical relevance of physical, chemical, and bonding properties of composite resins. Operative Dentistry 10:61–73, 1985.

This monograph, which was presented at the annual meeting of the Academy of Operative Dentistry in 1985, focuses on the relationship between the properties and clinical performance of composites. The importance of certain properties as predictors of clinical performance is discussed, as are many aspects concerning the bonding of composites to tooth structure.

Bayne SC, Heymann HO, Swift EJ Jr. Update on dental composite restorations. Journal of the American Dental Association 125:687–701, 1994.

This article describes the types and compositions of dental composites and explains the complex steps involved in placing them to avoid problems and enhance the likelihood of clinical success.

McLean JW. Cermet cements. Journal of the American Dental Association 120:43–47, 1990.

This article compares the properties of alloy-reinforced glass ionomers to conventional glass ionomers and describes their clinical applications.

Pashley DH. Dentin bonding: Overview of the substrate with respect to adhesive material. Journal of Esthetic Dentistry 3(2):46–50, 1991.

This article reviews the effects of several variables, including the smear layer, polymerization shrinkage of resins, and contamination on dentin bonding. Dentin sensitivity also is discussed.

Qvist V, Qvist J, Mjor IA. Placement and longevity of tooth-colored restorations in Denmark. Acta Odontologica Scandinavica 48:305–311, 1989.

This article describes the results of a survey on the reasons for replacement of 2542 tooth-colored filling materials in adults and children in Denmark. The average longevity of class III composites was 7 years and was 5 years for class IV and V composites. The primary reason for replacement was secondary caries.

Rueggeberg F. Contemporary issues in photocuring. Compendium of Continuing Education in Dentistry 20(Supplement 25):S4–S15, 1999.

This article discusses the mechanism of photopolymerization of dental composites and adhesives and the importance of such factors as light intensity and exposure time on depth of cure. In addition, a comparison of the many different types of curing lamps is presented.

Smith DC. Development of glass-ionomer cement systems. Biomaterials 19:467–478, 1998.

This article provides a comprehensive review of the development and properties of glass ionomer materials.

Tyas MJ. The Class V lesion—aetiology and restoration. Australian Dental Journal 40:167–170, 1995.

This article describes the materials and techniques used to restore cervical defects, such as glass ionomer, resin-modified glass ionomer, and bonded composite, highlighting the advantages and disadvantages of each. The results of clinical trials of these materials are discussed.

Van Meerbeek B, Perdigao J, Lambrechts P, Vanherle G. The clinical performance of adhesives. Journal of Dentistry 26:1–20, 1998.

This excellent article reviews the many types of adhesive systems available and their mechanism for achieving adhesion to the tooth. A simplified and useful classification system for modern dentin-bonding agents is described. The factors that contribute to clinical success with these materials are discussed, as are the results of clinical trials to date.

Willems G, Lambrechts P, Braem M, Celis JP, Vanherle G. A classification of dental composites according to their morphological and mechanical characteristics. Dental Materials 8:310–319, 1992.

This article suggests a system for classifying dental composites according to their filler particle sizes and amounts, as well as their properties. It includes scanning electron photomicrographs of many types of commercial composites.

Chapter 6

Direct Posterior Restoratives

Amalgam
  Uses
  Types and Composition
  Mixing and Handling
  Setting Reaction
  Characteristics and Properties
  Clinical Success
Composites

  Uses
  Types and Composition
  Mixing and Handling
  Setting Reaction
  Characteristics and Properties
  Clinical Success
Direct Filling Gold
Summary

Objectives

- Compare the elemental compositions and setting reactions of low-copper and high-copper amalgams.
- Compare the handling characteristics of lathe-cut, spherical, and admixed amalgams, and describe the placement procedure for each.
- Compare the creep, strength, and corrosion resistance of low-copper and high-copper amalgams and discuss the reasons for the differences in their clinical performance.
- Explain the effect of mercury-to-alloy (Hg/alloy) ratio and trituration time and speed on the working and setting time of dental amalgam.
- Explain the effect of Hg/alloy ratio and plasticity of the mix on the mechanical properties and clinical performance of amalgams.
- Compare abrasion wear to attrition wear for posterior composites.
- Describe the placement technique for a class II light-activated composite.
- Compare and contrast the indications for the use of posterior composites and amalgams.
- Describe the compositions and uses of the different types of direct gold restoratives.
- Briefly describe the technique for the placement of a direct gold restoration.

Direct gold was one of the first materials used to restore cavities in posterior teeth. Because placement of **gold foil** is a difficult, time-consuming, and costly procedure, its applications have always been limited; this is especially true in modern dentistry. The material that revolutionized the restorative treatment of caries was dental **amalgam**. Since approximately the beginning of the 20th century, amalgam has been the material of choice for restoring posterior teeth. Amalgam has several characteristics that contribute to its popularity, including excellent clinical longevity, familiarity, relative ease of use, and low cost. Perhaps its major drawback is its lack of true esthetic potential. The development of the resin composite was seen as a means to achieve esthetic results in a posterior restoration at a reasonable cost. For many years, the realization of this goal remained elusive because the available materials were vastly inferior to amalgam. In recent years, however, changes in the formulation of composites have led to significant improvements in clinical behavior, and posterior composites have become a viable alternative to amalgam for many restorations and at only a slightly higher cost. Because of the greater difficulty in placing them, however, as well as their more limited durability under heavy masticatory stresses, composites have not replaced amalgam as a posterior restorative.

■ *Amalgam*

Amalgam is defined as an **alloy** of mercury. An alloy is a combination of two or more metals; therefore, amalgam is a metal alloy containing mercury. The word "amalgam" also is used to describe a combination or mixture of things, and dental amalgam is a mixture of mercury, silver, tin, copper, and other elements. The use of this type of mercury alloy is relatively unique to dentistry and is dictated by the fact that the clinician must handle the material in a plastic or moldable state and place it into a cavity before it hardens into a rigid restorative material. Mercury is the only pure metal that is liquid at room temperature. Mercury became important to dentistry when it was discovered that, mixed with a powder of silver and tin, it formed an alloy with physical properties that were suitable for a dental restorative. The material has been studied and examined for over 100 years, yet it remains of interest to dental researchers because of its fascinating complexity. One of the areas of study that has received a tremendous amount of attention in recent years is the issue of biocompatibility—specifically, the toxic and allergenic potential of mercury, its main constituent.

A full treatment of this issue is beyond the scope of this book, and the reader is referred to several important review articles in the list of Selected Readings. Although controversy continues to surround the use of this material, the fact remains that no study has ever proven a link between dental amalgam restorations and any disease in dental patients. The issue of the safety of amalgam has been reviewed by nearly every health organization (i.e., WHO, NIH, FDI, FDA), and none has suggested that the material poses a significant health concern or that evidence exists to discontinue its use. In recent years, however, a new concern has arisen over the environmental consequences of the use of mercury. As the industrial use of mercury compounds decreases in many countries to minimize the production of mercury-contaminated wastes, dentally derived mercury waste is becoming a larger issue. This concern has resulted in a drastic reduction in amalgam use in some countries. Again, it is important to emphasize that it is the environmental issue that has largely driven this change in policy. In most countries, amalgam continues to be considered a safe and effective restorative material.

Uses

Because of its versatility, amalgam probably has been used in nearly every application in restorative dentistry. Its main use has been in the restoration of class I and II cavities, as a filling for buccal pits, and as a buildup material or core for teeth being prepared for crown and bridge dentistry. The material also has been used in posterior and anterior teeth to repair class V lesions and is a common material for the filling of the apices of roots after apicoectomies (i.e., removal of the apex of the tooth root). The latter application is a consequence of amalgam's ability to form a bacterial seal, despite the fact that it does not adhere to tooth structure. The mechanism will be discussed shortly.

Types and Composition

Amalgams are classified according to composition and particle shape. Composition will be addressed first. The conventional amalgam, commonly referred to as *low-copper amalgam*, is produced by mixing mercury with a powdered alloy containing silver (approximately 70%), tin (approximately 27%), and copper (approximately 5%). In some formulations, zinc (approximately 1% or less) is added to the alloy. The usual mixture contains 45 to 50% of mercury by weight. This provides a mercury-to-alloy (Hg/alloy) ratio (i.e., weight of Hg divided by weight of alloy used in the mix) equal to or slightly less than 0.5. In the 1960s, it was determined that increasing the amount of copper in the alloy produced an amalgam with significantly improved clinical performance. These *high-copper amalgams* were produced by mixing mercury with a powder containing silver (approximately 40 to 60%), tin (approximately 27%), and copper (approximately 13 to 30%). Most high-copper amalgams require less mercury in the mix and, therefore, have lower Hg/alloy ratios. Today, almost all of the amalgams that are placed are made from the high-copper alloy (Display 6-1).

Because of concerns over the use of mercury, an alternative "amalgam-like" silver restorative was developed in the early 1990s. These filling materials were made by mixing an alloy of silver and tin with a liquid of gallium, indium, and palladium in the same way as amalgams are mixed. This non–mercury-containing restorative is handled and placed in the same way as is amalgam, but its properties and corrosion are severely affected by contamination with moisture. For this reason, the cavity preparation is sealed with an adhesive prior to condensation into the cavity. Although the strength and creep of these gallium-alloy restoratives are probably adequate, clinical studies have shown poor long-term performance as a result of corrosion and expansion, often resulting in cuspal fracture.

Amalgams are supplied either in predosed disposable capsules or in bulk as powder or tablets (powder pressed together to look like aspirin tablets) that must be mixed in a reusable capsule with a precisely measured amount of mercury (Fig. 6-1). Reusable capsules are either screwed together or simply pressed closed to seal them during mixing. The preencapsulated form is the most popular because of its convenience and the fact that mercury is not openly handled, thus minimizing the chance of a spill or contamination of the operatory. The powder resides in one end of the capsule separated from the liquid mercury by a breakable diaphragm. In others, the mercury is sealed in a plastic diaphragm that breaks once

DISPLAY 6-1

Comparison of the Compositions of Low-Copper and High-Copper Amalgams

Low Copper			Examples
Silver	(68–70%)		New True Dentalloy
Tin	(26–27%)	+ Mercury (45–50%)	Spheraloy
Copper	(4–5%)		Velvalloy
Zinc	(0–1%)		
High Copper			
Silver	(40–70%)		Contour
Tin	(22–30%	+ Mercury (40–45%)	Dispersalloy
Copper	(13–30%)		Tytin
Zinc	(0–1%)		Valiant PhD

high-speed mixing begins. In some cases, the capsule must be squeezed together by hand or with a special activator to release the diaphragm (Fig. 6-1).

Amalgams also are classified according to the shape of their alloy particles. The first amalgam alloy particles were made by filing silver coins to produce shavings. In time, the alloy particles were made by filing a silver-tin alloy on a lathe to produce the shavings. The amalgams that are produced from these alloys are, therefore, called *lathe-cut amalgams*. A lathe is a machine on which a cylindrical sample of a material can be held tightly and turned by a motor at relatively high speeds. A tool, such as a file, can then be used to shape the material while it is turning. As this is done, the debris, which is in the form of powder, can be collected. The particles are small in size, ranging from several to 200 μm, and are irregular in shape with sharp edges and rough surfaces (Fig. 6-2). Years later, a second technique to produce *spherical amalgam* alloy particles for use in amalgam was developed. In this process, the alloy of silver, tin, and copper is melted and then sprayed through a nozzle to form a mist of small droplets (several to 100 μm in diameter), which are then quickly cooled or frozen to preserve their spherical shape. By altering the processing condition, it is also possible to produce particles with a rounded but elongated shape for use in amalgams.

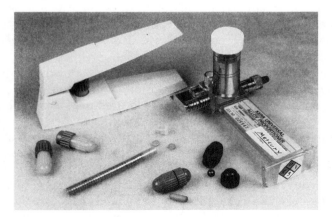

Figure 6–1 Amalgam capsules with pestles, individual alloy pellets, mercury dispenser, and preen-capsulated amalgam with its corresponding activator.

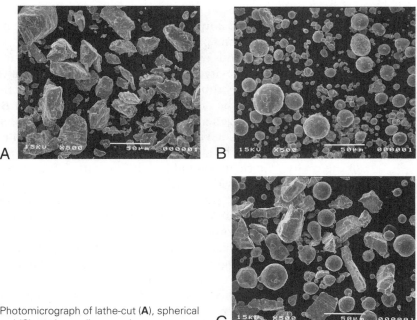

Figure 6–2 Photomicrograph of lathe-cut (**A**), spherical (**B**), and admixed (**C**) amalgam alloy powders.

The final classification of alloys for amalgams, *admixed*, is a mixture of lathe-cut and spherical alloys. The original high-copper amalgams were made by adding a spherical alloy powder containing only silver and copper to lathe-cut particles made with the conventional formulation of silver, tin, and copper. This was the birth of admixed amalgams. Today, high-copper amalgams can be made from a single composition of lathe-cut or spherical particles, or they may be admixtures of conventional or high-copper, lathe-cut particles with high-copper spherical particles.

> The properties of the amalgam depend largely on the alloy composition. The difference in the shape of the alloys, however, leads to significant differences in the handling characteristics.

Mixing and Handling

The primary goals in preparing an amalgam are to ensure that the mercury and low-copper or high-copper alloy are sufficiently mixed to allow the chemical reaction to proceed and to produce an amalgam mass with enough **plasticity**, or moldability, to allow it to be condensed into and adapted to a cavity with minimal porosity. The specific objectives for condensation are to adapt the amalgam intimately to the walls of the cavity, to minimize porosity within the amalgam, and to express excess mercury not needed for the chemical reaction. With this in mind, it is instructive to examine the many factors that influence the handling characteristics of amalgam. These include the shape of the alloy particle, the ratio of mercury to alloy powder in the mix, and the time and speed used to mix the two components.

The following example will help clarify the manner in which particle shape affects the handling properties of amalgam. Envision a small jar filled with aquarium rocks. Then envision taking a rod with a smaller diameter than the jar and trying to push the rod down through the rocks. When the rod is pushed into the rocks, the rocks pack and press together, resisting the forces of condensation pushing the rod down. This is essentially what happens to a lathe-cut amalgam during condensation into a cavity. The clinician notes a significant resistance to the condenser and must apply substantial force through the condenser tip, usually 4 to 6 pounds, to compact the amalgam and eliminate porosity. Because greater compacting stress can be generated with a smaller-tipped condenser (remember that stress equals force divided by area of application), it is most effective to use a condenser with a smaller head to begin the condensation into the depths and corners of the cavity. The cavity should be built up with increments of amalgam to avoid trapping large pores within thicker sections and to express excess mercury from the restoration at each step. As the cavity becomes filled, condensers with larger heads are used; a small condenser could be pushed through the deeper layers, which would create porosity in the amalgam. The restoration is overpacked with a slight excess of amalgam to ensure complete filling. When condensed correctly, the top layer will be slightly rich in mercury, but this is not a problem because this layer will be removed during carving.

The procedure for condensing spherical amalgams is similar, in that the cavity is filled in increments; larger-tipped condensers and lighter forces, however, are used throughout. The reason for this becomes obvious if one envisions pushing the condensing rod from the previous example through a jar containing small ball bearings instead of irregularly shaped rocks. A small-diameter condenser or rod would push through the balls, forcing them to roll out to the sides and away from the tip. Little resistance is offered by the spherical particles; therefore, lighter forces, perhaps only 2 to 3 pounds, are necessary for compacting the amalgam. Because the spheres roll away from the condenser, efficient packing can be accomplished only through the use of condensers with larger heads, which tend to trap the spheres instead of push them to the side. Thus, light forces and larger-diameter condensers are recommended for spherical amalgams, and heavy forces with small-diameter condensers are recommended for lathe-cut alloys. Admixed amalgams will lie somewhere between the two in their handling characteristics.

The next important consideration for handling is the moldability of the mix. This characteristic is termed **plasticity**; the amalgam, although metal, is often referred to as a "plastic mass." The plasticity is largely determined by the ratio of mercury to alloy used in the mix. Because mercury is the liquid portion, one would expect that adding more mercury would increase the plasticity of the material and make it less dry. The result of an increase in the Hg/alloy ratio is a more plastic mix with longer working and setting times (the latter will be discussed shortly). Because one of the most important aspects of an amalgam restoration is the manner in which it is adapted to the walls of the cavity, a slightly delayed set may be a small price to pay for the benefits reaped in handling characteristics by adding a little more mercury. Remember that if the amalgam is condensed properly, the extra mercury eventually will be expressed to the top layer of the restoration, which will be removed when the surface is carved to anatomic shape.

When amalgams were introduced, the alloy filings were mixed with mercury in a mortar and pestle, in much the same way a pharmacist produces a powdered form of a medication. This process requires the use of a large excess of mercury (i.e., much more than that required for the chemical reaction) to "wet" all of the powder and produce a plastic mass. The introduction of the high-speed amalgamator, or **triturator**, eliminated the need for hand mixing (Fig. 6-3). There are var-

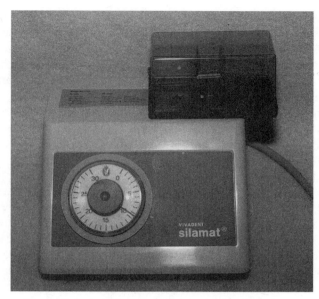

Figure 6–3 A single-speed triturator for dental amalgam.

ious types of triturators, but all work by the same basic premise. Mixing is accomplished by briefly shaking the alloy powder together with the liquid mercury in a closed plastic capsule at high speeds (i.e., triturating). Complete mixing usually is accomplished by triturating for 5 to 20 seconds at speeds of 2000 to 4500 cycles/minute. The exact conditions depend on the types of triturator and amalgam, and specific directions are supplied with each alloy. Faster speeds or longer trituration times generally hasten the setting of the amalgam and produce hotter mixes that tend to be shiny and sticky. The extra energy of mixing under these conditions is transferred to the amalgam, causing the reaction to take place faster. In contrast, undermixing with speeds that are too slow or times that are too short to "wet" all of the particles adequately with mercury produces amalgams that are not cohesive (i.e., crumbly) and look dull. Overtrituration or undertrituration can produce an amalgam that is difficult to condense and results in a porous restoration. A correctly triturated amalgam will appear shiny and cohesive (Fig. 6-4). It

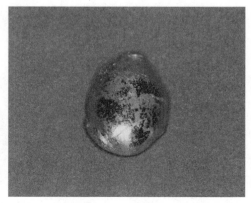

Figure 6–4 A correctly triturated amalgam mass. Note its cohesive nature and shiny appearance.

can be dropped onto a table from a height of 6 inches or so without breaking up; it also can be pressed out into a thin sheet without breaking.

After trituration, the capsule is opened and the amalgam mass is dispensed into a container. A common container is an amalgam well or a Dappen dish (Fig. 6-5). The material is then transferred to the cavity with an amalgam carrier. This instrument has two ends with different-sized cylindrical openings. The carrier is pushed into the mass, causing the amalgam to be forced up into the open end (Fig. 6-5*A*). Because the initial increments of amalgam should be small to fill the line angles and base of the cavity, the smaller end of the carrier is used first. The carrier is transferred directly to the patient's mouth by the clinician, and the amalgam is dispensed into the cavity by pressing down on the lever (Fig. 6-5*B*). While the first increment is being condensed (Fig. 6-6), the carrier is again filled with amalgam to provide the second increment. Once the base of the cavity has been placed, the larger head of the carrier is filled to supply the amalgam that will fill the bulk of the restoration (Fig. 6-7). The cavity should be overpacked with an excess of amalgam (Fig. 6-8). A burnisher is used to remove the excess, which contains extra mercury, and then the occlusal contours are carved into the restoration (Fig. 6-9). The surface of the restoration is then burnished with a ball burnisher to make it smoother (Fig. 6-10).

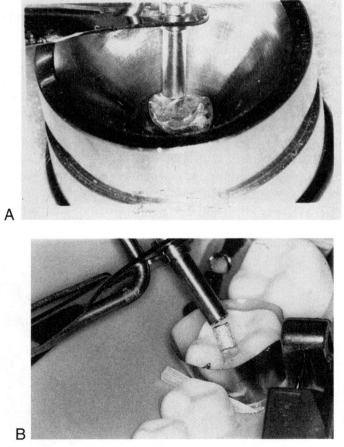

A

B

Figure 6–5 A. An amalgam carrier being forced into an amalgam mass in an amalgam well. **B.** Amalgam being dispensed into the cavity.

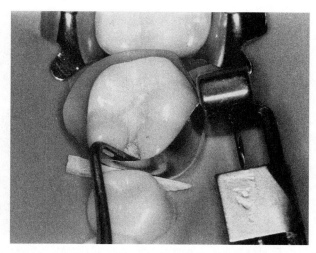

Figure 6–6 An amalgam being condensed into the line angles of the proximal box of a class II restoration. The metal matrix band contains the amalgam within the cavity.

The disposable capsules should be sealed in a plastic bag or sealed container to avoid even minimal contamination of the operatory air from any residual mercury in the capsule. When the bag or container is full, it should be taped shut and disposed of according to the local guidelines and regulations. Reusable capsules also should be sealed in plastic bags until their next use. Unused amalgam scrap should be placed into sealed containers and can be recycled by sending to an appropriate EPA (Environmental Protection Agency) refiner. Local dental societies and associations usually can supply information to help with this process.

Setting Reaction

There are similarities as well as differences between the chemical reactions for the low-copper and high-copper amalgams. The differences relate to the variations in composition of the materials and not to the differences in particle shape, although the rate at which setting occurs is dictated to some extent by particle size and shape. When mercury is mixed with the amalgam alloy, metal ions of silver, tin,

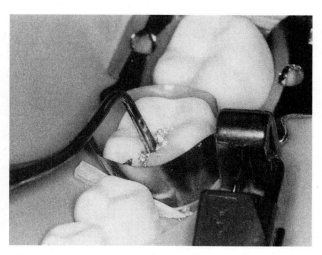

Figure 6–7 An amalgam being condensed into the bulk of a class II cavity preparation.

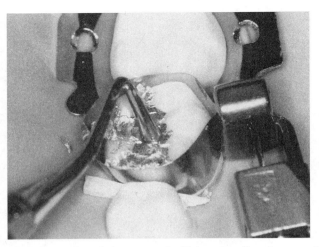

Figure 6–8 An amalgam being overpacked into a class II cavity preparation.

and copper dissolve from the outer surfaces of the particles into the mercury. The ions then react with the mercury to form new metal compounds. The most common reaction is between silver and mercury to form the crystalline matrix for the amalgam. This compound is called gamma-1 (γ_1). Gamma-1 eventually occupies nearly 40% of the total volume of the amalgam and holds the original alloy particles together. Because only the surfaces of the original alloy particles dissolve, most of the rest of the volume of amalgam is occupied by these particles. In addition, small amounts of other compounds also form; these "other" compounds highlight the differences between the low-copper and high-copper amalgams.

In the low-copper amalgams, tin reacts with mercury to form small areas of a tin-mercury compound referred to as gamma-2 (γ_2) (Display 6-2). In contrast, in the high-copper amalgams, tin reacts with copper to form tin-copper compounds. The different tin compounds that are formed are responsible for the differences in properties and clinical behavior between the two types of amalgams.

Immediately after trituration, the amalgam is somewhat plastic and condensable. The mixture remains condensable for 4 to 5 minutes from the start of trituration (i.e., its working time). Fresh increments of amalgam will bond to one an-

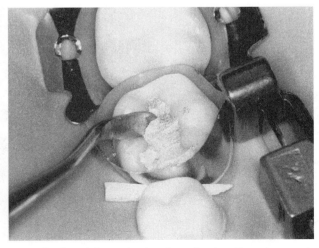

Figure 6–9 Carving of the occlusal surface of a class II amalgam restoration.

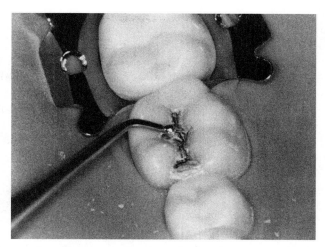

Figure 6–10 The margins and the occlusal surface of a class II amalgam restoration being burnished with a ball burnisher.

other during this period. It is important to realize this because if it becomes apparent that a single mix will not be enough to fill an entire cavity, a second mix must be initiated quickly before the end of the working time of the first mix. The actual working time varies among alloys, with most of the spherical, high-copper amalgams setting most rapidly. By approximately 5 minutes from the start of mixing, the restoration is ready to be carved for removal of excess and anatomic shaping. Carving should not be performed too soon because the carver will pull the amalgam mass away from the margins, leaving behind significant voids and defects. Once final carving is accomplished, a burnisher is used again to refine the occlusal margins of the restoration and enhance the adaptation of the amalgam to the cavity walls (Fig. 6-10). Final finishing should be delayed for 24 hours, or until a later appointment, to avoid damaging the margins. Although the amalgam has hardened substantially, it is still relatively weak at this point and should not be unduly stressed.

> Patients should be informed not to chew or grind on the new restoration for several hours because the amalgamation reaction continues for many hours and is not completed until several days have passed.

DISPLAY 6-2

Comparison of the Setting Reactions of Low-Copper and High-Copper Amalgams

Low Copper

Silver	(Ag)					Ag–Sn
Tin	(Sn)	+	Mercury (Hg)	$\longrightarrow$		Ag–Hg (γ_1 matrix)
						Sn–Hg (γ_2)

High Copper

Silver	(Ag)					Ag–Sn–Cu
Tin	(Sn)	+	Mercury (Hg)	$\longrightarrow$		Ag–Hg (γ_1 matrix)
Copper	(Cu)					Sn–Cu

For this reason, amalgams must demonstrate a minimal compressive strength of 80 MPa within 1 hour of trituration to be considered by the American Dental Association as acceptable restorative materials. For some applications, a faster set is desirable. When amalgam is used as a core material, where a crown preparation must be made and an impression taken in a single appointment, the amalgam must harden quickly so that it can be cut with the high-speed handpiece. Variations in alloy size and Hg/alloy ratio can be used to achieve this result. In any case, free mercury is no longer present in the amalgam after the first few hours post-trituration. After that point, all of it is bound within the amalgam and none is free at the surface of the restoration.

Any condition that hastens the rate at which the mercury is used up in the amalgamation reaction will cause a reduction in the working time and hasten the set. This includes the use of less mercury (i.e., just as much as is needed for the chemical reaction). As previously mentioned, a slight excess of mercury beyond that needed to complete the reaction usually is added to enhance the handling characteristics of the amalgam. This also slows the setting rate because more mercury must react. If this mercury is squeezed out during condensation, the setting time will not be appreciably lengthened, although the working time will have been adequately prolonged. This is the ideal case. Use of a lower Hg/alloy ratio (i.e., a slightly drier mix), however, will produce a shorter working time and a faster set. This may be desirable in certain instances. Because most modern amalgams are purchased as preencapsulated systems, the Hg/alloy ratio cannot be changed to achieve a faster set. The same result can be accomplished, however, by triturating for a slightly longer time or at a faster speed, if the triturator has variable speed settings. Generally, the manufacturer's recommendations have been designed to provide the best handling characteristics with a reasonable working and setting time and should be followed for the best results.

Characteristics and Properties

For an amalgam restoration to be successful, it must be stable and resistant to the solvents and stresses of the oral environment. At the same time, it must seal the tooth from bacterial penetration. Several characteristics of the material are important, therefore, because they dictate the extent to which these goals can be achieved. Properties such as susceptibility to corrosion influence the sealing capabilities of the material. Dimensional change as a result of contraction during setting, or creep deformation during service, also may influence marginal integrity. Other properties, such as strength, elastic modulus, and fracture resistance, determine the structural stability of the material. These characteristics are influenced by several factors, including Hg/alloy ratio, condensation technique (i.e., the amount of porosity), and trituration conditions. Furthermore, clinical factors such as cavity design and moisture contamination will have a profound effect on the performance of a given amalgam restoration. Strict attention to each aspect of the preparation and handling of the material is required to optimize clinical success.

Dimensional Change

As the mercury wets and begins to soak into the alloy particles, a more intimate contact is established between the two components, which results in an initial shrinkage of the amalgam. This shrinkage is slight but significant. Some of this shrinkage is compensated for by an expansion of the amalgam as the γ_1 matrix crystals grow, pushing out against one another and the original alloy particles. For most amalgams, the net result of these dimensional changes is a small contraction, which leaves a slight gap at the margins of the restoration. Studies using laboratory models have shown that there is an initial leakage of fluids between the amalgam and the wall of the cavity after placement but that this leakage stops within a period of months if amalgam is submerged in saliva. *What is the cause of this "self-sealing" behavior?*

In the oral cavity, the amalgam is subjected to the salinity and acidity of the oral fluids, which cause it to corrode. This happens on the surface of the amalgam, but the effects may not be readily apparent because tooth brushing removes the oxides that form during the process, leaving the surface relatively shiny. No abrasion occurs in the marginal gap, however, and corrosion products formed there can build up over time. These corrosion products eventually plug up the marginal crevice created by the setting shrinkage, thus effectively sealing the tooth from the oral environment. When the amalgam has not been well adapted to the cavity, it is more difficult to achieve this sealing because of the large size of the gap. In these cases, there may be lingering postoperative pain or sensitivity that does not readily subside. This pain is associated with the movement of fluids in the unsealed dentin tubules, which is made possible because the gap provides an open communication between the dentin and the oral cavity. In the worst case, the amalgam will require replacement.

A second form of dimensional change that may affect marginal integrity is called **creep**. Creep is defined as a flow or dimensional change produced in a material under a constant stress. The forces generated on the amalgam during chewing may cause it to creep into open areas, such as margins, and fracture. Evidence for these fractures can be seen in the marginal breakdown, or ditching, around amalgams in the oral cavity (Fig. 6-11). This process also is likely related to corrosion because the corroded amalgam at the margins may be weakened and more easily fractured. Clinical and laboratory studies with low-copper and high-copper amalgams have shown a good correlation between low-creep and low-marginal deterioration. Although this is probably not a cause and effect relationship, it suggests that anything that minimizes creep may help to minimize marginal breakdown in amalgams.

One factor that significantly influences creep is the presence of the γ_2 (tin-mercury) compound in the set amalgam. This compound is relatively soft com-

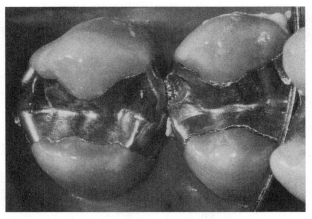

Figure 6–11 Minimal marginal fracture of a high-copper amalgam restoration (*left*) and moderate marginal deterioration of a low-copper amalgam (*right*), placed at the same appointment.

pared with the rest of the amalgam and, therefore, is easily deformed. Thus, amalgams with significant amounts of γ_2 (i.e., low-copper amalgams) are more prone to creep. In contrast, the tin-copper compounds that form in the high-copper amalgams are stronger than γ_2. Therefore, high-copper amalgams may be expected to be harder and undergo less creep than low-copper amalgams, and many research studies have confirmed this.

Amalgams made of certain specific alloys also have the potential to undergo dimensional change, with a clinically unacceptable result. There have been instances in which a delayed expansion has occurred in an amalgam, essentially forcing it out from the cavity. This is most easily observable in a class V or buccal pit lesion in which there are no biting stresses to force the material back or to wear down the protruding material. This delayed expansion phenomenon has been associated specifically with the use of low-copper amalgams containing zinc. Zinc is sometimes added during the manufacture of the alloy to produce a "clean" powder with good reaction characteristics. Moisture contamination during the placement of a zinc-containing amalgam may cause delayed expansion as the zinc and the water react to form a compound within the amalgam, forcing it to expand out of the cavity. This phenomenon provides further support for the use of a rubber dam during amalgam placement.

Strength and Stiffness

Dental amalgam is metal and has many of the characteristics of a metallic material. It is strong, especially in compression, and has a relatively high modulus of elasticity (Table 6-1). These two properties suggest that amalgam will not be appreciably deformed when placed in large cavities. Amalgam, however, has a much lower tensile than compressive strength, which is characteristic of a brittle material such as porcelain. Amalgam, therefore, should not be placed in thin layers where it will be exposed to tensile (i.e., pulling) or bending stresses. Bulk fractures of amalgam restorations are rare. When they do occur, it is usually because the amalgam was placed in a cavity preparation that was too shallow, i.e., not extending deeper than the dentin-enamel junction (Fig. 6-12). This is associated most often with a class II restoration. Forces applied to the interproximal ridge produce a bending stress across the restoration and, if the amalgam is too thin because of inadequate design, enhance the chance of failure.

TABLE 6-1. **Values for Various Properties of Amalgams and Dental Composites**

	Composites		Amalgam	
	Microfill	**Hybrids**	**Low-Cu**	**High-Cu**
Setting contraction (vol%)	2–4	1.5–4	0.6	0.3
Thermal expansion coefficient (α; $10^{-6}/°C$)	50–60	20–40	22–28	22–28
Thermal conductivity (cal · cm/cm^2 · sec · °C)	1–2	2–3	55	55
Tensile strength (MPa)	40–50	50–70	50–60	45–55
Flexural strength (MPa)	75–100	100–160	120–130	90–110
Flexural modulus (GPa)	5–7	8–14	20–25	25–40
Compressive strength (MPa)	400–475	375–475	300–400	400–500
Creep (%)	—	—	1.0–2.5	0.05–1.0

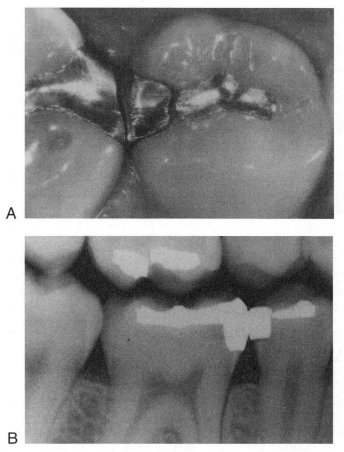

Figure 6–12 A. Amalgam fractured across the isthmus region. **B.** Radiographic image of the amalgam restoration, showing the shallow depth that led to the fracture.

Because the original alloy particles are the strongest and stiffest portion of the amalgam, anything that minimizes their content will decrease mechanical properties. Therefore, higher Hg/alloy ratios, which result in more γ_1 matrix formation, produce a weaker amalgam. Although handling characteristics are improved when more mercury is used in the mix, using too much produces an amalgam with poorer properties. *Is it obvious why there must be a trade-off between ideal handling characteristics and optimum physical properties for amalgams?*

The direct effect of trituration time and speed on amalgam properties is minimal. Because these variables can significantly influence working time and, therefore, handling, however, they can affect the strength of an amalgam by affecting the amount of porosity in the final material. Generally, the strength of a drier mix that sets too quickly will be low because it is more porous. This is especially true at the margins.

Other factors affect the properties of amalgam. As expected, because of the presence of the weak γ_2 phase, the low-copper amalgams are weaker in compression and are more easily deformed than the high-copper amalgams. Improvements in strength and corrosion resistance are achieved in other amalgams by adding small amounts of other elements, such as palladium.

Corrosion

Both low-copper and high-copper amalgams corrode in saline environments. The corrosion products that are formed are different, being predominately tin oxides in the former and copper oxides in the latter. The rate and extent of corrosion are greater for the low-copper amalgams, however, which is a factor contributing to their poorer clinical performance, compared with the high-copper amalgams. Low-copper amalgam corrosion is more significant because the attack is centered around the tin-mercury (γ_2) compound areas. These areas are the most susceptible to corrosion and are easily oxidized in the oral environment. As these areas deteriorate in the amalgam, they leave behind pores filled with corrosion products, which further weaken the amalgam. Corroded amalgams generally have a darkened surface, but much of this may be the result of tarnish of the silver as it contacts sulfides in foods. On rare occasions, a clinician may find an amalgam with a very pitted and deteriorated surface. This may be the result of galvanic corrosion from contact between the amalgam and a gold restoration, as discussed in Chapter 2.

As mentioned, a surface that has been poorly condensed and is porous is to be avoided because it will enhance corrosion. Therefore, it is generally considered more beneficial to polish amalgams than to leave the surface in the carved state. The smoother surface is less likely to trap plaque and is less susceptible to corrosion.

Clinical Success

The clinical success of dental amalgam has been evaluated and reviewed in numerous studies. As with many dental materials, when amalgam is evaluated in controlled clinical trials the success rate is extremely high, and longevity of 20 years and longer is predicted. Data gathered from private practice surveys, however, usually show a different tendency, with average lifetimes of 8 to 10 years for class I and II amalgam restorations. The major cause of failure for amalgam restorations is secondary decay. The second most common reason for replacing amalgams is marginal breakdown. The expectation is that marginal breakdown will lead to leakage and secondary decay, but the association is a tenuous one. Recent studies have attempted to determine how large a marginal gap needs to be to lead to secondary decay. The data from such studies suggest that because of the appearance of the margin and the difficulties in diagnosing secondary caries, many amalgam restorations probably are replaced unnecessarily. The third most common reason for failure is bulk fracture, which often is related to an inappropriate cavity design.

Many clinical studies have shown that when placed correctly, high-copper amalgams undergo less marginal deterioration than do low-copper amalgams over the same period of time. This clinical result can be predicted based on the higher strength, creep resistance, and corrosion resistance of the high-copper amalgams. Because marginal breakdown does not always correlate with caries, however, marginal breakdown in itself may not be the best indicator of amalgam failure. In fact, some studies have failed to show a correlation between amalgam longevity and the concentration of copper in the amalgam. Although these results are somewhat confusing, they point to the importance of the dental personnel in the success of a given amalgam restoration. Apparently, proper mixing, manipulation, and placement of an amalgam may be more important than composition in determining clinical success. Under identical conditions, however, the high-copper amalgams should outperform the low-copper formulations, and this is why they are the amalgams of choice. Subtle differences exist between the clinical performances of the various types of high-copper amalgams, but these comparisons are beyond the scope of this text.

Another common failure mode for an amalgam restoration is fracture of one of the tooth cusps. This usually occurs when the amalgam is large and the surrounding enamel is thin. Amalgam adhesives have been developed, in part, to address this issue. An adhesive that would bond to amalgam and tooth structure could potentially reinforce a tooth restored with amalgam, reducing the incidence of cusp fracture. The adhesive also should seal the dentin surfaces and reduce postoperative sensitivity. Several in vitro studies have shown that a tooth restored with a bonded composite is more resistant to fracture than one restored with unbonded amalgam. Because of the greater stiffness and strength of amalgam compared with composite, a tooth containing a bonded composite may be expected to be as strong as the natural, unrestored tooth. Furthermore, if the lack of adhesion at the enamel margin contributes to the marginal breakdown of amalgam because of a lack of support, bonding at the margins with amalgam adhesives may ameliorate marginal degradation, thus increasing the longevity of future amalgams. These matters remain conjectural, however, because the clinical success of amalgam adhesives is only now being established. To date, clinical studies have not shown reduced marginal fracture as a result of amalgam bonding. In addition, most controlled clinical studies evaluating amalgam bonding have not shown it to significantly reduce postoperative sensitivity. Because the experience of many private practitioners has been different in this regard, amalgam bonding continues to grow in popularity.

■ *Composites*

Uses

The uses for posterior composites are essentially the same as those for dental amalgam. Because they have not performed as well as amalgam, however, indications for their use have been more restricted. Although opinions differ and results vary from clinician to clinician, the results from general practice suggest that whenever possible, posterior composites should be limited to small to moderate class I and II restorations. In addition, they are most likely to be successful when the restorations are limited to those whose interproximal extensions do not exceed the cementum-enamel junction. Posterior composites are not recommended for patients who grind their teeth (i.e., bruxers) or for those with poor oral hygiene.

The major reasons for imposing limitations on the use of posterior composites revolve around the inadequate marginal and structural integrity of the material. The polymerization shrinkage of composites makes their placement a sensitive procedure in the hands of most clinicians. Second, their accelerated degradation in sites with heavy occlusal contacts makes them less suitable than amalgam for the restoration of large posterior lesions. The ability of composites to adhere to tooth structure, especially to enamel, however, allows for a more conservative cavity preparation than with amalgam. This benefit, in conjunction with their outstanding esthetic results, makes them a suitable alternative to amalgam for many patients, although at a slightly greater cost. At this point, however, most clinicians do not consider composites as a complete replacement for amalgam.

Many other composites are being marketed with alternative names, such as "ceromer" (ceramic-optimized polymer) and "polyglass" (polymer glass). These materials have slightly modified formulations, but their properties and characteristics are not significantly different from other minifill or midifill composites. Therefore, they will not be distinguished further in this chapter.

Types and Composition

Until recently, the types of composites used for posterior restorations differed little from those used in anterior restorations. These have been reviewed in Chapter 5. The separation between posterior and anterior composites became less distinct with the development of minifill composites, which are suggested to be universal restoratives. The demand for esthetically pleasing results, however, will necessarily leave room for the highly polishable microfills in certain anterior applications. In recent years, manufacturers have developed composite with a thicker consistency that can be packed into a cavity in a manner that is more similar to amalgam placement.

Mixing and Handling

The handling of posterior composites is essentially the same as that for anterior composites, except that special precautions must be taken during placement to minimize the negative effects of polymerization contraction. Most commercial products are light activated, but several brands are self-curing. One specific use for a self-curing formulation might be to fill the proximal box of a class II cavity (i.e., the deep portion between the two teeth). This is because light-curing of this region often is difficult. Because light penetration is not a concern, a metal matrix can be wedged between the teeth to provide the form for the interproximal portion of the restoration. The metal matrix has the advantage over a plastic strip of being **burnishable**. This enhances the clinician's ability to create tight contact between the composite and the adjacent tooth. The bulk of the restoration is then completed with a light-activated composite that can be cured from the occlusal surface.

Common procedures for placing class II composites involve the use of a dentin adhesive, a glass ionomer liner, or both to seal the dentin. In one technique, clear plastic matrices are used with aggressive wedging to enhance contact formation and allow the composite in the proximal box to be cured from the lingual, buccal, and occlusal directions (Fig. 6-13). It has been argued that this aids in directing the shrinkage stress toward the cavity wall instead of away from it, thus enhancing the marginal integrity of the restoration (Fig. 6-14). The procedure often includes the use of a light-reflecting wedge, whose purpose is to direct the light through the interproximal space and up at the gingival margin. Increments are placed to depths no thicker than 1.5 to 2 mm, and each is light cured for 40 seconds. Because some studies have reported an improvement in properties in composites whose surfaces were given additional light exposure, it is common to illuminate the occlusal surface an additional 60 seconds after the polishing is completed. Some investigators have suggested that it is beneficial to apply a surface-sealing resin after finishing, to fill in any cracks or gaps created during curing and finishing. The tooth surface is re-etched, and the low-viscosity resin surface sealer is applied and then light activated. This simultaneously polymerizes the resin and provides the additional light-curing of the composite surface. Clinical studies have shown some improvement in the marginal integrity of composite restorations as a result of surface sealing.

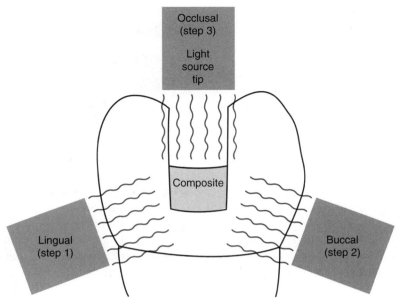

Figure 6–13 A light-curing sequence for the proximal box portion of a class II composite restoration. *Step 1* shows the light directed from the lingual surface, *step 2* shows the light directed from the buccal surface, and *step 3* shows the light directed from the occlusal surface.

Another common placement technique for class II composites is to use a sectional metal matrix with a special ring clamp. The teeth are wedged to achieve separation and the eventual production of a tight contact. After the adhesive is applied, the gingival increment of composite is added with a syringe. This increment, no more than 2 mm thick, is light activated for 40 seconds from the occlusal surface. The cavity is again built up in increments. After removal of the matrix, the restoration is again cured from the buccal and lingual directions to ensure sufficient polymerization of the composite.

This procedure can also be accomplished with a high-viscosity, packable composite (Fig. 6-15). Some clinicians feel that the heavy consistency aids to some ex-

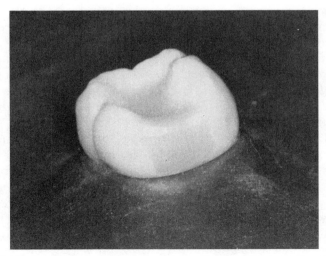

Figure 6–14 A well-adapted and well-cured class II composite restoration of a molar.

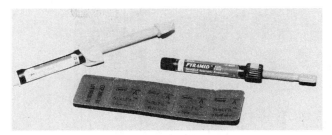

Figure 6–15 Packable composites, supplied in syringes and as individually wrapped pellets that are carried to the cavity preparation with an amalgam carrier.

tent in providing shape to the matrix for achieving the interproximal contact, although it is not nearly as proficient as packed amalgam in this regard. The heavy consistency also means that the packable composites will not flow and, therefore, filling the gingival margin is more difficult. For this reason, many clinicians place a low-viscosity, flowable composite as the first gingival increment to try to ensure good adaptation to the floor and margins of the cavity.

Setting Reaction

The curing of posterior composites is identical with that of anterior composites and is addressed in Chapter 5.

Characteristics and Properties

The physical and mechanical properties of composites are addressed in Chapter 5; they are reviewed, along with those for amalgam, in Table 6-1. Essentially, there is no difference in properties between hybrid and packable composites. There are, however, some specific properties that were not as important for posterior materials as for esthetic anterior composites. These include wear and marginal breakdown.

Generally, there are thought to be two different types of wear on posterior composites. The first, abrasive wear, takes place as a result of the movement of objects, such as food and toothpaste, across the entire surface of the restoration. It is distinguished from the more aggressive degradation experienced in the area in which the opposing tooth makes direct contact with the restoration. This latter form of wear is called contact or attrition wear. If there is no contact on the restoration, then wear is abrasive only and usually is of less concern. Studies have shown, however, that wear at the contact site is accelerated and may be three to four times more extensive than that occurring at noncontact sites. Therefore, the prognosis for the more conservative restoration that does not reside in "harm's way" is better than that of the restoration that includes the central holding area for the opposing tooth.

The abrasive wear characteristics for posterior composites have improved tremendously in recent years. Initial formulations would undergo wear, usually measured at the margins, in increments of 50 to 100 μm/year or more (i.e., a depth equal to one to two times the diameter of a human hair). After several years, the wear was clinically noticeable and unacceptable, even though the rate slowed and did not continue at such a fast pace. Because of the inclusion of smaller particles in their formulations, current materials undergo a much lower rate of wear. Abrasive wear rates of 10 to 15 μm/year in contact-free sites are common and are essentially equivalent to the wear rates of dental amalgam.

Abrasive wear occurs over the entire surface in a relatively uniform manner. First, the resin matrix, which is softest, is worn away, leaving the filler particles sticking out from the surface. As chewing continues, these exposed particles are eventually "plucked" or pulled out, leaving holes. The wear is accelerated because the fillers are continually being removed from the surface. The wear is most rapid for the composites having the largest fillers. As composites with smaller particle sizes were developed, wear rates were significantly reduced because it is more difficult to "pluck" a small filler particle from the matrix of a composite. The surface, therefore, remains smoother.

Although the wear in contact-free sites has been dramatically reduced by the development of composites with high levels of small fillers, concern remains over the relatively high rate of wear for posterior composites in direct contact with opposing cusps. Thus, the materials are not proven amalgam replacements, even though some studies suggest that composites undergo less marginal fracture than do amalgams.

Clinical Success

As one may suspect, clinical success with posterior composites is extremely variable. The clinician must pay strict attention to every detail during placement, making every effort to minimize the polymerization contraction forces that tend to pull the composite away from the tooth. Many clinicians have experienced poor results with posterior composites and do not choose them as their primary posterior restorative. Although numerous controlled clinical studies have shown that composites can serve as excellent restorations in conservative class I and II cavities (i.e., the occlusal dimensions are approximately one third or less of the intercuspal width), similar success has not always been reported by private practitioners. Although the data from private practice are limited, studies show that the average lifetime of a composite restoration in class I or II cavities is 3 to 5 years. This is only one third to one half of the lifetime of amalgams under similar conditions. The main reasons for failure have been reported to be secondary caries and loss of anatomic form or marginal failure. These reasons are similar to those reported for amalgam. Because much of the clinical data, to date, have been generated from older formulations of composites, expectations are that the minifill and midifill composites, which are more wear resistant than their predecessors, will show enhanced performance. A greater appreciation for the importance of technique also should help.

Although loss of anatomic form, or wear, has become much less of a problem with the new composite formulations, most of the data showing this improved performance have been generated from controlled studies in which the composites were used in smaller cavities. To date, there are few data on comparisons between composite and amalgam in similarly large restorations of posterior teeth. Generally, composites undergo minimal wear and degradation in premolars but greater amounts in molars, where the forces of mastication are higher. In addition, they are contraindicated for patients with bruxing and grinding habits because they cannot provide the same resistance as amalgam to attrition wear under such conditions. Because composites, unlike amalgam, do not have a self-sealing mechanism for marginal openings, their use in people with high caries rates and poor oral hygiene also is questionable. Finally, because composites contain hard, irregularly shaped reinforcing fillers, they may actually abrade the opposing dentition. Although this may not be a problem for a single restoration, extensive restoration of an arch that opposes natural teeth may result in accelerated wear of the dentition, leading to occlusal abnormalities. This has never been a problem with amalgams, which do not abrade enamel.

Thus, although the clinical behavior of composites in posterior teeth has not achieved the same level of success as has that of amalgams, recent evidence for newer formulations and the continual development of materials and techniques suggest a brighter future. At present, consideration of all factors, including the skill level of the dental personnel and the oral hygiene of the patient, is necessary before selecting posterior composites for specific cases.

■ *Direct Filling Gold*

Direct filling gold, also known as **gold foil**, has been used in the restoration of both anterior and posterior teeth. It is included in this chapter rather than in Chapter 5 because it is not an esthetic restoration. Although **direct gold** has a long history of clinical success, it is a difficult, time consuming, and costly restoration that is being used less frequently in dentistry because of the expanding roles of glass ionomers and composites. Therefore, the discussion of this material is pitched at an introductory level. The interested student is directed to other texts for more complete descriptions of the materials and techniques.

Pure gold is a soft, malleable metal with excellent resistance to tarnish and corrosion. It has a thermal expansion coefficient similar to that of tooth structure and, therefore, remains well adapted to a cavity when it is properly placed. Because it is biocompatible and can be finished to a very smooth surface, it does not cause periodontal problems. In fact, the gingival epithelium adjacent to direct gold restorations has been shown to be similar to that adjacent to enamel.

Although direct gold restorations claim many benefits, there also are significant drawbacks in addition to their lack of esthetics. As stated, they are difficult to place well and are costly. Pure gold has a very high thermal conductivity, even greater than that of amalgam. Because of the forces required to compact the material adequately into a cavity, there is a danger of pulpal damage during the procedure. Finally, the material has only minimal strength and resistance to abrasion, and thus its use is limited to restorations that encounter minimal stress. Hence, these materials are indicated mainly for posterior class V restorations (Fig. 6-16), buccal and lingual pits, and small occlusal lesions.

The theory behind the placement of direct gold has its roots in basic metallurgy. Pieces of pure, uncontaminated gold will weld together when compacted with sufficient pressure. One usually thinks of welding in terms of applying heat to bond two pieces of metal together, but in the case of pure gold, welding takes place at oral temperatures.

Direct gold may be supplied in several forms (Fig. 6-17). Typical examples of types of direct gold include thin gold foil (25-μm-thick sheets of smooth gold), mat gold (porous clumps of fine particles), mat foil (porous particles placed between smooth sheets of gold foil), and powdered gold (a blend of powders pressed together and cut into pieces). Although some forms contain pure gold, others are alloys or mixtures. The most common alloying elements for gold are platinum and calcium. When added to gold, both form alloys with increased strength and hardness, compared with pure gold. The various forms of direct gold are compatible with one another. *Why may more than one type of direct gold be used for a single cavity when one considers that the ultimate goal is to fill the cavity completely in a*

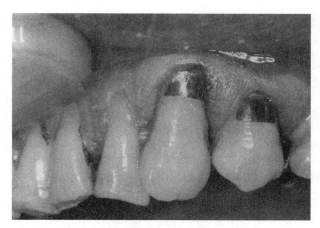

Figure 6–16 Class V gold foil restorations.

timely fashion, while producing a well-adapted restoration with excellent surface smoothness?

Filling of the cavity preparation is most easily achieved by using the bulk forms of the material. Therefore, it is common to use mat foil or chunks of mat or powdered gold. The surface must be smooth, however, so the clinician uses a thinner and smoother foil or mat foil to fill the last portion or outer surface of the preparation. In any case, the key parameter is that the gold be condensed with sufficient force to achieve excellent adaptation to the walls of the cavity and eliminate porosity, producing a dense, hard restoration.

Direct gold can be placed with hand condensers (like amalgam), by hammering pieces into the cavity with a small mallet and condenser, or with the aid of an electrically operated mechanical condenser. The latter produces small impact forces in rapid succession to compact the material. Regardless of the technique, the cavity must be built up in small increments to ensure that each increment is adapted and made dense. Remember that the hardness of pure gold is comparable to that of lead—in other words, it is very soft. If it were not this soft, it would not be malleable enough to be manipulated and welded together at oral temperatures. *If gold is so soft, why is it suitable for use as a permanent restoration?*

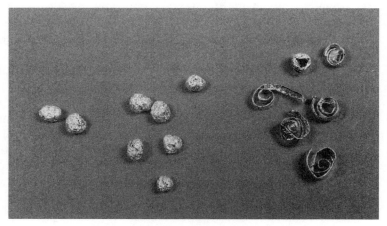

Figure 6–17 Various types of direct gold.

The answer to this question is based on another metallurgy principle that is discussed further in Chapter 7. Simply stated, when metals are bent, compressed, or hammered, they become harder. This process of imposing stress on the metal and inducing a dimensional change or strain is called **strain hardening**. A soft metal, such as gold, that is pounded or compacted well (estimated necessary force is 15 pounds) will undergo a 100% increase in hardness and strength. Thus, the soft gold may be used to produce an acceptable restorative, but only if it is handled correctly. There is a negative side to the use of high forces to place direct gold; when one remembers that amalgams usually are condensed with 2 to 6 pounds of force, the increased potential for trauma to the tooth during the condensation of direct gold is apparent.

Another factor concerns the oral environment and the use of a material that must be welded during placement. In this way, direct gold is similar to amalgam and composite, which also are placed in increments. The adhesion of one piece of gold to another will not take place in a cavity contaminated by moisture. Therefore, the maintenance of a dry field through rubber dam isolation is paramount during the placement of a direct gold filling. Furthermore, the material as supplied has been treated so it will not stick together during shipping and storage. Essentially, the foil or particles have been passed through a gas to adsorb a layer of ammonia onto their surfaces. The gas makes the surfaces nonadherent toward one another. The pieces will not weld together until this layer of contamination is removed, which usually is accomplished by passing the pieces of gold over the flame of an alcohol torch or by heating on an inert ceramic plate. Either treatment drives the adsorbed ammonia from the surface and makes the gold **cohesive**.

After placement, the direct gold restoration is finished by burnishing with a steel instrument to adapt the material better to the margins and smooth the surface. This burnishing also helps to harden the surface and improve its abrasion and scratch resistance.

Summary

Direct posterior restoratives are materials placed in a single dental appointment to repair or replace missing portions of bicuspids and molars. Direct gold (pure gold foil) is included in this chapter, although it is not generally used on surfaces subjected to heavy stresses. The most common posterior restoratives are dental amalgams and dental composites. Amalgam is a mixture of metals containing silver. The metal powder is mechanically mixed with mercury at high speeds and hardens within minutes to form a strong, hard material with excellent wear resistance and durability. The amalgams containing large amounts of copper are more corrosion resistant and generally are more clinically successful than those with lower amounts of copper. Both, however, are silver colored.

Dental composite is a paste mixture of polymer and reinforcing glass fillers that usually is hardened within the tooth by visible light illumination to produce an esthetic restoration suitable for use in anterior teeth as well. The materials are classified as microfill, minifill, and midifill, based on the size of their reinforcing filler. Composites with smaller particles generally are more polishable but weaker than those with higher concentrations of larger particles. Composite is reasonably strong but is less durable and wear resistant than amalgam. It also is difficult to place because its setting is accompanied by sub-

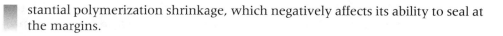

stantial polymerization shrinkage, which negatively affects its ability to seal at the margins.

STUDY QUESTIONS AND PROBLEM SOLVING

1. **Which element is most responsible for reacting with mercury to cause the hardening of dental amalgam?**
   a. Copper
   b. Silver
   c. Tin
   d. Zinc

2. **Good hand condensation of spherical amalgams requires:**
   a. Greater force than that used for admixed amalgams
   b. Approximately 2 to 3 pounds of force
   c. Less force than that used for lathe-cut amalgams
   d. The smallest-tipped condensers available

3. **A patient comes in with amalgams of equivalent age in both lower first molars, but the amalgam in tooth 19 shows much more extensive marginal degradation than that in tooth 30. Which statement(s) concerning these amalgams is (are) most likely true?**
   a. The amalgam in tooth 19 was made from a high-copper alloy
   b. The amalgam in tooth 30 contains a tin-mercury compound
   c. The amalgam in tooth 19 has higher creep than that in tooth 30
   d. The amalgam in tooth 19 is less corrosion resistant than that in tooth 30

4. **Which of the following is (are) a practical way(s) to speed the setting rate of the preencapsulated amalgam used in your office?**
   a. Triturate the capsule at a faster speed
   b. Chill the capsule before trituration
   c. Open the capsule and remove some of the mercury
   d. Triturate the capsule for a longer time

5. **Benefits directly derived from the use of a slightly higher Hg/alloy ratio than is necessary for an amalgam include:**
   a. Enhanced plasticity of the mix
   b. Better condensability
   c. Longer working time
   d. Greater strength

6. **A patient requests a posterior composite in a lower second molar, even though it will be in direct contact with the opposing cusp during biting. What are your expectations for this restoration?**
   a. Wear will be greater in the contact site than in the noncontact sites
   b. Wear in the contact site will be less than it would be for an amalgam
   c. The opposing tooth may show an accelerated rate of wear
   d. The composite cannot be placed with sealed margins

7. **A patient returns to the office complaining that the class II composite placed in a lower first molar 2 months ago remains very sensitive to hot and cold stimuli. It is determined that the restoration is leaking along the gingival margin, possibly as a result of:**
   a. Light-curing of the proximal box from the occlusal direction only
   b. Inadequate illumination of the increment in the proximal box
   c. Moisture contamination of the cavity preparation before placement
   d. Placing the light-cured restoration as a single increment

8. **Compared with conventional posterior composites, packable composites developed for posterior applications have improved:**
   a. Wear resistance
   b. Handling characteristics
   c. Esthetics
   d. Marginal adaptation

9. **Which of the following is (are) *not* a part(s) of the direct gold restoration procedure?**
   a. Dipping each piece of gold in alcohol to improve cohesion
   b. Condensing each piece of foil with 10 to 15 pounds of force
   c. Using cement to weld each increment to the next
   d. Isolating the tooth with a rubber dam

10. **It is common to use more than one type of direct gold material to fill a cavity because:**
    a. Some are manufactured with less density as bulk-filling materials only
    b. Smoothness is enhanced when dense foils are used on the surface
    c. Only alloys with calcium can be used in the final layer for optimal hardness
    d. It is not possible to truly condense certain materials in the base of cavities

SELECTED READINGS

ADA Council on Scientific Affairs. Dental mercury hygiene recommendations. Journal of the American Dental Association 130:1125–1126, 1999.
This short monograph presents current recommendations for handling mercury-containing compounds in the dental office.

Anusavice KJ. Phillips' Science of Dental Materials. 10th ed. Philadelphia: WB Saunders, 1996.
This classic text provides detailed information about the variables affecting the manipulation, placement, and performance of dental amalgams and composites. A detailed chapter on direct gold restorations is included.

Bayne SC, Heymann HO, Swift EJ Jr. Update on dental composite restorations. Journal of the American Dental Association 125:687–701, 1994.
This article provides a review of the composition and properties of dental composites.

Ferracane JL. Amalgam-derived mercury. General Dentistry 40:223–229, 1992.
This article summarizes the results of several studies dealing with the mechanism for mercury release and the quantity of mercury released from dental amalgams.

Geiger F, Reller U, Lutz F. Burnishing, finishing, and polishing amalgam restorations: A quantitative scanning electron microscopic study. Quintessence International 20:461–468, 1989.
This article compares the margins of amalgam restorations both before and after burnishing, finishing, and polishing procedures. The scanning electron microscope was used to show that burnishing is important for enhancing marginal integrity of fresh amalgams.

Hilton TJ. Direct posterior composite restorations. In: Schwartz RS, Summitt JB, Robbins JW, eds. Fundamentals of Operative Dentistry. A Contemporary Approach. Chicago: Quintessence Publishing, 1996.
This chapter provides an excellent and detailed overview of the important factors to consider during the placement of direct posterior composites.

Jokstad A, Mjor IA, Qvist V. The age of restorations in situ. Acta Odontologica Scandinavica 52(4):234–242, 1994.
This article presents a cross-sectional study and data that indicates 20 years for gold restorations, 12 to 14 years for amalgam restorations, and 7 to 8 years for composite resin restorations in clinical service. It cites the most common reasons for replacement of restorations as secondary caries, bulk fractures, and tooth fractures.

Mahler DB, Engle JH. Clinical evaluation of amalgam bonding in class I and II restorations. Journal of the American Dental Association 131(1):43–49, 2000.

This article presents the results of a 3-year-long clinical study comparing amalgams placed with and without resin adhesive dentin bonding. The study shows no difference in postoperative sensitivity, marginal degradation, or secondary caries when these two techniques were used.

Molin C. Amalgam: Fact and fiction. Scandinavian Journal of Dental Research 100:66–73, 1992.

This article provides a brief history of the development of amalgam and the controversy that has surrounded it. A review of its toxic and allergic effects is given.

Osborne JW, Albino JE. Psychological and medical effects of mercury intake from dental amalgam. A status report for the American Journal of Dentistry. American Journal of Dentistry 12:151–156, 1999.

This article reviews the literature regarding the safety of dental amalgam. The authors report that other studies have concluded that there is insufficient mercury released from amalgam restorations to cause a medical problem.

Roulet JF. Benefits and disadvantages of tooth-colored alternatives to amalgam. Journal of Dentistry 25:459–473, 1997.

This article reviews the alternatives to amalgam and describes their limitations. The clinical evidence for alternative materials is presented. The author concludes that all esthetic alternatives to amalgam are more difficult and time-consuming to place and that amalgam is still the most convenient restorative material for posterior teeth.

Chapter **7**

Materials for Inlays, Onlays, Crowns, and Bridges

Objectives

- List the major benefits and drawbacks of the various types of materials used for inlays, crowns, and bridges.

- Define the term *alloy* and compare the properties of an alloy with those of a pure metal.

- Define strain hardening and annealing and explain how they affect one's ability to bend an orthodontic arch wire.

- Identify metals as noble or base and explain the difference between the two.

- Compare the compositions, properties, and uses of the four types of American Dental Association gold alloys.

- Identify the major components in dental porcelains.

- Briefly describe the procedure for building up and firing a self-glazing porcelain restoration.

- Compare the composition and properties of cast and machinable ceramics to those of regular and aluminous porcelains.

- Describe the rationale for the various steps in the procedure for repair of a chipped porcelain restoration.

- Discuss the advantages and disadvantages of composite inlays and onlays to those of inlays and onlays made from ceramics and cast metals.

Types of Materials

Until recently, only metals were used as restorative materials for teeth requiring an inlay, onlay, crown, or bridge. In response to the demand for enhanced esthetic results, however, various materials are now used instead of metals for many of these restorations. The properties and characteristics of the available materials vary, and the choice for a given restoration must be based on a consideration of its type and size, its location in the mouth, the patient's oral habits, the patient's wishes, and the clinician's opinion.

The use of metals for restorations of a large portion of decayed or missing tooth structure is based on their high strength and durability. In addition, it is comparatively easy to make highly accurate metal restorations by using routine laboratory casting procedures (see Chapter 11). Cast metal restorations have two distinct drawbacks, however: high material and production costs and a lack of esthetics. Because most of the porcelains, glasses, and composites used in place of metals must also be processed by a laboratory, none offers a significant cost savings over cast metals. Compared with metals, the major benefit of these alternative materials is their superior esthetics, and their major drawbacks include poorer fit, lower fracture resistance, greater brittleness, and limited clinical track record.

The composition, properties, and methods of preparation for the various materials used in inlays, onlays, crowns, and bridges are discussed in this chapter. Some of the basic principles concerning metals and ceramics also are addressed to enhance the reader's understanding of these classes of materials.

Metals: Some Basic Concepts

Metals are materials composed of metallic elements that possess the characteristics of high thermal and electrical conductivity, ductility, opacity, and luster. They also have relatively high strengths and generally melt at high temperatures. Although the number of pure metals is limited to approximately 80, an almost unlimited number of different types of metals can be made by combining two or more metallic elements. This combination of metals is called alloying, and the resultant metals are known as **alloys**. Alloying allows one to produce a variety of metals with widely varying physical and mechanical properties. Although the list of alloys used daily in construction, machinery, etc. is enormous, relatively few alloys are used in dentistry. This is in large part because alloys for intraoral use must be compatible with the human body.

All metals dissolve to some extent in saline solutions, releasing positive ions. Dental alloys are basically resistant to this corrosion process, releasing only minute amounts of ions. Although there is little documentation of any toxic effects from dental alloys, a small percentage of the population is allergic to one or more types of metals, and even very small concentrations may cause them problems. There-fore, this problem must be considered when an alloy is being selected for a partic-ular patient.

Producing the Metallic Structure

Essentially all metals are **crystalline**. Recall that crystallinity implies a regular ar-rangement of atoms, similar to a stack of cannon balls. The production of a metal-lic object requires that at some point it must be heated beyond its melting range, molded, and subsequently cooled to form a crystalline solid. This stable solid struc-ture forms rapidly as the metal freezes. It is important to remember that the solid structure is more stable than the liquid **phase**; the metal can transform between liquid and solid simply through a change in its temperature. In the liquid state, the atoms are at a higher temperature and, therefore, have more energy than those in the solid state. Consider the following analogy of a large group of people milling around a movie theater before the movie starts. The people move around, often randomly, expending much energy. As the film starts, each person finds a seat and soon the arrangement of people takes on a regular appearance. Each person has ceased moving. In their seated and more stable positions, they are less energetic. The solidification of a metal is similar, except that the atoms do not make a con-scious effort to find their positions the way that theatergoers do. Instead, the atoms simply move into their final positions because of the attraction of other atoms and because much of their energy has been removed during cooling (Fig. 7-1). The crystalline arrangements of atoms differ from one type of metal or alloy to another because the different atoms are able to make different bonding ar-rangements on the basis of their electronic configurations. The process is always similar, however, regardless of the type of crystal structure formed.

To this point in this text, amalgam and gold are the only metallic dental ma-terials that have been discussed to any great extent. Amalgam is a bit different from other dental metals, in that it forms a solid at oral temperatures, as opposed to being cooled from a high temperature to solidity. Actually, a solid alloy con-sisting mainly of silver and tin is mixed with a liquid metal, mercury, and the mix-ture reacts to form additional solid metal phases. The process of solidification of

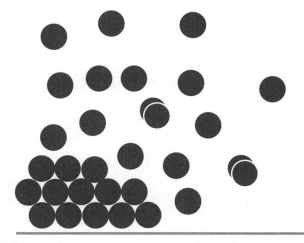

Figure 7–1 Solidification of a metal, showing the production of the regular crystalline arrangement of atoms.

amalgam is similar to that of a metal cooling from the melt. As the mercury is mixed with the silver and tin alloy, silver and tin dissolve into the mercury. There is a limit, however, to how much silver and tin can dissolve into mercury and stay in solution. *Have you ever noticed that you can dissolve only so much sugar or salt in water?*

When in amalgam this point, which is called the solubility limit, is reached, silver and mercury begin to react and precipitate out in a crystalline form. The silver and mercury atoms organize to form a regular crystalline arrangement (i.e., the μ_1 matrix phase).

The solidification of amalgam is similar to the way a cast metal solidifies or freezes from the molten state. **Casting** refers to the process of heating a metal and pouring or "flinging" it into a mold, where it can solidify into a specific shape. The solidification process begins simultaneously at many different locations within the cast metal. The crystals (or **grains**) grow larger as more atoms join them through the formation of primary metallic bonds. Eventually, each crystal meets up with other growing crystals, forming a boundary (i.e., a **grain boundary**) that prevents further growth in that direction. The final structure of the solid therefore contains millions of small crystals put together like the pieces of a jigsaw puzzle (Fig. 7-2).

The high stiffness and thermal stability of metals are the result of the strong metallic bonds formed between the atoms of the crystals. The great hardness and ductility of metals are, to a large extent, a product of the number and size of the crystals that form during solidification, as well as a product of the presence of additional types of atoms in the metal. Metals with many small crystals tend to be harder and have higher elastic limits than do metals with fewer, large crystals. In addition, alloys are harder and stronger than pure metals. The properties can be understood better by considering the manner in which metals deform in response to the application of stress.

Deformation of Metals

As is discussed in Chapter 2, when an object is bent or pulled, it may deform elastically (recoverable strain) or plastically (permanent strain). The result depends on

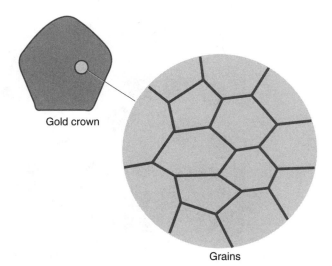

Gold crown

Grains

Figure 7–2 Grains or crystals of a solid metal, which fit together like the pieces of a jigsaw puzzle.

how much force (or stress) is applied. For example, if one bends a paper clip with only a small amount of force, it may bend but, when the force is removed, rebound to its original shape. In this case, the deformation was entirely elastic and completely recovered. On an atomic level, the planar layers of atoms (i.e., the rows of cannon balls) began to slide over one another, but they moved back into their original positions when the force was removed (Fig. 7-3*A*). The **elastic modulus** is the property that describes the stiffness of a material, i.e., how difficult it is to bend the metal elastically.

Something different occurs on the atomic level when a sufficiently high force is used to bend the wire and a permanent deformation or bend is produced. In this case, the atom planes have moved to new positions and do not rebound back to their original places when the stress is removed (Fig. 7-3*B*). The **elastic limit** is the property that describes the amount of stress required to make this happen. *What do grain boundaries and alloying elements have to do with sliding atom layers?*

Any impurity within the metal, such as other atoms and boundaries between crystals, makes it more difficult for the atom planes to slide over one another, thereby making it harder to permanently bend or change the shape of the metal. Therefore, metals with finer grains (smaller crystals) and more grain boundaries are harder to bend and shape.

In addition, each time a metal is bent, some movement of atom planes occurs and then stops, making it more difficult to move the next layer of atoms. This means that the act of bending or shaping a piece of metal makes it harder to bend it further, thus increasing its elastic limit (and hardness). This process of bending (i.e., straining) to increase the hardness of the metal is called **strain hardening**. Because it happens at room temperature, which is a low temperature for a metal, it is often called cold working. *Where is this process important in dentistry?*

Two good examples demonstrate the effect of strain hardening. One is the placement of a direct gold restoration. The pure gold is soft and **malleable** (i.e., easily compressed or condensed), allowing it to be packed into a cavity. How can such a soft metal possibly produce a useful restoration? Condensation is a form of strain hardening. As the gold is deformed and packed into the cavity, the foil is strained. On an atomic level, with each condensation it becomes more difficult to move the atom planes. Therefore, the gold becomes harder and harder during the process. When

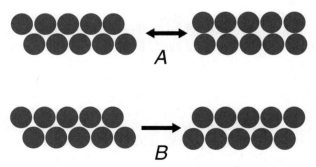

Figure 7–3 **A.** Atom planes sliding over one another and then returning to their original positions (*double-headed arrow*) in response to a low force that is within the elastic range of the material. **B.** A permanent shift in atomic planes (plastic deformation) (*arrow*) caused by the imposition of a stress that exceeds the elastic limit of the material.

condensation is performed correctly, the condensed direct gold has a hardness twice as great as that of the original material, thus making it a useful restorative.

A second example of strain hardening can be found in orthodontics. Wires often are bent into shapes to impose forces in specific directions so that teeth can be moved in a desired way. Complicated appliances may contain wires bent into springs and loops. Each time the wire is bent, the metal becomes harder and more difficult to bend because of strain hardening. If the clinician is not careful, he or she could cause the wire to fracture before achieving the desired shape. This danger exists because with each bend it becomes more difficult for the wire's shape to be changed permanently. In other words, the wire is losing its **ductility**, or its ability to be permanently deformed; it is becoming more brittle (i.e., like a ceramic). When this happens, further bending cannot be accommodated by the slipping of atomic layers. Instead, the imposition of more force causes atomic bonds to break, producing cracks within the metal at the site of bending. Continued application of stress causes the cracks to grow and ultimately fractures the piece of metal. This is readily seen by repeatedly bending a common paper clip. Because of strain hardening, the number of bends that can be completed is limited.

Strain hardening would create an insurmountable problem during the forming or shaping of metals if the process were irreversible. Fortunately, it is not. The effects of strain hardening can be eliminated, and the metal can be returned to its original condition without altering its shape. For this to happen, however, significant rearrangements of atoms must occur. Atoms are essentially frozen in place within a metal at room temperature and are difficult to move without applying force. At higher temperatures (although still far below the melting range), however, atomic rearrangements take place rapidly. These rearrangements relieve the stress imposed by the bending process, thus recovering the ductility of the metal and allowing further bending without the potential for fracture. This heating process, called *annealing*, can be used to eliminate the effects of strain hardening while maintaining the shape of the metal. An orthodontic wire that has been extensively shaped can be annealed by heating it in an oven or over a flame at several hundred degrees Celsius for several minutes, with resulting atomic rearrangement. After cooling, the wire can be subjected to further bending with little fear of fracture. If the wire is heated too long or at too high a temperature, however, it will soften and be less efficient at moving teeth. Therefore, this process must be carefully controlled and clearly defined for different types of metals.

Alloying

Most metals are not pure but are a combination of two or more metallic elements, called **alloys**. Alloys are popular because they are stronger and harder, usually less expensive, and often more easily fabricated than pure metals. They also have improved mechanical properties because the addition of a second element makes it harder for planes of atoms to slide over one another under stress. Consider sliding a large box across a floor; the bottom of the box represents a plane of atoms moving over a second plane of atoms, the floor. Then consider a bump in the floor, an impurity, which rises up from the floor and causes the box to catch on it, inhibiting its sliding motion. The box can still be moved, but it takes some extra force to move it past the bump. If the floor is full of bumps, it is easy to see how the process of sliding the box can become difficult. If each bump represents an impurity atom in a metal, the manner in which alloys are hardened, compared with pure metals, becomes more obvious.

There are many different types of alloys, some complicated and others relatively simple. Whatever their degree of complexity, alloys are formed when the atoms from one metal become dissolved within the atoms and crystals of a second metal. In much the same way salt dissolves in water, producing a liquid solution, two metals can be dissolved in one another, producing a **solid solution**. When the two metals are completely soluble in one another at all temperatures and compositions, the alloy is called a complete solid solution. Silver and palladium make such an alloy, commonly used in dentistry for crowns and bridges. When the two metals are not completely soluble in one another, precipitates are formed. These precipitates will have different compositions and coexist in the alloy. When the chef mixes oil and vinegar to make salad dressing, the liquid formed is a mixture of two separate liquid phases, with one being mostly oil and the other being mostly vinegar. This is because the two do not completely dissolve in one another. They are distinct and have different compositions, but they coexist in one liquid. The same thing happens when two metals that are not soluble in one another are mixed; the only difference is that the separate phases exist in a solid state instead of in a liquid state. Amalgam is a good example (Fig. 7-4); the alloy is heterogenous, and each phase has its own crystal structure.

In some alloys, the crystal structure consists of a random or disordered arrangement of the different types of atoms. In other alloys, the two types of metal atoms occupy very specific or ordered positions within the crystal, producing different mechanical properties than the randomly organized crystals. This **order-disorder transformation** can be controlled in certain types of gold-copper casting alloys used in dentistry to make crowns and bridges. If the restoration is cooled slowly after the casting process, the gold and copper atoms form in an ordered arrangement that is hard and slightly more difficult to finish. If the metal is **quenched** (i.e., plunged into cold water immediately after casting), however, the atoms will not have time to order themselves and will be frozen into a more random arrangement, thus leaving the metal in a more softened condition. The manner in which an alloy is heated and cooled often plays an important role in determining its physical and mechanical properties, but this is beyond the scope of this text.

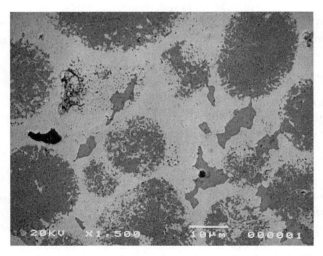

Figure 7–4 Scanning electron micrograph of amalgam phases, showing their different appearances as a result of differences in their compositions.

■ *Metals: Composition, Properties, and Preparation*

The requirements for metals and alloys in dentistry are specific. They must be strong enough and hard enough to withstand wear and occlusal forces, and they must be biologically compatible. They must also have a high resistance to corrosion and tarnish, and they must be relatively easy to cast into complicated shapes and structures by techniques that are not cost prohibitive. The metal alloys that best satisfy these requirements are based on the series of metals described as **noble**, sometimes called **precious**. The noble metals are gold (Au), platinum (Pt), palladium (Pd), iridium (Ir), ruthenium (Ru), niobium (Nb), and osmium (Os). They are called "noble" because they are resistant to corrosion and tarnish. Gold, palladium, and platinum are the ones most commonly used in dental alloys.

Noble Metal Alloys

Because of its excellent resistance to corrosion and tarnish, gold was the first metal successfully used in dentistry. The first cast inlays were made from pure gold. Pure gold, however, was not strong enough or hard enough to be used in stress-bearing restorations. To enhance its properties, gold was alloyed with copper (Cu) in a composition similar to that of gold coin (approximately 10% Cu).

All metals are silver colored (referred to as white), with the exception of gold and copper. The gold color was associated with wealth and quality and was desirable, whereas the reddish cast of copper was not. The original coin gold was not strong enough for dentistry and did not have ideal color quality because of the copper. Taking a cue from the jewelry business, dentists began adding silver (Ag) to the gold-copper alloy. This served two purposes. First, the silver further improved the strength and hardness of the alloy; second, the white silver metal partially offset the reddish cast of the copper, returning the alloy to a more acceptable gold color.

Pure gold is designated as 24 karat (K). All alloys of gold have a lower karat rating, depending on the percentage of alloying elements added. For example, the coin gold with 10% copper would be only 90% gold, or 0.9 × 24 K = 21.6 K. High-quality jewelry gold is 18 K (75% gold), whereas more common jewelry is 12 or 14 K (50 and 58%, respectively). Jewelry becomes less gold colored as the karat rating is reduced; this is most noticeable at 12 K or less. The original dental alloys were approximately 18 K, containing at least 75% gold to ensure tarnish and corrosion resistance.

American Dental Association Gold Alloys

Although today all alloys are produced by dental manufacturers, dentists commonly mixed their own metals to make castings in the early 1900s when the lost wax casting technique was first used for dental restorations. Dentists realized the need for alloys of differing strengths and ductility. Although alloys for inlays (see Fig. 2-3) did not need great strength, they required high ductility to allow the margins to be burnished for enhanced sealing. Crowns and bridges did not require ductility but needed a high elastic limit and hardness to remain stable and wear resistant during use (see Figs. 2-2 and 2-5). Partial denture frameworks needed exceptional rigidity and hardness (see Fig. 2-7). Therefore, many alloy compositions were developed, and these could be divided into four general classes.

Four different types of gold alloys became a part of a specification program developed by the American Dental Association (ADA) for certification purposes and

TABLE 7–1. **Properties of the Alloying Elements and Their Effect on Gold Casting Alloys**

	Gold	Platinum[a]	Palladium[a]	Copper[a]	Silver[a]
Elemental symbol	Au	Pt	Pd	Cu	Ag
Density (g/cm^3)	19.3	21.5 (like Au)	12.0 (lowers)	9.0 (lowers)	10.5 (lowers)
Color	Yellow	White (whitens)	White (whitens)	Red (reddens)	White (offsets Cu)
Melting point (°C)	1063	1769 (raises)	1552 (raises)	1083 (lowers)	961 (lowers slightly)
Chemical activity	Inert	Inert	Mild	Very active	Active
Tarnish resistance	Excellent	Excellent (none)	Very good (very little)	Fair (lowers)	Poor (lowers)
Effect on hardness	—	Increases	Increases	Increases	Increases
Approximate cost ($/oz, early 2001)	260.00	570.00	775.00	0.05	4.40

[a]Words in parentheses indicate effect in Au alloy.

quality control. As shown in Table 7-1, as the percentage of gold is reduced, the hardness of the alloy increases, and the alloy becomes useful for more stressful applications. The compositions in the table are examples for common alloys. In actuality, ADA-approved alloys can have any composition as long as they exceed certain minimal requirements for specific properties, such as strength, tarnish, and toxicity, as specified in ADA/ANSI specification no. 5. Type I (soft) and II (medium) gold alloys are predominantly used for inlays; type III (hard) alloys, for crowns and bridges; and type IV (extra hard) alloys, for **partial dentures**. Because of the high concentration of noble elements in these alloys, all are costly. Therefore, many less expensive but acceptable alternatives have been developed.

When considering the alternatives, consider the effect of each element on the resultant alloy. These effects are summarized in Table 7-1, along with an estimate of cost in early 2001. Note that most alloys contain some palladium and platinum because they considerably strengthen and harden the alloys without diminishing corrosion resistance, tarnish resistance, or biocompatibility. The amount of platinum or palladium that can be added is limited, however, because these elements greatly increase the melting point of the alloy, making it more difficult to cast. They also have a strong tendency to whiten the alloy. Palladium is an especially good whitener, several times more effective than platinum. Any gold alloy containing more than 6% palladium will be white—hence the term "white gold." The high cost of platinum and palladium is another reason their use is limited.

Alternative Alloys

As the price of gold rose dramatically in the 1970s, dentists and dental manufacturers created alternatives to the original formulation of type III ADA golds. These alternatives were less expensive than the ADA gold because they contained lesser amounts of gold or no gold at all. Table 7-2 lists the characteristics of representative alternative alloys. Note that the hardness of these alloys is equal to or better than that of type III gold. The same can be said of the elastic modulus and elastic limit. Although they contain less gold, corrosion and tarnish resistance is still very good for these alloys. Clinical studies have demonstrated a slightly greater inci-

TABLE 7–2. **Typical Compositions and Properties of ADA Gold Alloys and Alternatives**

	Au (%)	Cu (%)	Ag (%)	Pd (%)	VHN (kg/mm^2)	Elongation (%)	Color	Uses
Type I	83	6	10	0.5	60–90	30	Gold	Small inlays
Type II	77	7	14	1.0	90–120	25	Gold	Inlays
Type III	75	9	11	3.5	120–150	10–20	Gold	Crowns and bridges
Type IV	70	10	11	3.5 (+1% Pt)	150–200	5–10	Gold	Partial dentures
Medium Au	46	8	40	6	180–200	5–10	Gold	Crowns and bridges
Low Au	15	14	45	25	170–200	5–10	White	Crowns and bridges
Ag-Pd	—	—	70	25	150	5–10	White	Crowns and bridges

ADA, American Dental Association; VHN, Vicker's hardness number.

dence of tarnish on medium-gold and Ag-Pd alloys compared with the alloys with higher gold contents, as expected. These alternative alloys are, however, clinically acceptable and appropriate replacements for the original formulation of type III gold.

The current classification system for ADA alloys uses three categories. High noble metals contain greater than 40 weight percent gold and at least 60 weight percent of noble metal elements. Noble metals contain greater than 25 weight percent of noble elements. Predominantly base metal alloys contain less than 25 weight percent of noble metal elements.

Porcelain-Fused-to-Metal Alloys

The baking (firing) of porcelain coatings onto gold alloys for enhanced esthetic results began in the 1950s. Porcelain was fired onto metal in ovens set at approximately 850 to 1000°C. This temperature was in the melting range of the metals in use at the time, which meant that the casting would either melt or become severely distorted during the baking of the porcelain coating or veneer. The process could not become commonplace unless the melting point of the metal was raised. *Based on the information in Table 7-1, can you predict the manner in which the melting point of a gold alloy was raised to deal with this problem without sacrificing corrosion or tarnish resistance?*

The melting point of the alloys for porcelain-fused-to-metal (PFM) restorations was raised by increasing the concentration of Pd and Pt and reducing or eliminating Ag and Cu (Table 7-3). Instead of melting at approximately 1000°C like the type III golds and their alternatives, these alloys have melting points of 1200 to 1300°C. They also are hard and have high elastic limits. Although the fact that they melt at such high temperatures makes it more difficult to produce accurately fitting cast restorations, most of the problems have been overcome through the development of improved techniques specific to these metals.

There were two other concerns over the production of PFMs. When used for long bridges, those spanning six teeth or so, there was a significant potential for the center of the bridge to sag slightly under its own weight because of the high temperatures used for the porcelain baking procedure. In response to this prob-

	Au (%)	Pt (%)	Pd (%)	Cu (%)	Ag (%)	Other (%)	Color
High Au	86	9	5	—	—	—	Light gold
Low Au	52	38	—	—	—	9% In	White
Pd-Ag	—	—	65	—	35	—	White
Pd-Cu	—	—	80	15	—	5% others	White
Ni-Cr	—	—	—	—	—	65% Ni; 17% Cr	White

TABLE 7–3. **Typical Composition of Alloys for PFM Restorations**

lem, alloys were developed with very high elastic properties, resulting in greater resistance to sagging. Second, when the restoration cooled down after the porcelain firing process, the metal, possessing a thermal expansion coefficient approximately 2.5 times greater than that of the porcelain, would undergo more dimensional change than would the porcelain. This produced stress within the porcelain coating, causing it to crack, or "check." This was a problem from the standpoint of esthetics and bonding. Therefore, the existing porcelains were modified to obtain thermal expansion coefficients that were more closely matched to the alloys. There are extensive tables showing the compatibilities between the various alloys and porcelains produced by dental manufacturers. Dental laboratories must pay close attention to this information because even slight differences in thermal expansion coefficients can have disastrous results.

The compositions of the various types of PFM metals are shown in Table 7-3. Note that the high-gold alloys do not contain Ag or Cu. It was determined that Cu in the alloy caused discoloration of the porcelain, as well as disrupting its bond to the metal. Indium (In) or tin (Sn) commonly is added to these alloys in place of Cu to produce oxide surfaces on the metal that enhance its chemical bonding with porcelain. Likewise, Ag caused severe discoloration of certain porcelains, best described as a "greening" effect. It was even determined that porcelain baked onto a silver-free metal could discolor if the walls of the oven had previously been contaminated with Ag. Therefore, Ag was deleted from most alloys until specific porcelains were developed that would not discolor in the presence of Ag.

Although alloys containing mostly Ag seem to have a color problem, when Pd is the major metal used for the alloy neither Ag nor Cu seem to discolor the porcelain. The reason for this is not known, but this discovery led to the development of Pd-Ag and Pd-Cu alloys for PFMs (Table 7-3). Although there is a cost savings in moving from the high-gold to the low-gold and Pd-based alloys, one of the most common alloys used for PFMs is a non-noble, or base metal, alloy.

Base Metal Alloys

A metal that does not contain noble elements is referred to as a base metal. Steels, brasses, and aluminum alloys are base metals. Base metal does not necessarily imply poor corrosion resistance. As described in Chapter 2, corrosion resistance also may be achieved by the formation of a passive, protective oxide film, such as is found on stainless steel and aluminum alloys. The base metal alternative for PFM restorations in dentistry is similar to stainless steel in that its corrosion resistance is achieved through the formation of a protective surface oxide film composed of chromium. The main element in this base metal is nickel (Ni), although other elements are added for strengthening and improved handling properties (Table 7-3). One such element is beryllium (Be), which is added in small amounts to improve casting and the bonding of porcelain to Ni-Cr alloys. Beryllium dust is toxic and carcinogenic, however, and laboratory personnel must take extreme caution to grind Be-containing alloys only under well-ventilated conditions. The addition of beryllium poses no health problem to the patient or to dental office personnel, but because of these concerns, many non–Be-containing Ni-Cr alloys have been developed.

The Ni-Cr alloys were successful because of their extremely low cost, which is a fraction of that of even the most inexpensive noble metal PFMs. After the initial casting difficulties were overcome, the use of Ni-Cr alloys for PFMs became widespread. They have excellent sag resistance and outstanding stability under occlusal loads. Both of these characteristics make them ideal for bridges spanning many teeth. Despite these benefits, concern remains over the biocompatibility of these alloys, based on their high Ni content. Nickel is a known allergen; it has been estimated that nearly 10% of women and approximately 1% of men may be allergic to it. The allergy often is caused or manifested by the wearing of costume jewelry or pierced earrings made with stainless steel or nickel-plated alloys instead of noble metal posts. This characteristic limits the use of these alloys, but only to a minimal extent.

An even greater concern, however, has been raised over the use of these alloys. Nickel is a suspected carcinogen. There are no reports of dental restorations containing Ni causing cancers in patients, but the results of certain animal tests have given rise to concerns not unlike those with regard to saccharin, the artificial sweetener. No restriction exists on the use of Ni-Cr alloy in dentistry in the United States; a few other countries have taken a more rigid approach, however, establishing more specific guidelines.

In any event, the high hardness and elastic limit, as well as the more difficult casting procedures, limit the use of Ni-Cr alloys to PFM restorations. In addition, they are white in color, which still is considered to be a negative trait for all metal restorations.

Most recently, titanium and titanium alloys have been developed as dental casting alloys. These metals are used with porcelain. Titanium is very reactive to oxygen and has a very high melting point. Therefore, it requires special casting equipment to produce dental prostheses. Although titanium has excellent biocompatibility, the extra effort and cost required to cast this metal have limited its use as a dental restorative.

■ Ceramics: Some Basic Concepts

Ceramics as a class of materials possess such characteristics as a high melting point, low thermal and electrical conductivity, high compressive strength and stiffness, low tensile strength, brittleness, and optical qualities varying from clear to translucent to opaque. They are also relatively inert and insoluble. Ceramics, predominantly porcelains, have been used in dentistry for at least 200 years. One of their first uses was for dentures, a purpose for which they are still used today. Porcelains are also used as single-unit anterior crowns, often called porcelain jacket crowns, as an esthetic veneer for anterior teeth or metallic crowns and bridges, and as inlays.

Because of their outstanding esthetic appeal, there has been a strong emphasis on improving ceramics to make them suitable for stress-bearing applications, such as full-coverage crown and bridge restorations that do not have a metal substrate for support. The main problem with ceramics has been a lack of adequate fracture resistance, attributed to their brittle nature. Reinforced porcelains and glass ceramics have been developed to address this problem, with variable results.

Ceramics can be defined as a class of materials composed of metallic oxide compounds such as feldspar, quartz, and clay. Therefore, all ceramics have similar compositions. This is especially interesting given that ceramics include such diverse materials as fine china, crystal, pottery, earthenware, cookware, and common drinking glasses. Some ceramics, such as fine crystal glasses, are like metals, in that they have a crystalline structure. Others, such as common drinking glasses, have a completely amorphous structure more similar to polymers. In any case, the main building block of ceramics is the silicon dioxide molecule (silica or SiO_2). Silicon forms a tetrahedron (like a prism) with oxygen, such that each silicon atom is capable of forming a covalent bond through electron sharing with four oxygen atoms. Therefore, the oxygens occupy the space between silicon atoms, forming what can be regular crystals or an amorphous structure that resembles a cross-linked polymer. These silica-based materials also contain other primary additives that greatly influence and alter their solubility, melting point, and thermal expansion, all of which are important for dental restorative materials.

The components of dental ceramics are mined from the earth, although industrial methods of synthesizing silica-based compounds from other materials have been developed. The composition of porcelains and other ceramics used in dental applications are described in the next section. During the discussion, keep in mind that ceramic objects are formed from powders of the various components that have been blended together. The blend of powders is mixed with water and then heated at very high temperatures to eliminate the water and produce a hard, cohesive material. The process, referred to as baking or firing, is not unlike the process used to produce pottery. Pottery production is an art form, as is the formation of ceramic dental restorations.

■ *Ceramics: Composition, Properties, and Preparation*

Dental Porcelains

Composition

Porcelains are generally white, translucent ceramics. The translucency is a function of its composition and level of porosity, with the latter being determined by the method of preparation. Porcelains contain three main components: quartz or flint (silica), feldspar (a potassium-aluminum silicate), and kaolin clay (aluminum silicate). In dental feldspathic porcelain, feldspar makes up 75 to 85% of the porcelain and serves as the amorphous, glassy phase that holds the silica mineral crystals together. Kaolin, added at only 3 to 5% serves as an opaquing agent and enhances the workability of porcelain. In contrast to dental porcelains, fine porcelain used in decorative figurines contains high concentrations of kaolin and low concentrations of feldspar. Porcelains contain other additives to produce desirable properties. For example, many contain sodium oxide (Na_2O) and potassium oxide (K_2O). These additives are called glass modifiers because they react with the oxygen atoms instead of the silicon atoms, thus reducing the number of bonds or cross-links formed within the glassy silicate structure. This is possible because Si can make four bonds, whereas Na or K can make only one. Therefore, a bond to Na or K means a dead end in the chain with no further bonding possible. This has a pronounced influence on properties because it makes the matrix network less stable.

Another important component of porcelain is **leucite**. Leucite is a crystalline potassium-aluminum-silicate mineral that forms when feldspar and glass are melted together within the porcelain. Leucite is often also an added component because it strengthens, toughens, and raises the thermal expansion coefficient of normal feldspathic porcelain. Many new porcelains have been developed with high leucite content to enhance their strength and usefulness in stress-bearing restorations.

In addition to glass modifiers, pigments (metallic oxides) are added to porcelains for color, and fluorescing agents (such as cerium oxide) are added to cause porcelain to **fluoresce** like natural teeth under ultraviolet lighting (e.g., fluorescent bulbs and sunlight). Fluorescence is the phenomenon in which an object emits light when it is illuminated by a specific light source; in the case of teeth, this gives an increased appearance of vitality.

Properties

Three types of porcelains are commonly used in dentistry. One particular type is used to make denture teeth (Fig. 7-5). This porcelain is called "high fusing" because it fuses (or melts) at approximately 1300 to 1350°C. The high melting point is achieved by minimizing the additives such as sodium and potassium, which maximizes the silicate cross-links to produce a porcelain with low solubility, high strength, and high stability. A second type of porcelain is the low-fusing porcelain, which has a fusion range of 850 to 1050°C and is used as a veneer for metal in PFM restorations (Fig. 7-5). The lower fusion point is produced by increasing the amount of additives in the porcelain, thus reducing the number of cross-links within the silicate network. Using a low-fusing porcelain for a PFM is important because it helps to avoid overheating the metal framework during the process of baking the porcelain. These porcelains are only slightly weaker and less stable than the high-fusing types and are only slightly more soluble in the oral environment. A medium-fusing porcelain (fusion point of 1100 to 1250°C) is used for anterior porcelain jacket crowns and has properties intermediate between those of the low- and high-fusing porcelains.

The hardness of high-fusing porcelain exceeds that of enamel by approximately 30%. This property ensures excellent wear resistance but also causes many problems, in that porcelain will rapidly abrade enamel. This limits the use of

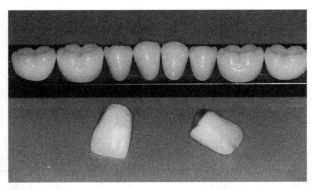

Figure 7–5 Denture teeth made from a high-fusing porcelain, a jacket crown made from a medium-fusing porcelain, and a PFM restoration made with a low-fusing porcelain.

porcelain in posterior teeth and is the rationale for using porcelain only on the labial or facial aspects of bridges involving several posterior teeth, especially when they are in opposition to natural dentition. The wear of a single tooth may present only a minor problem in terms of occlusion, but the simultaneous abrasion of several posterior teeth in one arch could be disastrous. Therefore, such restorations often contain metal occlusal surfaces and porcelain facings (see Figs. 2-6 and 7-5).

Recently, a new type of low-fusing porcelain has been developed for veneering gold-colored alloys. These porcelains are made with a very small particle size powder. In preliminary studies, they have been shown to be less abrasive toward natural teeth than conventional feldspathic porcelains. The low-fusing point of the porcelain allows it to be baked onto alloys with high gold content and a rich gold color, thus providing more ideal esthetics in a PFM restoration.

Porcelains are very stiff, possessing elastic moduli of approximately 70 GPa (10 million psi), which is slightly lower than that of gold alloys. They have a high elastic limit and very low percent elongation (less than 1%); in other words, they are not ductile. Like most brittle materials, porcelains are strong in compression but relatively weak when subjected to tensile stresses. In fact, the tensile strength of porcelain (35 MPa; 5000 psi) is only approximately 4% of its compressive strength (875 MPa). Thus, porcelains are brittle and subject to fracture during cementation or chewing. They also have low impact strength and low fatigue resistance. All of these deficiencies explain why porcelains often are used to veneer metal structures rather than as the support structure for restorations, especially in regions of considerable stress.

Porcelains have a density of 2.2 to 2.3 g/cm^3. This property is controlled to some extent by porosity and contraction accompanying firing. Linear shrinkages of 11 to 14% are common for porcelains, and this large contraction explains the difficulties encountered in fitting porcelain restorations.

Preparation of Porcelain

The blend of quartz, feldspar, and clay powders (plus additives) is mixed with water and painted onto the die (replica of the prepared tooth) or onto the metallic framework in the case of a PFM. The excess water is removed by vibration or repeated brushing of the porcelain mix. This process is essential for condensing or tightly packing the powder particles together. As the water is eliminated and blotted from the surface, the particles are drawn closer together. Once the core layer or bottom "dentin" replacement layer of the restoration has been added, the die is transferred to a porcelain oven and heated slowly to a temperature slightly below the fusion point of the porcelain. This process causes the porcelain to shrink as all of the water is removed and the particles begin to coalesce, or **sinter**, together at their edges. Sintering refers to the process of fusing particles together without completely melting them. This first heat treatment, also called a "biscuit bake," is performed slowly to ensure that a visually homogenous product is formed. In addition, the firing often is done in a vacuum oven. ***What benefit would be derived from firing the porcelain in a vacuum oven?***

If the porcelain is heated slowly under vacuum, water will be drawn out before the fusing takes place. This is possible because the mixture is still somewhat plastic at this point. The elimination of water results in a denser final product, and one with enhanced optical and mechanical characteristics. The vacuum is an effective way to draw air from the porcelain, thus increasing its density and ultimately its esthetic qualities.

In a porcelain jacket crown, the first porcelain layer forms the bulk of the restoration, and its strength is of primary importance. Therefore, this "core" porcelain is usually of a different composition than the applied surface porcelain. The core porcelain may be either an **aluminous porcelain** or a **magnesia core porcelain**. The former is a porcelain the composition of which is 40 to 50% alumina (aluminum oxide) crystals. The second type of core contains magnesia crystals instead of alumina. Both core porcelains are approximately twice as strong as the normal feldspathic porcelain. Their strength is adequate for anterior teeth, and studies have shown that restorations made from these materials undergo only a 2% failure rate over a 7-year period. The failure rate increases as the restorations are placed more distally in the mouth, to a rate of 6% in premolars and 15% in molars. Clearly, these restorations are unacceptable for posterior teeth because of the high rate of fracture and chipping.

After the first bake of porcelain (or core porcelain) is cooled, the "enamel replacement" or outer portion is added in a manner similar to that of the dentin portion. It also is fired slowly. After cooling, stains are added, and the porcelain is given a final, high-temperature firing. This completes the fusion of the powders and produces a smooth, glass-like surface called a **glaze**. This final firing temperature may be in the range of 950 to 1060°C. A porcelain that is glazed in this manner is called self-glazing. For other, non–self-glazing porcelains, a separate low-fusing porcelain is applied before the final bake to produce a glazed surface. The surfaces produced on self-glazing porcelains are usually considered to be more stable than are those from applied glazes, but both are common.

After glazing, the porcelain is slowly cooled to room temperature. *What ill effects could be produced by a rapid cooling of the porcelain?*

Because the porcelain has a low coefficient of thermal conductivity, it must be cooled slowly to avoid the formation of stresses that would cause it to crack. A similar problem arises when it is fired onto a metal substructure (i.e., in a PFM) because the metal cools at a different rate as a result of its higher coefficient of thermal expansion. Therefore, the thermal expansion coefficients of the metal and porcelain must be precisely matched to avoid this differential in thermal contraction after firing. The original porcelains used in dentistry had very low coefficients of thermal expansion, approximately half that of the alloys used in prosthetics. The development of PFM restorations necessitated the invention of new porcelains with much higher thermal expansion coefficients to eliminate this potential problem. The addition of sodium oxide or other fluxes is one way to increase the thermal expansion coefficient for PFM porcelains.

Other Dental Ceramics

Although popular because of their excellent clinical performance, PFM restorations are not esthetically ideal. Natural teeth are composed of regions of varying composition and appearance, but all are translucent to some extent. Metal is opaque, and although porcelain can enhance its appearance, a PFM restoration is less similar to a natural tooth than is an all-porcelain restoration. This dilemma has led to intensive efforts to produce more fracture-resistant ceramics to be used by themselves for dental restorations (Fig. 7-6). Ceramics similar to those used in cookware have been developed for dentistry. These ceramics are produced in a variety of manners, including casting through a lost wax casting process like that used for gold alloys, injection molding, infiltration, and machining with the aid of a computer. A full description of these ceramics is beyond the scope of this text,

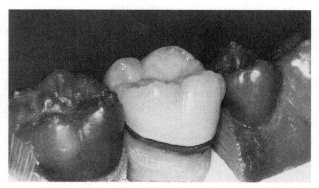

Figure 7–6 A cast glass ceramic molar crown on a die.

but a brief description of their composition and properties is presented, and the different types are listed in Table 7-4.

Description of All-Ceramic Systems

As shown in Table 7-4, all-ceramic restorations can be made from a variety of reinforced porcelains, glass ceramics, alumina or magnesia materials, or zirconia. Various procedures for producing a dental restoration have been developed for use in conjunction with these materials. Changes in the composition and internal structure of the ceramics produce materials with greater resistance to cracking, thus allowing many of them to be machined or milled like metals. In addition, many of the glass ceramics can be cast like metals by using the lost wax casting process (see Chapter 11).

Glass ceramics begin with an amorphous (or glassy) structure. In dentistry, they are composed basically of silica. One example is a product that is cast by using the lost wax technique into a phosphate investment mold by using the lost wax technique. The cast glass initially has an amorphous silicate structure, but on subsequent heating for several hours at approximately 1075°C, the glass transforms into a crystalline solid containing tiny, thin sheets of crystalline mica. The sheets stack on one another like a deck of cards, so the material is very dense. Because the ceramic is white, color is added externally by applying feldspathic porcelain to the surface of the restoration. This is not as durable as the internal col-

TABLE 7–4. Types of All-Ceramic Materials for Dental Restorations

Types	Composition	Flexure Strength (MPa)
Feldspathic porcelain	Porcelain	65–75
Reinforced porcelain	Added leucite or alumina	110–150
Castable glass	Glass ceramic (contains mica)	125–150
Machinable—CAD/CAM	Feldspathic porcelain or glass ceramic	100–200
Machinable—copy-milling	Fine-grained feldspathic porcelain or alumina	150
Injection-molded	Leucite-reinforced feldspathic porcelain	160–180
Infiltrated	Alumina or magnesia core infiltrated with glass	450

orization produced by using different-colored feldspathic porcelains. The development of internally colorized glass ceramics should produce more esthetic restorations.

The success rate for anterior crowns made from machinable or cast ceramics has been equivalent to that for aluminous porcelain jacket crowns. Early studies for posterior crowns did not show good results, in part because the restorations were cemented with brittle zinc phosphate or glass ionomer cements. More recent studies have reported improved results (2 to 3% failure rate per year) for posterior crowns cemented with composite cements capable of bonding to the ceramic and the tooth surface when used in conjunction with a dental adhesive. Further strengthening and toughening of these ceramics may be required before they are acceptable for a full range of posterior restorations. At least one material has been used to make three-unit bridges, but because of the preliminary nature of the studies, the efficacy of this procedure is not yet established. Initial results are encouraging, however.

The glass ceramics have strengths equal to or greater than those of the aluminous porcelain cores. In addition, they are virtually free of porosity as a result of their manufacturing method. They are hard but not as abrasive as porcelains and, therefore, are kinder to the opposing dentition than are feldspathic porcelains. When they must be coated with feldspathic porcelain to be made more tooth-like in appearance, however, the benefits of their lower abrasiveness are not realized. The development of glasses with improved internal colorization could solve this abrasion problem.

Another aspect of certain ceramics is that they can be machined like metals. The presence of small crystals dispersed throughout their glassy matrix minimizes cracking and chipping when they are drilled, milled, or ground. Although they still are somewhat brittle, they do not crack like other glasses and porcelains. This machinability allows them to be made into dental restorations by using a technique called CAD/CAM.

CAD is an acronym for computer-assisted (or aided) design; CAM is an acronym for computer-assisted machining (or manufacture). Basically, a computer is used to design and cut a restoration, such as a veneer, inlay, onlay, or crown. In one commercial technique, a small, handheld camera is used intraorally to make a video image of a prepared tooth. The image of the tooth is displayed on a computer monitor, and appropriate computer software is used to design a restoration by defining the outlines of the margins and line angles. The information for this computer-generated restoration is then sent to an attached milling machine. The milling machine uses diamond-edged disks and tools that precisely cut away the machinable ceramic to the specifications ordered by the computer, within a period of 4 to 7 minutes. This can be accomplished in the dental office. The final restoration is then polished and cemented into the cavity with a composite luting cement in the same appointment. A typical time for producing an inlay may be 2 hours or so. The equipment is expensive, but clinical trials with inlay restorations have shown good results, with failure rates of 1 to 3%.

In an alternative technique, called copy-milling, a composite restoration is fashioned on a die, which is then used as a master to mill the restoration from a ceramic block. A tracing device is first used to digitize the surface of the die with the aid of a computer. This information is then sent to the mill, which then faithfully replicates the surface contours of the die by milling the ceramic. This method is somewhat similar to that used to duplicate a key and is usually performed in a dental laboratory.

Another laboratory technique for producing all-ceramic restorations involves the process of infiltration of a high strength, porous alumina core with a glass. The core is produced by a slip-casting process and then slightly sintered to produce a porous structure. A molten glass is then infused in the core, filling up all of the pores to produce a dense ceramic on solidification. Feldspathic porcelain is next applied to the surface to optimize esthetics. This process produces a material with very high strength.

All-ceramic restorations can also be produced in a laboratory through an injection molding process. A mold is produced by the lost wax technique in which a wax pattern of the restoration is fashioned and then invested in a ceramic mold. The mold is heated to eliminate the wax. A cylindrical piece of glass, porcelain, or an alternative glass ceramic is then heated and injected into the mold under pressure. During this process, the material transforms into a highly crystalline restoration. Feldspathic porcelain is then applied to the surface to achieve an esthetic outcome. Clinical studies of inlays made from this injection-molded or pressable ceramic show low failure rates of 1 to 2% per year. Results for crowns have shown higher failure rates, both in anterior and posterior applications.

Repair of Porcelain and Ceramic Restorations

That ceramic inlays, onlays, veneers, or crowns can be cemented into or onto the tooth with a composite cement suggests that intraoral repairs of such restorations also are possible. Although they are never as good as the original restoration, composite repairs may function quite well if carried out correctly, especially if the chip or fracture is not too large. The key is to produce a rough surface for enhanced mechanical bonding. The first step is to isolate the chipped or fractured region with a rubber dam. Subsequently, the fractured surface is roughened with a diamond bur. Another option is to sandblast the surface with an intraoral sandblaster using aluminum oxide particles (50 μm in diameter). After roughening, the surface is etched for 2 to 3 minutes with hydrofluoric acid, which etches or dissolves glass. A 10% solution works well on porcelain or ceramics, although it is caustic and extreme care must be taken to avoid burning the gingiva. An alternative is to apply an acidulated phosphate fluoride gel (fluoride treatment solution). This has much lower acidic activity and must be left in contact with the surface for approximately 10 minutes. Afterward, if enamel is showing, it must be etched with phosphoric acid to allow for bonding with the composite repair.

Next, a silane solution is applied to the porcelain. The silane serves the same purpose as the silane coupling agent that bonds the resin matrix to the glass fillers in the dental composite restorative material. An adhesive primer is then applied to the silanated surface, as well as to any exposed metal, if the restoration is a PFM, and to any exposed enamel. An unfilled resin is then applied and light cured. Finally, the composite is applied. If there is any metal showing, it should first be covered with an opaque composite to avoid metal "show through," which makes the composite appear gray.

■ Composites: Composition, Properties, and Preparation

As discussed, the placement of large posterior composites is challenging because of the polymerization contraction that accompanies the curing of the material. In response to these difficulties, composite inlays were introduced as an alternative.

By processing the composite extraorally, concerns over polymerization shrinkage are essentially eliminated. Also, the composite can be cured more fully in the laboratory, which produces materials with superior physical and mechanical properties compared with those cured intraorally. Because the strength and stiffness of composites cured in the laboratory are still inferior to those of metal and ceramics, these materials usually are not indicated for onlay or full-coverage restorations. Composites are increasingly used as inlay materials, however, and many manufacturers produce materials designed specifically for this application (Fig. 7-7). The composition of the composites used for inlays is essentially the same as that of many of the composites used for direct posterior restorations. The main difference is in the manner in which the materials are processed.

There are two types of composite inlay materials. The most popular type is the indirect composite inlay, which is made in a manner similar to that of a metal or ceramic inlay. After the tooth is prepared for the inlay (Fig. 7-8A), an impression is made and a die is poured. A temporary restoration is placed, and the patient leaves. The composite inlay is later fashioned on the die and cured by either light or heat application in the laboratory; some systems use both light and heat and apply pressure in a nitrogen gas environment. The polished restoration is cemented into the prepared tooth (Fig. 7-8B) with a dual-cure composite cement at a second appointment (Figs. 7-9 and 7-10). This cementation procedure is identical with that used for a ceramic inlay.

The second type of composite inlay is produced by a direct technique. The prepared tooth is lubricated, and the composite is placed and cured. The cured composite inlay is removed from the tooth, given a secondary cure with heat to maximize its properties, and then cemented within the tooth with a composite cement during the same appointment. This second type is more labor intensive on the part of the dentist but does not require the placement of a temporary restoration.

Whether the inlay is cured within the tooth or on a gypsum die, polymerization shrinkage causes it to be smaller than the cavity preparation. In the direct technique, this shrinkage facilitates the removal of the cured inlay from the tooth. The difference between the inlay technique and the direct composite placement technique is that in the latter, the shrinkage takes place while the composite is attempting to bond to the cavity walls. As was discussed, this imposes stress on the

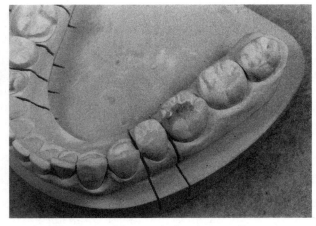

Figure 7–7 A composite inlay prepared for a molar in a heat- and/or pressure-curing oven, demonstrating its fit on a stone model.

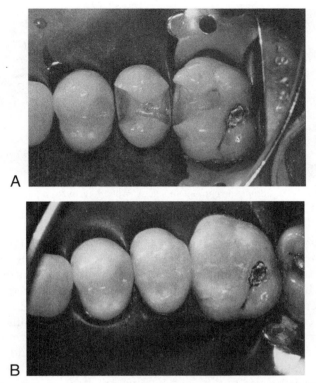

A

B

Figure 7–8 A. Two posterior teeth prepared for composite inlays. **B.** Same teeth after the inlays have been cemented in place and polished.

bond between the tooth and the composite, potentially creating marginal gaps. For the inlay, the space that is left between the tooth and the inlay will be filled by a composite cement. Although the composite cement also shrinks during polymerization, the amount of material that shrinks is very small because it is equivalent only to the volume of the cement. The film thickness of the cement usually is in the range of 50 to 200 μm. Therefore, the stresses imposed on the tooth-inlay bond are reduced, and the quality of the restoration margins should be excellent. In vitro studies show that compared with leakage around direct composite, leak-

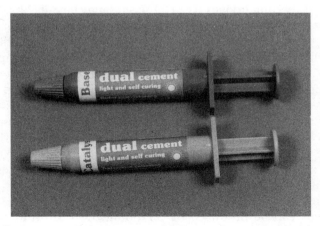

Figure 7–9 Dual-cure composite cement used for cementing a composite inlay into a tooth.

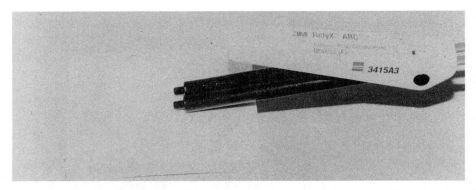

Figure 7–10 Composite cement supplied in a cartridge system that facilitates the dispensing of equal lengths of the two component pastes.

age around inlays may still occur when the margins extend below the cementum-enamel junction, where adhesion is most difficult, but that it is significantly reduced. The clinical evaluation of such restorations is incomplete, however.

The second major benefit of the inlay technique relates to the mechanical properties of the inlay. Because the inlay can be cured in the laboratory, it may be subjected to heat treatments at elevated temperatures after the initial light-curing. These treatments have been shown to enhance the degree of cure and the mechanical properties of composites. Although some brands of composite inlays are processed by a heat-curing procedure, inlays that initially have been light cured may be subjected to the same heat treatment to enhance their properties. A typical post–light-cured heat treatment is 7 to 10 minutes at 120°C.

Clinical results suggest that compared with direct composites, inlays show an improved marginal integrity over the same 3-year period but may not provide improved wear resistance. Evidence suggests that improvement in the properties of the composite inlays as a result of heat treatment may be transient, declining to lower levels as the polymer absorbs water over time and becomes softened. There appears to be no negative effect from the heat treatment, however, and the procedure is simple and quick.

Reinforced Composites

More recently, composites have been developed to produce onlays, crowns, and even three-unit bridges. The composites may be called by different names, such as ceromer or polyglass, but they are composites nonetheless. The properties of these new composites are similar to typical minifills and midifills. One difference is in the use of reinforced composites containing glass or polymer fibers.

Composites can be reinforced with glass or polyethylene fibers, used in either straight fiber bundles or as woven meshes. A typical example of a woven polyethylene fiber is shown in Figures 7-11 and 7-12. The glass or polyethylene may be provided preimpregnated with a resin or composite, or this process may be accomplished by the lab technician or the clinician during the process of fabricating the restoration. The glass fibers have high elastic modulus and therefore stiffen as well as strengthen the composite. The polyethylene fibers provide added strength and toughness (it is more difficult to fracture the prosthesis) but, because of their low elastic modulus, do not stiffen the structure. Reinforced composite crowns can be produced by wrapping the resin-impregnated mesh or fibers

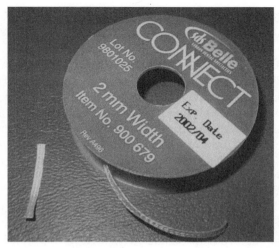

Figure 7–11 Woven polyethylene fiber supplied on a spool and used to reinforce composites for crown and bridge applications.

around the die of the prepared tooth to provide a supportive substructure. The structure is light cured and usually heat processed. Composite is then applied to the substructure to produce the anatomical surfaces of the crown. The composite is also light cured and heat processed. Three-unit bridges can similarly be produced by wrapping the fibers around the prepared abutment teeth on a die, with the fibers spanning the pontic region. The surfaces of the abutment teeth and the pontic tooth are then built up on the fibrous support by using a composite with good strength and wear characteristics.

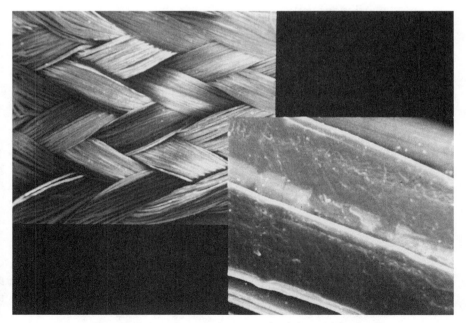

Figure 7–12 Magnified view of a typical woven polyethylene reinforcing fiber system.

Summary

The materials described in this chapter are used for teeth that have experienced extensive deterioration. Therefore, the materials must have very good mechanical properties and structural durability. Metal alloys (mixtures of metals), ceramics, porcelains, and, to a lesser extent, laboratory-processed composites are used for these applications. Alloys of noble metals such as gold, platinum, and palladium mixed with silver and copper are the oldest and most commonly used metals for these types of restorations. They are melted and cast into molds to form dental restorations and appliances, are adequately strong, and have excellent corrosion resistance. They are the most costly, however.

Alternative alloys contain base metals such as nickel and cobalt mixed with chromium. The chromium provides corrosion resistance. Porcelains are silica-based powders that are heated to high temperatures to fuse them into dense structures such as denture teeth, veneers, and other restorations. Their low strength and brittle nature, however, prohibit their extensive use in stress-bearing areas. Therefore, numerous ceramics with improved fracture resistance have been developed for dental applications. Some of these ceramics can be cast like metals, and others can be machined to the correct shape and size. In general, metal restorations are the most durable, although they are not esthetic. A common approach is to cover metal restorations, such as crowns, with porcelain to combine structural support with esthetics.

STUDY QUESTIONS AND PROBLEM SOLVING

1. **Which of the following is (are) a reason(s) for making dental bridges from alloys rather than from ceramics?**
    a. Alloys are much less expensive
    b. Alloys are more biocompatible
    c. Alloys are much less brittle
    d. Alloys are less abrasive to teeth

2. **Compared with pure gold, dental gold alloys are:**
    a. Less expensive
    b. Harder
    c. More corrosion resistant
    d. More malleable

3. **The orthodontist bends a wire six times and unintentionally fractures it. What could have been done after a few bends had been completed to avoid this?**
    a. Heat the wire
    b. Anneal the wire
    c. Strain harden the wire
    d. Quench the wire

4. **A patient presents in need of a PFM restoration and has a known allergy to costume jewelry and certain pierced earrings. Which of the following alloys would be the least acceptable for this patient?**
    a. Nickel-chromium
    b. Palladium-silver

   c. High-gold PFM

   d. Low-gold PFM

5. **Which one of the following statements concerning type III ADA gold alloys is true?**
   a. They have more gold than type II
   b. They are harder than type IV
   c. Their main use is for small inlays
   d. They are less burnishable than type I

6. **Which of the following is *not* one of the major components of dental porcelain?**
   a. Clay
   b. Feldspar
   c. Cerium oxide
   d. Quartz

7. **Which of the following is *not* a step normally recommended for the intraoral repair of a chipped anterior PFM restoration?**
   a. Etch the porcelain surface with hydrofluoric acid
   b. Place a glass ionomer liner over any exposed metal
   c. Roughen the surfaces with an intraoral sandblaster
   d. Make the repair with a light-cured composite

8. **A patient who continually clenches and grinds his teeth has fractured a cusp from a class II amalgam restoration in a second molar. The most logical choice would be to replace it with an onlay made of:**
   a. Resin composite
   b. A gold alloy
   c. Porcelain
   d. A cast ceramic

9. **If strength requirements are taken into consideration, which of the following ceramics would be the least ideal choice for an onlay on a first molar for a patient demanding that no metal be used?**
   a. Infiltrated ceramic
   b. Feldspathic porcelain
   c. Injection molded ceramic
   d. Leucite-reinforced porcelain

10. **Composites used for indirect restorations, such as three-unit bridges, differ from composites used as direct posterior fillings, in that the former:**
    a. Are twice as strong
    b. Have 10 times the wear resistance
    c. Are often heat processed after initial light-curing
    d. Are often reinforced with woven fibers

SELECTED READINGS

Anusavice KJ. Noble metal alloys for metal-ceramic restorations. Dental Clinics of North America 29:789–803, 1985.

   This article provides detailed information about the composition and factors that affect the clinical performance of PFM alloy restorations.

Bertolotti RL. Casting metals, Part I. Compendium of Continuing Education in Dentistry 11:300–308, 1990 (see also Casting metals, Part II: High-fusing alloys. Compendium of Continuing Education in Dentistry 11:370–378, 1990).

This two-part article describes the status of casting alloys used in dentistry. It follows the development of the materials and compares them in terms of cost, composition, properties, and ease of use.

Christensen GJ. Buonocore Memorial Lecture: Tooth-colored posterior restorations. Operative Dentistry 22:146–148, 1997.

This article provides a review of the many different types of esthetic restoratives for inlays and onlays, including ceramics and composites. The article emphasizes the clinical aspects of patient selection, tooth preparation, and restorative procedures.

Leinfelder KF, Isenberg BP, Essig ME. A new method for generating ceramic restorations: A CAD-CAM system. Journal of the American Dental Association 118:703–707, 1989.

The procedure for the production of CAD-CAM dental restorations is described in a pictorial format.

McLean JW. The science and art of dental ceramics. Operative Dentistry 16:149–156, 1991.

This article is from the Buonocore Memorial Lecture series. It describes the general characteristics of ceramics, including methods for strengthening. The clinical advantages and shortcomings of dental ceramics used in veneers and crowns are discussed.

Rosenblum MA, Schulman A. A review of all-ceramic restorations. Journal of the American Dental Association 128:297–307, 1997.

This article provides a comparison of the properties and processing methods used for five types of all-ceramic materials, including conventional porcelain, castable ceramics, machinable ceramics, pressable ceramics, and infiltrated ceramics.

Shellard E, Duke ES. Indirect composite resin materials for posterior applications. Compendium of Continuing Education in Dentistry 20:1166–1171, 1999.

This article provides a comparison of the properties, composition, and uses of dental composites used for indirect restorations, such as inlays and onlays. Results from clinical evaluations of several of the existing systems are described.

Touati B, Aidan N. Second-generation laboratory composite resins for indirect restorations. Journal of Esthetic Dentistry 9:108–118, 1997.

This article describes composites used alone or as a veneer over metal for inlays, onlays, and implant-supported bridges. The clinical factors affecting the success and failure of these materials are discussed.

van Dijken JWV. All-ceramic restorations: Classification and clinical evaluations. Compendium of Continuing Education in Dentistry 20:1115–1134, 1999.

This article provides a comparison of the properties, composition, and uses of commonly used dental ceramics. Data from clinical evaluations of many of the different types of ceramics are also provided.

Chapter 8

Impression Materials

Uses of Impression Materials in Dentistry

Composition of Impression Materials
Inelastic Materials
Elastic Materials: The Hydrocolloids
Elastic Materials: The Elastomers

Mixing and Handling of Impression Materials
Inelastic Materials
Elastic Materials: The Hydrocolloids
Elastic Materials: The Elastomers

Characteristics of Impression Materials
Flexibility
Accuracy
Tear Strength
Stability
Dimensional Change
Surface Wetting
Working and Setting Time

Disinfection of Impression Materials

Summary

Objectives

- Describe the ideal requirements for a dental impression material for dentulous patients.

- Define inelastic and elastic impression materials and contrast their uses.

- Identify examples of inelastic and elastic impression materials.

- Contrast the composition and setting behavior of different inelastic impression materials.

- Compare the composition, setting behavior, and uses of the two different hydrocolloid impression materials.

- Compare the composition, dimensional stability, and physical properties of the elastomeric impression materials.

- Describe the clinical technique for the appropriate mixing and taking of an alginate impression.

- Describe the equipment used and the procedures followed when taking an impression with agar hydrocolloid.

- Describe the clinical technique for the appropriate mixing and taking of an additional silicone impression, using the regular and putty-wash techniques.

- Indicate an appropriate disinfecting regimen for each type of impression material.

It would be virtually impossible to perform high-quality restorative and prosthetic dentistry without impression materials. An **impression** is essentially a
"negative" replica of some structure. In dentistry, this replica usually is made of
the teeth or gingival tissues of the mandibular or maxillary arch. From the impression, it is possible to produce an exact **replica** of the dental structures by using a cast or die material, such as dental stone or some type of plastic. The replica
thus is a "positive" reproduction that can be used in treatment planning or in the
production of a restoration. These activities can take place in the absence of the
patient; the dental staff makes an impression of a tooth prepared for a crown while
the patient sits in the dental chair, but the actual process of producing the crown
takes place in a dental laboratory using an exact replica of the prepared tooth. This
example underscores the need for accuracy and stability in dental impression materials. The final restoration fits only as accurately as the initial impression allows,
based on its accurate rendition of the oral structure.

Different types of impression materials have been developed for different applications, but all have similar requirements. These requirements can be summarized as follows:

1. Impression materials must be fluid enough to flow into or around the area
   of interest to reproduce accurately all of the fine structural details.
2. Once placed, they must harden within a few minutes to form a semirigid
   material that does not distort on removal from the mouth (distortion
   would lead to inaccuracies in the final restoration).
3. They must not produce any harmful effects on the host's tissues during
   their short stay in the oral cavity.
4. They should be relatively tasteless and odorless so as not to be offensive to
   the patient.
5. The impression should be dimensionally stable to allow time for a positive
   replica to be made in die stone or some other material.

Obviously, the materials also should be easy to handle and relatively inexpensive. One further requirement is that the clinician, using appropriate solutions,
must be able to disinfect the impression in the dental office, without compromising its accuracy or stability.

■ Uses of Impression Materials in Dentistry

The wide variety of available impression materials falls into either of two categories: **inelastic** (i.e., rigid) and **elastic** (i.e., rubbery) (Table 8-1). As the names
imply, inelastic materials are not elastic and exhibit little to no "spring-like" quality when deformed. In other words, they are rigid materials with a low maximum
flexibility (see Chapter 2); any significant deformation produces a permanent
change in their shape. In contrast, elastic materials behave in a manner more similar to that of a rubber band. They can be bent and stretched appreciably without
suffering a permanent change in dimension. It is obvious that these two classes
have been developed for different purposes. *Can you imagine making an impression of a dentulous patient with an impression material that does not deform elastically when being removed from around the teeth?*

Inelastic impression materials are used to make impressions of edentulous patients—for example, during the preliminary stages of making a full-arch denture. To
ensure the fit of the denture, it is necessary to work with an accurate replica of the
patient's arch. The impression material makes this possible. The inelastic materials

TABLE 8–1. **Types of Impression Materials**	
Inelastic	**Elastic**
Impression compound	Hydrocolloids
Zinc oxide eugenol	Agar (reversible)
Plaster	Alginate (irreversible)
	Elastomeric
	Polysulfide
	Condensation silicone
	Polyether
	Addition silicone (polyvinylsiloxane)

discussed in this chapter include *impression compound* and **zinc oxide eugenol (ZOE)** impression paste. Historically, *impression plaster* also has been used (see Chapter 9).

Compound has been used in the past to make impressions of edentulous arches, but it is used more commonly for other applications. It can serve as an impression tray to carry some other impression material, such as ZOE, and can be used to make impressions of single-tooth preparations that do not have significant **undercut** areas. Undercuts are areas that curve under, like the cervical portion of the tooth (Fig. 8-1). An inelastic impression material can be locked into

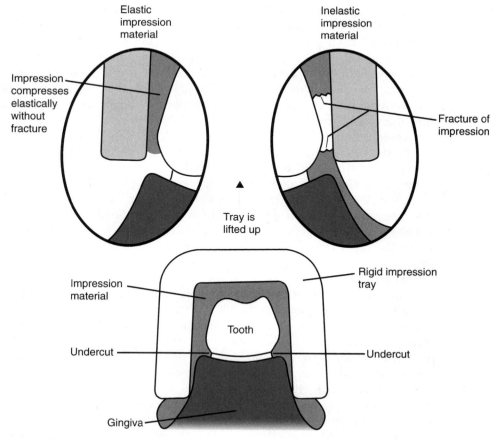

Figure 8–1 An undercut at the cervical portion of a tooth being locked into by an inelastic impression material.

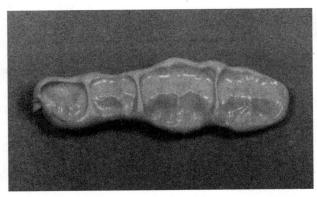

Figure 8–2 A bite registration impression used to establish the correct relationship between the upper and lower arch casts when they are mounted on an articulator.

undercuts, making it difficult to remove from the mouth without fracturing the impression.

ZOE often is used to make impressions of edentulous arches and for **bite registrations** of occlusal relationships. Bite registrations are thin impressions of the biting surfaces of the teeth used to set gypsum casts in the correct occlusal relationship when the casts are mounted on an **articulator** (a mechanical hinge device that works like the temporomandibular joint) (Fig. 8-2).

In contrast, elastic impression materials are used to make impressions of both dentulous and edentulous patients. This is possible because elastic materials can be removed from undercuts without undergoing any permanent distortion in shape (Fig. 8-1). The impressions can be used to make gypsum study casts for treatment planning or for assessing the progress of orthodontic treatment. They are accurate enough to be used in the first step of the process of making cast restorations, such as inlays, onlays, crowns, and bridges, as well as fixed and removable partial dentures. These procedures have already been discussed or will be addressed in subsequent chapters.

Elastic impression materials are subdivided into two types. One type comprises the **hydrocolloids**. These impression materials contain large amounts of water, even after they have set. Because water can evaporate rapidly under normal conditions, impressions made from these materials have only limited stability once they are removed from the mouth. One type of hydrocolloid sets by an irreversible chemical reaction and, therefore, is called *irreversible hydrocolloid* (alginate); the other transforms from a fluid paste to a rubber-like solid by a physical process that can be reversed simply by altering its temperature. It is called *reversible hydrocolloid* (agar).

The second type of elastic impression materials comprises the **elastomers**. Elastomers set by irreversible chemical reactions and do not have water as a main component. Therefore, they are more dimensionally stable over long periods of time than the hydrocolloids. The choice between the reversible hydrocolloid and an elastomer for crown and bridge impressions often is based solely on personal preference, in that accurate impressions can be made with either. Some clinicians find the reversible hydrocolloids less convenient, however. Because of their high water content and instability, they must be poured up immediately. Also, additional equipment is necessary for the agar hydrocolloid.

As is true for many other materials, the accuracy and the quality of the impression material depend completely on the manner in which it is mixed and handled. Therefore, the dental assistant may have a direct effect on the outcome of the final product. The accuracy of the final restoration depends completely on making a good impression.

■ *Composition of Impression Materials*

This section is divided into two parts. The first part considers the inelastic impression materials, and the second considers the elastic impression materials. The manner in which each impression material is packaged by the manufacturer and the general composition of each type of material are discussed.

Inelastic Materials

Impression Compound

Impression compound demonstrates **thermoplastic** behavior. Thermoplastic solids can be transformed from a hard, solid material into a softened, moldable material simply by raising their temperature to an appropriate level. The process can be reversed by cooling to room temperature. Because the change is purely physical (i.e., no chemical reaction occurs), there is no need to mix components.

Impression compound is distributed in several forms. There are plates that are shaped like the dental arch for making custom trays for edentulous patients, and there are sticks that are used to make final impressions (Fig. 8-3). Impression compound is composed of natural resins, such as shellac, that soften when heated above a specific temperature. These materials also contain other components such as various waxes, fillers, and pigments. The wax provides the necessary plasticity to allow the material to be manipulated and formed into shapes. The fillers, usually chalk or talc, give compound the "body" and stability it requires to hold its shape and take an accurate impression. The pigments provide color.

Zinc Oxide Eugenol Impression Paste

ZOE is used in dentistry as an impression material as well as a periodontal dressing, cavity base, temporary cement, and temporary restorative material (see Chapter 4). The chemical composition for each application is generally the same. The

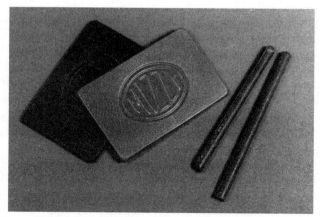

Figure 8–3 Impression compound in the form of plates and sticks.

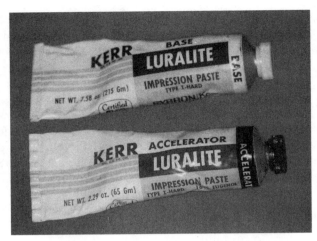

Figure 8–4 Tubes of ZOE impression paste.

impression material is manufactured in two forms, a two-paste system and a paste-liquid formulation (Fig. 8-4). Both are sold in tubes. In the two-paste system, the base paste contains zinc oxide powder mixed with various oils and a natural resin called rosin. Mixing the powder with the oils makes the material paste-like in consistency. Only the zinc oxide is needed for the chemical reaction, however. The catalyst paste contains 12 to 15% of an organic liquid called eugenol (the main component in oil of cloves), in addition to various oils and rosin to enhance the mixing and flow characteristics. Silica particles are added as fillers to make the catalyst paste-like. Finally, a catalyst (usually zinc acetate) is added to accelerate the chemical reaction between eugenol and zinc oxide. The chemical reaction takes place when equal portions of the two pastes are mixed on a mixing pad. The zinc oxide and the eugenol react to produce a matrix of zinc eugenolate that holds the unreacted particles together. The catalyst paste usually is colored brown, whereas the base paste is white. The eugenol gives the catalyst paste the characteristic smell often associated with dental offices. In addition, because of its analgesic nature, eugenol in oil of cloves often is used to ease the pain of a toothache.

The difference between the two-paste and the paste-liquid systems is that the liquid in the latter simply contains the eugenol and oils and does not contain the filler particles. This material is mixed like the two-paste formulation except that a specific number of drops of liquid is dispensed for a specific length of paste (e.g., 1 drop per each 1-inch length of paste). The setting reaction is the same.

Elastic Materials: The Hydrocolloids

A **colloid** is a suspension of fine particles (less than 1 μm) within a liquid. When the liquid is water, the colloid is known as a hydrocolloid. Two colloidal impression materials made from polysaccharide particles suspended in water are used in dentistry. The particles are derived from seaweed and kelp.

Reversible Hydrocolloid (Agar)

Agar is called the reversible hydrocolloid because it can be changed from a liquid solution, or **sol**, into a rubber-like **gel** simply by raising or lowering its temperature. The transformation is a physical change and is not accompanied by a chemical reaction; therefore, it is reversible. Agar is supplied either in plastic tubes, from

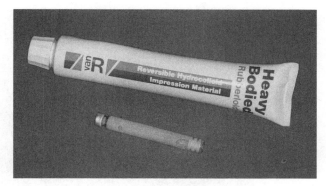

Figure 8–5 Agar hydrocolloid tray and syringe material.

which impression trays can be filled, or in the form of cylindrical sticks, which can be placed conveniently into special syringes for direct use in the mouth (Fig. 8-5). At room temperature, agar is in a gelled or solid rubber form. The agar molecules take the form of long, thin fibrils that interlock to produce the partially rigid but elastic gel. Water is the main component of the material, occupying all of the space between the fibrils. In addition, small amounts of borax and potassium sulfate are added to improve the strength of the agar and to ensure that the stone cast or die poured from the agar impression will have a smooth, hard surface.

Irreversible Hydrocolloid (Alginate)

The second type of hydrocolloid is called **alginate**. Alginate is also a seaweed derivative, but it is supplied as a powder. It differs from agar in that it sets by a chemical reaction when mixed with the appropriate amount of water and other components. The powder is a sodium alginate, to which are added a small amount of calcium sulfate, which causes the reaction; silica fillers, which provide "body" and rigidity; sodium phosphate, which retards the chemical reaction to provide ample working time; and potassium sulfate, which ensures that the surfaces of the stone casts poured in the alginate impression will be of good quality. The sodium alginate is soluble in water and when the two are mixed, a sol is formed, similar to the agar sol. In time, the sol forms a gel as the alginate polymer chains become cross-linked by calcium ions. The sodium phosphate slows down the reaction to provide adequate working time.

Alginate is supplied in two different forms. Bulk alginate is supplied in containers about the size of 2-pound coffee cans. The material is also supplied in small packages that are used for individual impressions (Fig. 8-6). The material commonly contains an additive, such as a quaternary ammonium compound, that theoretically aids in the disinfection process. Because alginate powder contains silica dust, a potential biohazard when inhaled, modern alginate powders are coated with a special compound that keeps them from generating dust when the can or package is shaken just before being opened.

Elastic Materials: The Elastomers

There are four basic types of elastomers: the *polysulfides*, the *condensation silicones*, the *polyethers*, and the *addition silicones*. Addition silicones are also known as *polyvinylsiloxanes*. A fifth material, a light-cured impression material based on a urethane polymer, also is commercially available.

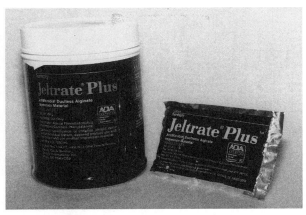

Figure 8–6 Alginate irreversible hydrocolloid impression material supplied in bulk containers and in individual premeasured packages.

The elastomers are supplied in several different consistencies that are used for different applications. For a given type of elastomer, the composition of the different consistencies is similar, and the pastes differ basically in terms of the amount of filler particles that are added to increase their viscosity. As more fillers are added, the consistency of the paste increases and the fluidity decreases. The fillers also serve to reduce the shrinkage that accompanies the setting reaction. The different viscosities are light, medium, and heavy in body. The *light-body* materials are best suited for syringing around prepared teeth to register the finest details, but when held in a tray, they are too fluid to support themselves. In contrast, the *heavy-body* materials are used to fill the tray and provide support for the less viscous and ultimately more flexible light-body materials. *Medium-body* materials are of intermediate viscosity. They can be syringed like light-body materials but also are viscous enough to fill and remain within a tray. A fourth type of material, called a *putty*, is discussed shortly.

Many of the elastomers, especially the polyvinylsiloxanes, are also supplied with different setting times. These materials are often labeled with a numbering system (such as 1:3) that designates the end of working time (first number) and setting time in the mouth (second number). A clinician then has the option of choosing a material with a specified setting time, depending on the application. For example, more complicated impressions of several teeth require more time for placement than does an impression for a single inlay or onlay.

Polysulfide

Polysulfide impression material is the oldest and most economic of the elastomers, although it is not the most accurate or stable. It is supplied in two tubes, one containing the base paste and the other containing the catalyst paste (Fig. 8-7). Both tubes contain the liquid polysulfide polymer. These long-chain, organic polymers contain many sulfhydryl (—SH) groups. This chemical group is also known as a **mercaptan**, and therefore, **mercaptan** and the polysulfides are commonly referred to as mercaptans. The liquid polymer is made into a paste by mixing it with fillers, such as silica particles, and various oils that improve the handling and mixing characteristics of the paste. The catalyst paste differs from the base in that it contains a lead dioxide catalyst and some additional sulfur, both of which enhance the chemical reaction responsible for transforming the paste into an elastic rubber.

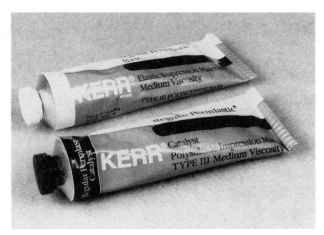

Figure 8–7 Polysulfide impression material supplied in tubes containing the base and catalyst pastes.

The chemical reaction cross-links the polymers through a condensation reaction between sulfhydryl groups (i.e., —SH + —SH → —S—S—), thus producing a rubber. Rubber tires are made in a similar manner. The industrial term for this type of reaction is *vulcanization*, as in vulcanized rubber.

Because of the color of the lead dioxide, the catalyst paste is brown. This paste provides the characteristic odor of the polysulfide impression material and is also responsible for staining clothing and skin with which it comes in contact. The base paste usually is pigmented white, but it too can stain clothing. Because polysulfide is more difficult to use and has more objectionable characteristics than other elastomeric impression materials have, its popularity has diminished substantially. Polysulfide, however, has a slightly greater tear strength than the other elastomers have, which makes it a useful material for impression of teeth with deep undercuts.

Condensation Silicone

The condensation silicon impression materials are made from a silicone polymer. They are supplied either as two-paste systems or as a paste-liquid system similar to the ZOE impression paste. Both pastes of the two-paste system contain the liquid silicone polymer made from polydimethylsiloxane molecules, which contain many hydroxyl (—OH) groups. As with the polysulfide material, fillers are added to the liquid to produce a paste. The base paste also contains a very important organic molecule called an orthoalkylsilicate; addition of this molecule causes the polymer chains to become cross-linked, thus transforming the paste into a fairly rigid and dimensionally stable rubber. The catalyst paste contains the same components as the base, in addition to a tin octoate catalyst. The two pastes are pigmented with different colors to enhance the clinician's ability to discern when the material has been mixed adequately. In the paste-liquid system, the liquid component is labeled as the catalyst. It contains the tin octoate catalyst in a pigmented oil base. Dental-grade and medical-grade silicone rubbers are formulated with tin octoate catalyst so that the materials are relatively nontoxic. In contrast, commercial grades of silicone rubber, such as bathroom caulking, may be extremely toxic.

Polyether

The polyether impression materials are the stiffest of the elastomers when set. Their name derives from the fact that they are composed of polyether polymer

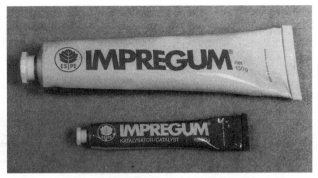

Figure 8–8 Base and catalyst for a two-paste polyether impression material.

molecules. The liquid polymers are mixed with fillers to provide rigidity. Oils are added as plasticizers to enhance the mixing and handling characteristics of the material. These materials also are distributed as two-paste systems (Fig. 8-8). The catalyst paste differs from the base paste in that the former contains an aromatic sulfonic acid ester that enhances the further polymerization and cross-linking of the polymer chains during the chemical reaction. This reaction is responsible for transforming the paste into a stiff polyether rubber. Because of its tremendous stiffness, full-arch impressions made from these materials may be difficult to remove from the mouth. Therefore, some clinicians suggest using them for impressions of a few teeth or a quadrant.

Addition Silicone

Addition silicone impression materials are also known as polyvinylsiloxanes because they contain silicone polymers that have many vinyl ($C{=}C$) groups. These vinyl molecules engage in further polymerization and cross-linking during the setting reaction. They are supplied in three different forms. One form is the typical two-paste system (Fig. 8-9). The second form is a gun-and-cartridge system in which the base and catalyst are dispensed from side-by-side cylinders directly through a series of alpha helices (or propeller blades) that act as a mixing device (Fig. 8-9). The mixed impression paste can be injected directly into the mouth or into an impression tray. The pastes contain fillers to provide rigidity to the set material, and the catalyst paste contains chloroplatinic acid. The third form in which these materials are supplied is as a heavy putty used in the **putty-wash** technique. The base and catalyst putties are supplied in plastic tubs (Fig. 8-9). They are scooped out and mixed together by hand, by kneading. Certain compounds present in latex examination gloves inhibit the setting of these materials, so vinyl

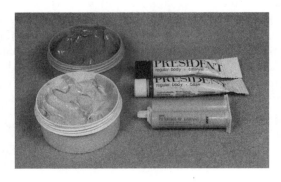

Figure 8–9 Addition silicone (polyvinyl-siloxane) impression materials supplied as a putty-wash system, as two pastes, and as an automix cartridge.

gloves should be worn. An initial impression is made of the tissues by loading a stock plastic impression tray with the material and placing it into the mouth. Once it hardens to a rigid but elastic material, it is removed from the mouth. Subsequently, the more fluid wash material (light body) is injected or dispensed around the prepared teeth as well as into the initial putty impression. The impression is then reinserted into the mouth to acquire the fine detail of the oral structures. Both the putty and wash set by the same chemical reaction and are pigmented differently for easy identification. Because they have the same composition, they adhere well to one another and are not easily separated.

The addition silicones are hydrophobic materials. This characteristic has led to some problems with air bubbles trapped on the surface of the impression when pouring gypsum casts and dies. **Surfactant** molecules such as soap have been added to the materials to make them more hydrophilic, thus achieving a lower contact angle with water-based materials such as gypsum. Recall that a lower contact angle denotes better wetting, a condition that is desirable when trying to pour "bubble-free" casts. Many manufacturers produce these newer "hydrophilic" elastomeric impression materials.

■ Mixing and Handling of Impression Materials

Because of their differences in both composition and setting reactions, not all of the impression materials are mixed and handled in the same way. In this section, the proper techniques to be used for each type are outlined for all of the impression materials.

Inelastic Materials

Impression Compound

Compound is very hard and brittle at room temperature; therefore, it must be softened and made to flow to be useful as an impression material. This can be done by heating the compound to a temperature only 8 to 10°C above oral temperatures. *Why should this temperature be significant?*

> The compound will flow best at higher temperatures, where it becomes more fluid. Temperatures above 45 to 50°C, however, cause burns and damage oral tissues.

Therefore, it is important to minimize the heating of the compound. The goal is to produce flow properties adequate to make an accurate replica of the important tissues while not harming the patient. In addition, the material must be rigid when cooled down to mouth temperature; otherwise, it would distort on removal from the tissues. The material is used most effectively over a narrow range of temperatures, and the dental personnel have complete control over this behavior.

Tray compound usually is softened in a water bath that can be accurately controlled. Although compound also can be softened directly over the flame of a Bunsen burner or alcohol torch, more uniform heating of large pieces is accomplished in a water bath. Because the thermal conductivity of the compound is very low, the outside will soften first and the inside last, so sufficient time must be taken to ensure a uniform heating. After it is softened, it is placed into a stock metal tray and applied to the tissues. It is allowed to cool and harden, thus forming the custom tray directly in the mouth. It also is possible to form the tray on a plaster cast in the same way that acrylic custom trays are made (see Chapter 12).

Compound also can be used to make an impression of a prepared tooth. The stick form of the material usually is softened over a flame and then pressed into a copper matrix band that has been adapted to the tooth in such a way that all undercuts are excluded. Water can be sprayed onto the warm material to hasten its cooling, but the clinician must hold the material firmly in place during this process to avoid distorting the impression.

Zinc Oxide Eugenol

In contrast to compound, ZOE pastes harden by a chemical reaction. Therefore, the two components must be adequately mixed to ensure uniformity. Because the oils present in the pastes have a tendency to be absorbed by ordinary paper pads, these impression materials, like the cements and bases discussed in Chapter 4, must be mixed on glass slabs or special pads made with oil-impervious coatings. Loss of oil from the paste would change the setting behavior of the material.

The base and catalyst pastes are squeezed from the tubes in equal lengths and diameters. The brown paste is then picked up onto a stiff-bladed steel spatula and added to the white paste. The two pastes are mixed with sweeping strokes across the entire area of the pad or slab. The material at the bottom of the mix routinely should be scraped from the pad or slab to ensure that all of the paste gets mixed together. Mixing is completed when the mix takes on a homogeneous color, devoid of streaks from the individual pastes. The procedure should take 30 to 45 seconds.

After mixing, the paste is spread in a uniform, thin layer into the impression tray (which is made from either dental acrylic or impression compound). The tray is then seated in the mouth and held firmly in place for approximately 4 to 5 minutes, until the material hardens. The edges of the material can be probed to determine whether setting is complete. The impression is washed with cold water (warm or hot water may distort the impression or tray) and then disinfected before pouring a stone or plaster cast (see the section on disinfection at the end of this chapter).

As is the case for the ZOE cements, the impression material sets faster when the operatory is warm. More important, moisture contamination hastens the set of the material; therefore, the tubes should always be tightly sealed and stored in a cool and dry place.

The eugenol in the material can be irritating and may cause tissue burns under certain conditions. Any eugenol that is left on tissues can be removed with a solvent, such as oil of orange or spearmint. Coating the lips with petroleum jelly before taking the impression will inhibit the paste from adhering and facilitate cleanup. As an alternative, zinc oxide impression pastes without eugenol have been produced. They are similar to the noneugenol temporary cements described in Chapter 4.

Elastic Materials: The Hydrocolloids

Alginate (Irreversible Hydrocolloid)

Alginate is called an irreversible hydrocolloid because it forms an elastic material through a chemical reaction that cross-links its polymer chains. Because the strength and stability of the material come from the polymeric alginate, correct water-to-powder ratios and proper mixing technique are important. When the material is supplied in bulk, a special scoop is provided for accurate dispensing.

Likewise, a plastic cylinder with special markings is provided for measuring the correct amount of water. Because the powder will harden in the presence of water, the container needs to be sealed after each use. This is one reason why individual packages may be more desirable.

Alginates are mixed by hand in rubber bowls with stiff, wide-bladed steel spatulas (Procedure Display 8-1). The same type of rubber bowl is used to mix plaster

PROCEDURE DISPLAY 8-1

Mixing Alginate Impression Material

Equipment checklist
- Alginate (bulk container or individual package)
- Plastic measuring cylinder for water
- Supplied scoop for powder (if using bulk material)
- Rubber mixing bowl
- Stiff, wide-bladed steel spatula
- Prepared metal or plastic impression tray
- Disinfectant and plastic bag

STEP 1: **Proportioning**
- Measure cool (20°C; 70°F) water for required number of scoops
- Fluff container or package
- Measure appropriate number of scoops of powder; level with spatula blade
- Add powder to bowl
- Add water to powder

STEP 2: **Mixing**
- Stir powder and water vigorously to wet powder completely
- Strop (wipe) mix against side of bowl for 60 seconds to homogenize and remove bubbles
- Visually inspect mix for creamy, thick consistency

STEP 3: **Filling tray and taking impression**
- Wipe alginate into tray with spatula from posterior region forward
- Continue wiping in from posterior until tray is full with uniform layer and minimal material is left in the posterior region
- Smooth alginate surface with moistened finger (at this point, the operator may take some alginate from the bowl and wipe it onto the occlusal surfaces of the teeth with a finger to help get a better impression)
- Seat tray from posterior region first to displace material in anterior direction
- Press middle and front of tray against tissue to produce uniform layer of material
- Hold tray in place until alginate is set, as determined by probing with finger (4 to 5 minutes)
- To remove impression, lift lips and cheek away with fingers to break seal
- Grasp handle and pull tray away from teeth with quick motion

STEP 4: **Cleanup and disinfection**
- Wash impression under cool running water to eliminate saliva and blood
- Spray impression with disinfectant and seal in plastic bag for 10 minutes
- Peel rubbery alginate from bowl and spatula and dispose of in trash
- Pour impression as soon as possible (if waiting up to 1 hour, store in moist paper towels in container)

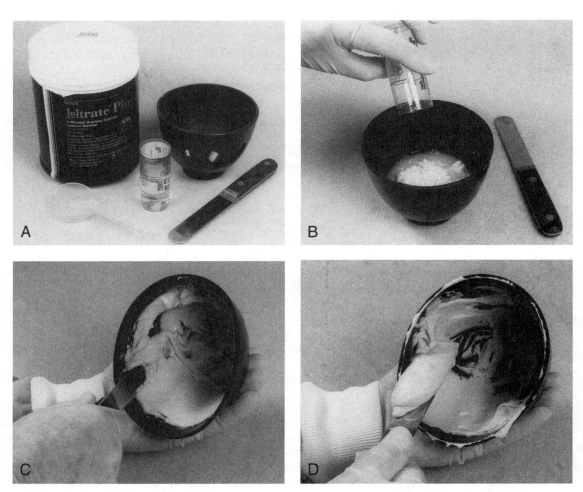

Figure 8–10 A. Bulk container of powder, rubber mixing bowl, spatula, special graduated cylinder filled with water, and measuring scoop for the preparation of an alginate impression. **B.** Premeasured cool water being poured into the bowl containing the alginate impression powder. **C.** Stropping motion used to mix the alginate impression material and eliminate air bubbles by wiping the mix against the side of the rubber bowl. **D.** Final alginate impression material mix displaying the appropriate creamy texture and uniform consistency. **E.** Stock metal rimlock tray (*right*) and a metal tray (*center*) and plastic tray (*left*) containing holes to hold the alginate impression material within the tray during removal from the mouth. **F.** Alginate impression material being loaded into the tray. **G.** Alginate impression after removal from the mouth and trimming of the posterior region with a knife.

or stone. The manufacturer's recommendations are followed for the powder-to-liquid ratio. First, the plastic cylinder is filled to the appropriate level with water at room temperature (i.e., 68 to 72°C) (Fig. 8-10*A*). The temperature of the water is important because warm water will hasten the set of the alginate and cold water will delay it more than is desirable. A mix made with water at room temperature also is most comfortable for the patient. The cylinder has two or three markings on its side. Usually, the first marking provides enough water for one scoop, the second for two scoops, and so on. The powder container is then shaken, or "fluffed," to loosen the powder and prevent clumping. This also ensures that a consistent amount of powder is dispensed each time. The scoop is then used to remove the appropriate amount of powder by filling it and leveling it with the blade of the spatula. The powder is then poured directly into the bowl (Fig. 8-10*B*). The

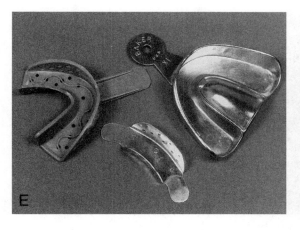

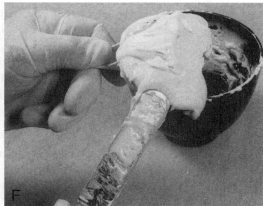

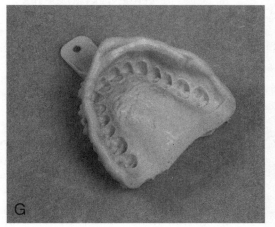

Figure 8–10 *(Continued)*

powder and water are vigorously spatulated (at a rate of approximately 100 turns/minute) for 1 full minute. During the process, the mixture is "stropped," or wiped along the sides of the bowl, to push air bubbles out and produce a homogeneous mix (Fig. 8-10C). Care is taken not to overmix, because this limits the working time and breaks up the gel that is forming, thus reducing the strength of the final alginate. Likewise, inadequate mixing produces a grainy material with low strength. The final mix should appear creamy and smooth and remain on the spatula when lifted from the bowl (Fig. 8-10D).

Metal or plastic trays are used to carry alginate impression materials to the mouth. Adhesives are not required to hold the impression in the tray. Instead, the trays contain either holes or a metal rim to lock the impression in (Fig. 8-10E). The trays come in stock sizes, and the proper one should be selected and tried in the patient before mixing the material. Immediately after mixing, the alginate is quickly wiped into the metal impression tray from the posterior portion of one side and pushed anteriorly (Fig. 8-10F). Subsequent additions are made in the same manner to avoid trapping large regions of air bubbles in the impression. After loading the tray, the surface of the material is smoothed out with a wet finger, with care taken to ensure that only the minimal amount is present in the posterior region. ***What is the reason for being concerned about the amount of material in the tray?***

It is important to have a uniform layer of impression material in the tray to avoid missing any of the tissues. Also, the amount of material in the posterior region is important because on seating the tray, the impression material in the posterior portion of the tray may be displaced down the patient's throat, stimulating a gag reflex. Therefore, the tray is seated in the patient's mouth from the posterior region first, to displace the material anteriorly in the patient's mouth.

Once the back is seated, the tray is pressed up (or down) against the tissues, with care taken to leave a uniform layer throughout the tray. The tray must be held steady for an additional 2 to 3 minutes (total time from start of mix is about 4 to 5 minutes), until the alginate is completely set. The edges can be probed with the finger to determine whether complete gelation has occurred. The alginate will no longer be tacky to the touch, and the impression will feel stiff and spring back rapidly after probing.

The impression is removed from the mouth by first breaking the peripheral seal of the impression with the gingiva by lifting away the lips and cheek with the fingers in areas away from the critical regions. The handle of the tray is then grasped tightly, and the impression is removed with a rapid thrust perpendicular to the occlusal plane. The material is stronger and more resistant to distortion when removed quickly, hence the importance of this rapid removal technique. Subsequently, the impression is washed well in cool water to remove debris or blood (Fig. 8-10*G*). The excess water is shaken out, and the impression is then disinfected (see section at the end of this chapter).

As soon as is possible, the impression should be poured with plaster or stone. The alginate will lose water quickly, so immediate pouring is important. If pouring is delayed for any reason, the impression should be wrapped in wet paper toweling to minimize water loss and distortion. Any distortion of the impression will render it inaccurate and useless. A rule of thumb is that pouring of the impression should never be delayed for longer than 1 hour. The steps for pouring the gypsum cast are detailed in Chapter 9.

Agar (Reversible Hydrocolloid)

Agar is a reversible hydrocolloid because the physical state of the material can be changed back and forth between a liquid sol and a rubbery gel simply by altering temperature. Agar is an accurate impression material but, because it requires the use of additional equipment, has largely been replaced by the other elastic impression materials. It is still used successfully by some clinicians, however.

Agar is not mixed and does not undergo a chemical reaction. Instead, it is treated much like impression compound. It is heated in a special piece of equipment to make it liquid and is cooled in the mouth with special trays that can be attached to the dental unit so that cold water can be circulated through them. The heating to produce the sol takes place in one section of a hydrocolloid unit (Fig. 8-11). Its separate chambers are designed to accomplish three different tasks. First, tubes of agar and the carpules containing the syringeable agar are placed into the conditioning chamber, which contains boiling water at 100°C (212°F). After approximately 10 minutes, the stiff agar gel transforms into the fluid sol state. When the gel has already been liquefied and cooled at some earlier time, it usually is necessary to heat it in the conditioning bath longer (i.e., 20 minutes) to break down the gel structure completely.

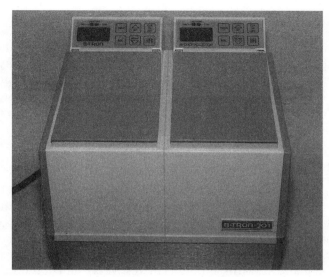

Figure 8–11 Hydrocolloid unit showing the compartments for the conditioning bath, held at 100°C, to produce the gel-to-sol transformation and then serve as the storage bath, held at 65°C, and the tempering bath, held at 45°C, to cool the agar hydrocolloid before placing it into the mouth.

After the sol has been created, the tubes and the syringe material (still in the syringe) can be transferred into the storage bath, which contains water at 65°C (150°F). At this temperature, the sol will not transform to gel, and the tubes can be stored until needed, up to several days. Even if the material is needed right away, the tube should be left in the storage bath for at least 10 minutes to allow all of the agar in the tube to cool down to that temperature. Agar, like compound, has a low thermal conductivity, so adequate time must be allotted for its temperature to equilibrate throughout its mass.

When the dental personnel are ready to take the impression, the tube of agar can be removed from the storage bath and placed into the tempering bath, which contains water at 45°C (110°F). The tube is kept in this bath for approximately 5 minutes. *What might be the purpose of the third bath?*

> The tempering bath reduces the temperature of the agar to a level that will not burn the patient. Although the agar will not immediately form a gel at this temperature, it will become rubbery in time, so care must be taken not to leave the agar in this bath too long.

Just before the tray is removed from the tempering bath, the syringeable form of the agar in the carpule is removed from the storage bath, the syringe is loaded, and the material is injected around the prepared tooth. Note that the syringe material is never placed into the tempering bath. Any cooling of the syringe material inhibits its ability to flow out of the small opening of the syringe and around the prepared teeth, resulting in a loss of accuracy. Because the material is being dispensed in small amounts from a small orifice, it cools to a tolerable temperature rapidly and does not harm the tissues when taken directly from the storage bath.

While the syringe material is being applied, the tube of tempered agar is removed from the bath and used to fill the special tray. (Note that an alternative is to temper the material in the tray while the syringe material is being loaded and applied to the prepared tooth. On removal from the tempering bath, however, the agar will have a surface skin that must be scraped off before seating the tray.)

When the tray is ready, the hoses from the dental unit are attached, and the tray is seated against the tissue and held firmly in place. Cool water is then circulated through the tray to chill and gel the impression material quickly. Once it completely gels, as determined by probing for elasticity, the tray is removed in a manner similar to that used for an alginate impression. The impression is treated in the same manner as the alginate impression and is equally unstable because of its high water content. Therefore, agar impressions should be poured in stone or plaster as soon as possible.

Elastic Materials: The Elastomers

All of the elastomers are supplied as two-paste systems that are mixed in a similar manner. All undergo chemical reactions, and therefore, their setting can be hastened by higher temperatures. This is especially true of the polysulfide materials. In addition, the set of the polysulfide can be hastened inadvertently by the presence of a small amount of moisture, which makes the use of these materials very problematic in warm, humid climates where air conditioning is not always available. The polyvinylsiloxanes (addition silicones) and polyethers also are supplied as automix systems. As mentioned, the two pastes are mixed together in a propeller mixer attached to the cartridge of the gun from which they are dispensed, thereby lengthening the working time of the materials by eliminating the mixing period. Some manufacturers also produce motor-driven mechanical mixing systems for impression materials. These may be in the form of a bench-top model or an electric-powered handheld gun device. This section discusses the mixing procedure for all two-paste, elastomeric impression materials (Procedure Display 8-2), and the use of the gun-and-cartridge system is described in more detail.

Two-Paste Systems

Equal lengths of the base and catalyst pastes are dispensed next to one another (but not touching) on the pad supplied by the manufacturer (Fig. 8-12A). These pads are large, providing an appropriate surface over which to mix. Because of its viscous nature, a stiff, tapered steel spatula is used to mix the material. First, the catalyst paste is picked up on the spatula and added to the base paste, and the two are mixed together for about 10 seconds with a circular stirring motion (Fig. 8-12B). The material is then wiped across the entire surface of the pad with a pressing motion, with the aim of producing a homogeneous, creamy consistency (Fig. 8-12C). Frequent scraping of the material from the pad will help to ensure a proper mix. The entire mixing procedure should take about 45 to 60 seconds. Subsequently, the material can be loaded into a syringe or the impression tray for seating.

Elastomers often are used with acrylic custom trays. An adhesive must be applied to the inside surface of the custom tray to retain the impression on removal from the mouth. The volatile adhesive is painted onto the inside surface of the tray and then allowed to dry so that it is tacky but not wet. Note that each material has a different composition; therefore, each is supplied with a different adhesive, and they cannot be used interchangeably. When an adhesive is not available, it is possible to drill holes in the tray to retain the impression.

Elastomeric impressions should be removed from the mouth with a steady force. It is not so important to remove them quickly, as is the case for the hydrocolloids. These polymer systems have much greater tear resistance than the hydrocolloids, and thus removal is less of a concern. The one exception might be the polyether material, which is very rigid but has a relatively poor tear resistance.

PROCEDURE DISPLAY 8-2

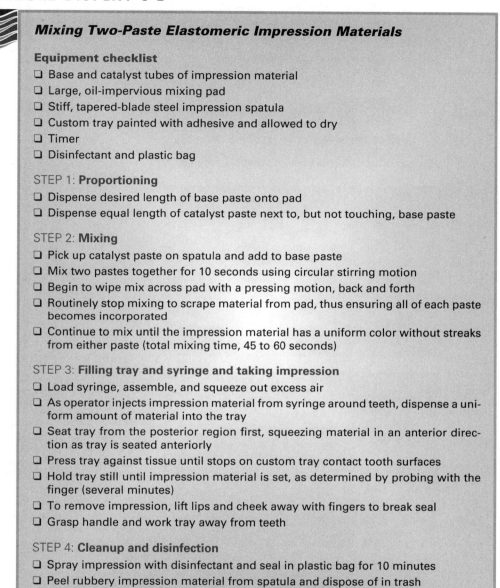

Mixing Two-Paste Elastomeric Impression Materials

Equipment checklist
❑ Base and catalyst tubes of impression material
❑ Large, oil-impervious mixing pad
❑ Stiff, tapered-blade steel impression spatula
❑ Custom tray painted with adhesive and allowed to dry
❑ Timer
❑ Disinfectant and plastic bag

STEP 1: **Proportioning**
❑ Dispense desired length of base paste onto pad
❑ Dispense equal length of catalyst paste next to, but not touching, base paste

STEP 2: **Mixing**
❑ Pick up catalyst paste on spatula and add to base paste
❑ Mix two pastes together for 10 seconds using circular stirring motion
❑ Begin to wipe mix across pad with a pressing motion, back and forth
❑ Routinely stop mixing to scrape material from pad, thus ensuring all of each paste becomes incorporated
❑ Continue to mix until the impression material has a uniform color without streaks from either paste (total mixing time, 45 to 60 seconds)

STEP 3: **Filling tray and syringe and taking impression**
❑ Load syringe, assemble, and squeeze out excess air
❑ As operator injects impression material from syringe around teeth, dispense a uniform amount of material into the tray
❑ Seat tray from the posterior region first, squeezing material in an anterior direction as tray is seated anteriorly
❑ Press tray against tissue until stops on custom tray contact tooth surfaces
❑ Hold tray still until impression material is set, as determined by probing with the finger (several minutes)
❑ To remove impression, lift lips and cheek away with fingers to break seal
❑ Grasp handle and work tray away from teeth

STEP 4: **Cleanup and disinfection**
❑ Spray impression with disinfectant and seal in plastic bag for 10 minutes
❑ Peel rubbery impression material from spatula and dispose of in trash
❑ Pour impression after about 1 hour (time can be extended for many days when using addition silicone and polyether materials

Contact with the materials should be avoided because the oils and pigments used in all of the elastomers stain clothing. Cleanup of the spatula is easy, however; simply waiting for the material to set and become rubbery allows one to peel it off the blade. Disinfection of elastomeric impressions is addressed at the end of this chapter.

Although certain elastomeric impressions should be poured as soon as possible, this is not a concern for the polyethers and addition silicones. In fact, it is ideal to delay pouring of the addition silicones for at least 45 minutes to 1 hour after

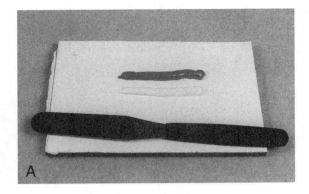

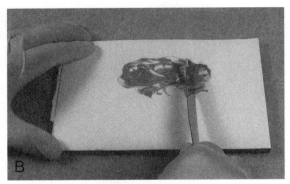

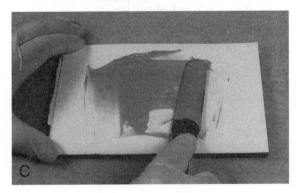

Figure 8–12 A. Equal lengths of the base and catalyst of a two-paste polyvinylsiloxane impression material dispensed onto a pad for mixing. **B.** Circular motion used in the initial stages of mixing the two-paste elastomeric impression materials. **C.** Wiping motion used to mix completely the two-paste elastomeric impression materials to a uniform, streak-free color.

taking the impression. Many of these materials release hydrogen gas during the setting reaction. If the impression is poured too soon, this "outgassing" will produce tiny bubbles on the surface of the model or die material. The delay in pouring has no effect on the dimensional stability of these materials; because both polyethers and polyvinylsiloxanes have excellent dimensional stability, they can be poured up with no loss of accuracy even after a delay of several days and probably several weeks.

Gun-and-Cartridge System

The gun-and-cartridge system offers a simple and effective way to mix and dispense impression materials. The pastes are supplied in two cylinders mounted side by side in a gun similar to the one used to apply caulking around bathroom

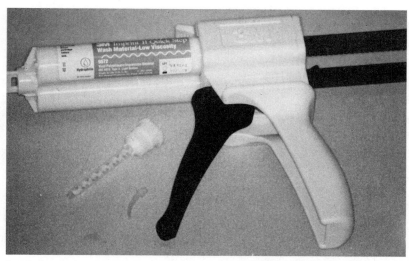

Figure 8–13 Gun-and-cartridge system for mixing and dispensing elastomeric impression materials. Note the fine tip that allows for direct intraoral injection of the impression material.

fixtures or windows (Fig. 8-13). In this case, however, a second tube containing a plastic propeller-type assembly is attached to the end of the cylinders. As the impression material is extruded into the mixing tube and travels down its length, the two different pastes are mixed together to produce a homogeneous material (Fig. 8-14*A*). Special tips are supplied to allow the clinician to dispense the material directly into the mouth. The material can also be extruded directly into a plastic syringe, filling from the front first to avoid leaving a large bolus of air at the back (Fig. 8-14*B* and *C*). This syringe then is used to inject the impression material around the prepared teeth in the mouth. During this procedure, the assistant can load the impression tray with material dispensed directly from the gun (Fig. 8-14*D*).

Although polyvinylsiloxane impression materials have become the materials of choice because of their excellent physical characteristics and accuracy, some care must be taken when manipulating them. It has long been known that the setting of these materials is inhibited when they contact latex examination gloves, rubber dams, or any surface that has had recent contact with these products. It has been suggested that washing the gloves before touching the material will eliminate the problem, but evidence to the contrary exists; the sulfur compounds believed to be responsible for the inhibition of setting probably are not completely extracted from the gloves during washing. Therefore, it is prudent to avoid touching the impression material with a glove, as well as to avoid touching any surface to be impressed with the gloves. The use of vinyl gloves is another option. Similarly, many of these materials may experience an inhibition of setting on surfaces that have come into contact with various organic chemicals, such as methacrylates from temporary restorative materials. Therefore, it is recommended that the impression be made of a prepared tooth before making the temporary. Otherwise, the surface of the impression material in contact with the prepared tooth may not completely set and may have a wrinkled appearance.

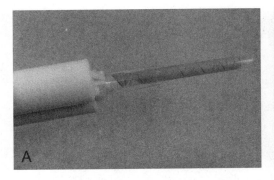

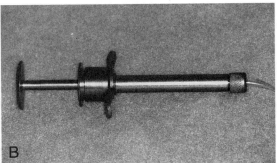

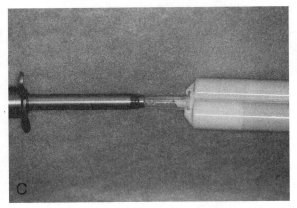

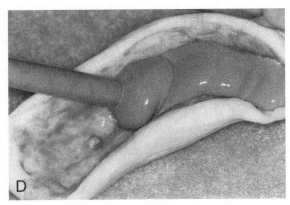

Figure 8–14 A. Gun-and-cartridge system used to mix and dispense a polyvinylsiloxane impression material. Note the uniform mixing taking place in the propeller tip as the material is discharged. **B.** Syringe for the intraoral application of an elastomeric impression material. **C.** Syringe being filled directly from the cartridge gun. **D.** Impression tray being filled directly from the cartridge gun. Note the adhesive covering the inside of the tray and the occlusal stop protruding from the bottom of the tray.

■ *Characteristics of Impression Materials*

Because of their different compositions, impression materials have a broad range of properties and characteristics. Many of these are summarized for the elastic impression materials in Table 8-2 and are discussed in this section. When appropriate, the properties of the inelastic materials are also discussed.

Flexibility

Flexibility is an important property for an impression material because it is a measure of stiffness. In the discussion of mechanical properties in Chapter 2, it was mentioned that maximum flexibility was a measure of the extent to which a material could be strained or deformed while remaining in its elastic region. It also

TABLE 8-2. **Comparison of the Properties of Elastic Impression Materials**						
	Alg	**Agar**	**PS**	**CS**	**PE**	**AS**
Flexibility (%)	12	11	7	5	3	4
Elastic recovery (%)	97.3	98.8	97.9	99.5	98.5	99.8
Tear resistance	Good	Poor	Good	Good	Good	Good
Flow (%)	—	—	0.50–2.00	0.08–0.14	0.02–0.05	0.01–0.04
Relative stability	Poor	Poor	Fair	Fair	Good	Good
Setting shrinkage (%)	—	—	0.25	0.6	0.1	0.05
Relative setting time	Slow	Slow	Slow	Slow	Fast	Fast
Wettability by gypsum	Excellent	Excellent	Good	Poor	Good	Poor/good

Alg, alginate (irreversible hydrocolloid); agar (reversible hydrocolloid); PS, polysulfide (mercaptan); CS, condensation silicone; PE, polyether; AS, addition silicone (polyvinylsiloxane).

was stated that this was an important property for an impression material that would be deformed by some small amount during removal from the tissues. The maximum flexibility of the elastic impression materials is sufficient to allow this deformation without recording a permanent change in shape (i.e., a distortion). In contrast, the inelastic impression materials have virtually no flexibility. They are rigid, do not flex, and fracture when deformed. Because they have no flexibility, inelastic materials cannot be removed from undercuts and, therefore, are inappropriate for dentulous patients (Fig. 8-1). Clearly, the lower the percent flexibility of an elastic impression material, the more difficult it will be to remove the material from the mouth.

The data in Table 8-2 demonstrate that the polyether material is the least flexible of the elastic impression materials, making it the stiffest and most difficult to remove from the mouth. Because of their stiffness, these materials are recommended only for quadrant impressions instead of full-arch impressions. The addition silicone materials are only slightly less stiff than the polyethers. Although both of these materials are relatively rigid, their flexibility is sufficient to allow removal from undercuts without permanent deformation or distortion. The hydrocolloid materials are the most flexible of the elastic impression materials and, therefore, the easiest to remove from around teeth. The agar material is chilled before removal, however, significantly increasing its stiffness, compared with the same material at oral temperatures.

Accuracy

Elastic recovery is a measure of an impression material's accuracy. This property is of the utmost importance because the primary function of an impression material is to reproduce accurately and reliably the relationships between oral tissues. Therefore, the higher the value for elastic recovery, the more accurate the material. Simply stated, this property describes the ability of the material to spring back to its original shape when it is distorted by pulling it from undercuts. Another term used to describe this property is **permanent set**, which describes the percentage of permanent change in shape that occurs during removal from undercuts. In the latter usage, materials with low values are most ideal. Because inelastic impression materials do not possess any significant elasticity, this property is not applicable to them. The elastic impression materials with the greatest elastic recovery are the silicones, but there is virtually no clinical difference between materials with an elastic recovery of 98.5% or more. Table 8-2 shows that the polysulfide materials are not as accurate as the other elastic materials, with the exception of alginates. Alginates have the poorest accuracy and, therefore, are not used as the final impression material for crown and bridge prosthetics.

Tear Strength

The tear resistance of an impression material is an important consideration during its removal from the mouth. Obviously, distortion will occur and detail may be lost if the material tears in critical areas. Tears may be noticed in the interproximal areas of nonprepared teeth where contacts are tight, but such tears usually are not a problem. Table 8-2 shows that with the exception of the agar hydrocolloid, there is little difference in the tear strength of the elastic impression materials, though the polysulfides are slightly stronger. Although the rigidity of the polyethers may suggest a lower tear strength, studies have not shown this to be the case. The agar, however, is easily torn compared with the other materials. It is not a tough material, and care should be taken during handling of a final impression to avoid tearing and distortion.

Stability

Stability is an important property for an impression material, but only from the standpoint of convenience. For example, if an accurate impression is poured up in gypsum immediately after it is made, it is not important if several hours later the impression has severely distorted and is no longer useful. This property is assessed by measuring the amount of flow, or change in shape, that takes place in an impression material within some period of time after making an impression, usually 1 hour. A smaller value for flow is most ideal. The data in Table 8-2 show that the addition silicones and polyethers have the least flow and are, therefore, the most stable of the impression materials. The benefit of this stability is that these impressions can be sent to a laboratory to be poured up instead of pouring them up in the office. These impressions are stable for weeks and perhaps longer, although it would seem prudent to use them within a day or so. In contrast, polysulfides exhibit significant flow and have only fair dimensional stability. Therefore, impressions made from this material should be poured up within hours.

The least stable materials are the hydrocolloids. Because they contain such a large amount of water, they are terribly unstable and must be poured immediately. As mentioned, they can be wrapped in wet towels (to maintain a 100% humidity environment) and poured within an hour or so, but longer waiting times are contraindicated. Therefore, the hydrocolloids are the least convenient of the elastic impression materials. The inelastic materials are stable as long as they are kept at room temperature. Because compound is a thermoplastic material, exposure to elevated temperatures will result in distortions and a loss of accuracy.

Dimensional Change

Another characteristic of the impression material has a profound influence on accuracy: Because the materials transform from a liquid paste to an elastic solid, often by polymerization, there is a dimensional change accompanying the reaction. Of the elastic impression materials, the addition silicones are the least affected by setting shrinkage. Table 8-2 shows that these materials undergo only a small setting shrinkage. The shrinkage of the polyethers, although slightly higher than that of the addition silicones, also is low. The polysulfides shrink by about five times the amount of the addition silicones, but this change is clinically insignificant. The high shrinkage of the condensation silicones is of some concern, however. A shrinkage of this magnitude negates to a great extent the outstanding elastic properties of these materials, causing them to be the least accurate of the group. This is one reason why these materials never were as popular as the polysulfides. This large dimensional change also was the driving force behind the development of the putty-wash technique. The polymerization shrinkage problem is minimized by the use of a very stiff putty for a first impression, followed by a wash that uses the bare minimum of material to record the final impression. Total shrinkage is related to the quantity of material, and use of the smallest amount of material feasible therefore limits the overall dimensional change to a clinically insignificant level.

Surface Wetting

Another important property for making accurate castings is the ability to produce accurate models and dies from the impression. To reproduce clearly and accurately all of the sharp angles and irregularities of the impression material, the water-based gypsum material must wet the impression material well. The idea is not to adhere the stone or plaster to the impression but to allow intimate contact between the two so that the detail of the impression is recorded in the gypsum. Therefore, one might expect that water-based impression materials would be best wet by gypsum and create the best dies and models. Table 8-2 shows that this is the case. The hydrocolloids have the best wettability by gypsum and can be poured with the fewest bubbles.

This does not mean that accurate models and dies cannot be produced from the other materials, but the procedure is a bit more demanding. Often, a surfactant, such as a dilute detergent solution supplied usually in a spray bottle, is used to coat the impression before pouring the stone or plaster. This surfactant reduces the contact angle between the gypsum product and the hydrophobic impression surface, thus enhancing wetting. The wettability of the polysulfide and polyether materials is good, so bubble formation is less of a problem than for the silicones. Certain addition silicones, however, have been modified by incorporating surfactants to make them more hydrophilic expressly for this purpose.

Working and Setting Time

Generally, the set of the addition silicones and polyethers is rapid, compared with that of the other materials. Normal working times for these materials are 1 to 2 minutes, with setting occurring within 4 to 5 minutes in the mouth. The ideal material would have a long working time and a fast set once placed into the mouth. The higher temperature of the oral cavity, compared with the office temperature, is responsible for some acceleration in setting. The development of gun-and-cartridge mixing systems has greatly facilitated the use of the faster setting impression materials by increasing the usable working time. These mixing systems also minimize the number of air bubbles produced in the mix.

■ *Disinfection of Impression Materials*

The American Dental Association has developed general recommendations for infection control in the dental office that include specific recommendations for impression materials. The recommendations are based on studies showing no significant loss in accuracy as a result of an effective disinfection procedure. The impression should be rinsed first, to remove blood, debris, and saliva, and then treated as outlined next:

- *ZOE and compound impressions:* ZOE impressions may be disinfected by immersing them in a glutaraldehyde (e.g., Banicide and Cidex) or an iodophor (e.g., Biocide) for a minimum of 10 minutes and a maximum of 30 minutes. Compound can be treated the same way, except that hypochlorite compounds (e.g., commercial bleach) should be substituted for glutaraldehydes.
- *Alginate:* Alginate impressions can be immersed or sprayed with a disinfectant, but the resultant casts may be optimal when a spray technique is used. Therefore, a typical procedure is to spray the alginate impression with an iodophor or hypochlorite compound and then place it into a sealed plastic bag for approximately 10 minutes.
- *Agar:* Agar impressions usually are immersed for 10 minutes or so in an iodophor or glutaraldehyde. Agar can also be disinfected with a hypochlorite solution, such as common bleach.
- *Elastomers:* Because these materials do not contain water and, therefore, are more stable, it is less critical that they be disinfected for only 10 minutes. All types can be immersed in appropriate solutions, such as the glutaraldehydes or iodophors. Shorter immersions (i.e., 2 to 3 minutes) in chlorine solutions may be best for polyethers, however. Another option is to treat the elastomers like alginate and spray them with the disinfectant before placing them into a sealed plastic bag for 10 minutes.

Summary

An impression is a negative replica of a dental structure, such as a prepared tooth. Dental impression materials are classified as inelastic (rigid) or elastic (flexible). Inelastic impression materials, such as plaster, ZOE, and compound, are used mainly to make impressions of edentulous patients. Elastic impression materials are used for all applications and are subdivided into hydrocolloids (agar and alginate) or elastomers (polysulfide, condensation silicone, addition silicone or polyvinylsiloxane, and polyether). The hydrocolloid, agar, is a reversible material that transforms between a paste and solid rubber through temperature change. It is an accurate but unstable material that is used for crown and bridge preparations. Alginate is similar to agar, being a seaweed derivative, but it is irreversible because it sets by a chemical reaction. This water-based material is also unstable; it also is less accurate and is used mainly to make study models and impressions with less stringent requirements for accuracy.

The elastomers are all fairly stable polymeric materials that transform from a paste to a solid by irreversible chemical reactions. The polyvinylsiloxanes and polyethers are the most accurate and most stable. They are also very stiff and rigid materials. Most elastomers are sold as two different-colored pastes that must be adequately mixed mechanically or by hand to produce a homogeneously colored and streak-free material to ensure ideal accuracy and handling and setting characteristics. Disinfection of impressions is accomplished by spraying with or immersing in a variety of suitable agents.

STUDY QUESTIONS AND PROBLEM SOLVING

1. **Which of the following is (are) a difference(s) between inelastic and elastic impression materials?**
   a. Ability to reproduce fine detail
   b. Set in a reasonable time
   c. Can be removed from undercuts
   d. Can be successfully disinfected

2. **Which impression material(s) could theoretically be disinfected and used to make another impression?**
   a. Polyether
   b. Agar
   c. Alginate
   d. Compound

3. **Agar hydrocolloid can be used for accurate crown and bridge impression taking, whereas alginate cannot because:**
   a. Alginate is less stable
   b. Alginate is less accurate
   c. Agar is faster setting
   d. Agar is more flexible

4. **The setting rate of which inelastic impression material can be accidentally accelerated by exposure to moisture during preparation?**
   a. Alginate
   b. ZOE paste
   c. Compound
   d. Addition silicone

5. **Which of the following is *not* a correct step during the preparation of an alginate impression?**
   a. Wiping the mix against the side of the bowl to remove air bubbles
   b. Mixing for 60 seconds to provide ample working time
   c. Loading a water-cooled tray from the posterior to eliminate trapped air
   d. Holding the tray in the mouth for several minutes to ensure accuracy

6. **Which of the following statements applies best to the polyvinylsiloxane impression materials?**
   a. Stiffest elastomeric impression material
   b. Most dimensionally stable elastomeric impression material
   c. Could not be used for edentulous arches
   d. Pouring within 1 hour is most critical

7. **Failure to place a tray filled with agar impression material into the last bath before seating in the patient could cause:**
   a. A significant loss of accuracy
   b. Burning of the patient's tissues
   c. The material to remain unset
   d. A reduction in working time

8. **Complete mixing of an addition silicone impression material is achieved when the material:**
   a. Begins to feel rubbery
   b. Can be poured into a syringe
   c. Has a uniform color
   d. No longer sticks to the pad or spatula

9. **A polyvinylsiloxane impression is taken of a tooth prepared for a crown. On removal from the mouth, the impression is inspected, and it is noted that the tooth surface and gingival areas around the tooth have a wrinkled appearance and seem moist. The most likely reason for this defect is the:**
   a. Impression material was not mixed properly
   b. Manufacturers packaged base pastes in both tubes of the cartridge
   c. Impression was removed from the mouth too soon
   d. Impression area was contacted by gloved fingers prior to taking the impression

10. **Which of the following is recommended as an appropriate disinfection procedure for an alginate impression?**
   a. Complete immersion in bleach in a plastic bag for 1 hour
   b. Spraying for 30 seconds with an iodophor and then wiping dry
   c. Placing in an autoclave on low temperature for 3 minutes
   d. Spraying with glutaraldehyde and sealing in a bag for 10 minutes

SELECTED READINGS

Craig RG, Sun Z. Trends in elastomeric impression materials. Operative Dentistry 19:138–145, 1994.
   This article compares the physical and mechanical properties of many different types of commercial elastomeric impression materials. Practical information about factors affecting clinical performance, such as working time and dimensional stability, is provided, as is a comparison of available delivery systems.

Dounis GS, Ziebert GJ, Dounis KS. A comparison of impression materials for complete-arch fixed partial dentures. Journal of Prosthetic Dentistry 65:165–169, 1991.
   This article compares a polyether, two polyvinylsiloxanes, and an agar hydrocolloid impression material in terms of their abilities to produce accurate single-tooth castings as well as fixed partial dentures. The authors conclude that the materials are equally effective in producing single crowns but that the hydrocolloid is not as suitable as the other for producing a complete-arch, fixed partial denture.

Fan PL. Disinfection of impressions. Council on Dental Materials, Instruments and Equipment. Journal of the American Dental Association 122:124, 126, 128–130, 1991.
   Recommendations for the disinfection of various types of impression materials are given in this short article.

Kahn RL, Donovan TE. A pilot study of polymerization inhibition of poly (vinyl siloxane) materials by latex gloves. International Journal of Prosthodontics 2:128–130, 1989.
   This is a report on the inhibition of setting of an addition silicone impression material contacted by a latex glove. Inhibition of setting was noted even after the gloves were washed with soap and water.

Mandikos MN. Polyvinyl siloxane impression materials: An update on clinical use. Australian Dental Journal 43:428–434, 1998.
   This article provides a review of the polyvinylsiloxane impression materials, including their chemistry, properties, and important clinical factors for their use.

Merchant VA. Infection control in the dental laboratory: Concerns for the dentist. Compendium of Continuing Education in Dentistry 14:382–391, 1993.
   This article provides appropriate disinfection protocols for dental impressions, as well as casts, prostheses, and waxes.

Mitchem JC. Impression materials and techniques. In: Clark JW, ed. Clinical Dentistry. Vol 4. 9th ed. Philadelphia: Harper & Row, 1984;1–10.

This treatise provides general guidelines for the mixing and handling of hydrocolloid and elastomeric impression materials. Step-by-step descriptions are given for loading impression trays and taking impressions.

Thouati A, Deveaux E, Lost A, Behin P. Dimensional stability of seven elastomeric impression materials immersed in disinfectants. Journal of Prosthetic Dentistry 76:8–14, 1996.

This article describes an experiment in which three disinfectant solutions were tested for their effect on the dimensional accuracy of seven elastomeric impression materials. The study showed that glutaraldehyde had little effect on the dimensions of the impressions. Hypochlorite, however, often caused a slight expansion that the authors suggested could be beneficial for prosthodontic procedures.

Dental Plaster and Stone

Objectives

- Compare the chemical and physical structure of plaster, stone, die stone, and gypsum.
- Describe the manner in which plaster, stone, and die stone are produced from gypsum.
- Compare the strength and setting expansion of the different types of plaster and stone.
- Given a specific dental use, select one of the American Dental Association types of plasters and stones appropriate for that use.
- Describe the manner in which plaster or stone form gypsum and what physical phenomenon is responsible for the expansion and strength of the material.
- Explain the effect of water-to-powder ratio, additives, gypsum contaminants, temperature, and mixing on the setting time of plaster or stone.
- Identify the items needed to mix gypsum products.
- Identify the correct water-to-powder ratio for the different types of gypsum products.

- Describe the correct way to mix plaster or stone to minimize porosity.
- Describe the correct procedure for pouring a gypsum cast from an impression and explain the rationale for this method.
- Describe the correct procedure for trimming a full-arch gypsum cast with regard to the objectives of the exercise.
- Identify possible ways to disinfect a stone cast or die.

Plaster and **stone** are chemically identical but physically distinct forms of the compound, calcium sulfate. When mixed with water, plaster or stone forms **gypsum**, a naturally occurring mineral that is mined in many parts of the world. Plaster is used extensively in home construction to make wall boards, is routinely used in the health care profession to make casts to immobilize and protect arms and legs, and is used extensively in artistic circles, where it is known as plaster of Paris. Plaster has also been used as a dental material for several hundreds of years, principally to make **casts** of objects on which dental appliances, such as dentures carved from ivory, can be fashioned. Today, plaster and stone are used in dentistry in a variety of ways.

■ Uses of Gypsum Products in Dentistry

In dentistry, plaster and stone are used mostly outside of the oral cavity. For example, plaster is used to make study casts for treatment planning and orthodontics and to mount casts to a dental **articulator** (Fig. 9-1). Stone is also used to produce study casts and to form **dies** on which wax patterns of restorations can be fashioned (Fig. 9-1). An additional use of stone is as an additive to dental casting investments, where it serves as a binder. Plaster, however, also is occasionally used intraorally to make impressions of the gums of patients who are completely edentulous.

There are different forms of plaster and stone, and each form has specific uses in dentistry, based on its specific properties and behaviors; these forms are introduced later in the chapter. The limited strength, abrasion resistance, solubility, and esthetic qualities of these ceramic materials, however, restrict their usefulness to a preparatory rather than a restorative role in dentistry. For example, one would not consider manufacturing a dental bridge from gypsum, but the use of stone to produce a dimensionally accurate and stable cast on which the wax pattern for the bridge is fashioned is nonetheless essential to the success of the final restoration. Therefore, as with many other materials, the operator has a direct influence on the ultimate usefulness of plaster and stone through appropriate manipulation and handling of these materials.

■ Composition of Plaster, Stone, and Gypsum

Chemically, gypsum is known as calcium sulfate dihydrate; the chemical formula is $CaSO_4 2H_2O$. After it is mined, it is ground to a powder and then heated in an oven to dry. This procedure, called calcining, is accomplished in a variety of ways by varying the temperature and pressure under which the heating takes place. If the gypsum is heated to between 110 and 130°C without adding pressure, the di-

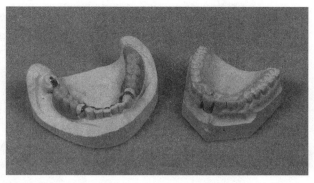

Figure 9–1 Plaster used as a cast on which to mount a partial denture (*left*) and a stone cast and die used to make an anterior porcelain crown (*right*).

hydrate powder (dihydrate means there are two water molecules for each molecule of calcium sulfate) is transformed to a hemihydrate powder (one water molecule for every two molecules of calcium sulfate), which is known as plaster. The reaction is as follows:

$$CaSO_4 \cdot 2H_2O + heat \rightarrow CaSO_4 \cdot {}^{1}/_{2}H_2O + water$$

The plaster particles have an irregular shape and appear somewhat "fluffy" (Fig. 9-2*A*).

In contrast, if the gypsum powder is heated under pressure to similar temperatures, the dihydrate is transformed to a different hemihydrate called stone. Stone has exactly the same chemical formula as plaster but possesses a much denser, regular shape (Fig. 9-2*B*). If even greater pressures are applied during the heating, an even denser form of stone is formed. This denser version is called "improved stone" or *die stone* because it is used to make dies on which to wax patterns for restorations. Compared with stone, the denser die stone is harder and stronger and less likely to be chipped or abraded by metal waxing instruments during fabrication of the wax pattern.

Plaster and stone are both white in color. To make it easier to distinguish between them, pigments often are added to stone to make it yellow or pink. The materials often are packaged in bulk in plastic bags in large cardboard containers or in single-use foil packages. Sealing in plastic or foil containers ensures that the material will not become contaminated by moisture, which would likely affect its setting behavior and properties. *What would you expect to happen if water came in contact with the hemihydrate?*

■ *Handling and Mixing*

Adding water to plaster or stone powder causes a chemical reaction that transforms the hemihydrate back to the dihydrate, gypsum. There is a significant evolution of heat during this reaction; remember that it took heat to break down the gypsum into plaster or stone. Therefore, the impression, die, or cast is actually made of gypsum. The chemist can examine the reaction equation and calculate that it is necessary to add 18.6 g of water to 100 g of plaster or stone to transform all of the powder to gypsum. Because the density of water is 1 g/mL, 18.6 g is essentially 18.6 mL. One would have great difficulty, however, attempting to mix 100 g of plaster or stone with this small an amount of water because there is an

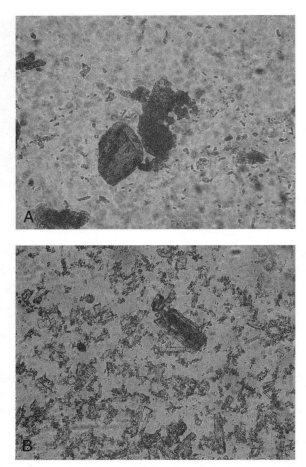

Figure 9–2 A. Photomicrograph of plaster particles. Note their irregular shape. **B.** Photomicrograph of stone particles. They have a more crystalline shape than do plaster particles.

insufficient amount to wet all of the particles completely and produce a flowable mix. Therefore, an excess of water is required, solely to make handling possible.

Because plaster particles are more irregularly shaped than are stone particles, they have a greater surface area and require more water for complete **wetting** during mixing. The typical ratio of water to powder (W/P) for plaster is 50 mL of water to 100 g of powder, or 50 g/100 g equals 0.5. Stone particles, being much denser and having a much smoother surface, require only 30 mL of water for 100 g of powder, or a W/P ratio of 0.3, for adequate wetting and mixing characteristics. Die stones are denser yet and can be mixed with a W/P ratio of 0.24. Figure 9-3 shows the relative densities of plaster, stone, and die stone, illustrated by measuring out equal weights of each and placing them into graduated cylinders. Obviously, the lower density of plaster causes it to fill up a greater volume of the cylinder, compared with stone, and it is easy to see why more water is needed to mix plaster. *What happens to the excess water in the gypsum if only 18.6 g is needed to react completely with 100 g of powder?*

At this point it is instructive to discuss the ways in which plaster, stone, and die stone are mixed to produce gypsum products for dental use. Typically, plaster and stone are mixed in rubber bowls by using stiff steel spatulas. There are two reasons for this. The stiff spatula allows the viscous material to be stirred efficiently

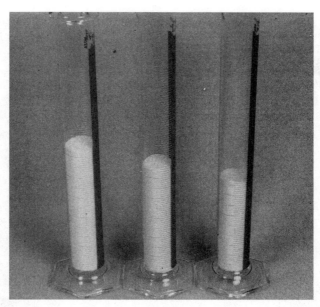

Figure 9–3 Equal weights of plaster (*left*), stone (*middle*), and die stone (*right*) in graduated cylinders, demonstrating the differences in the volume they occupy and, therefore, their different densities.

and pressed against the side of the bowl in a wiping motion to squeeze out air bubbles incorporated during the procedure. The rubber bowl is easily cleaned by squeezing and bending the sides to break up the unused gypsum that may have been allowed to harden in the bowl. The set material crumbles and can be tossed into the wastebasket. It is always a good idea to use the spatula to remove as much of the excess material as possible from the bowl before the material hardens. In any event, remember to throw all gypsum residue into the trash instead of down the sink, where it may clog the drainpipes. Even if the drain contains a plaster trap, only a bowl that has been scraped clean of most of the unset material should be cleaned in the sink.

Dispensing

For the most reproducible mixes, the powder should be weighed out on a laboratory balance, and the water should be measured in a graduated cylinder or similar device (Fig. 9-4*A*). The water should be near room temperature, but cool water from the faucet is usually fine. The water is placed into the mixing bowl first, and then the powder is *slowly* sifted into the water (Fig. 9-4*B*). This process should take 30 to 60 seconds to prevent the powder from clumping together excessively, which hinders the wetting of all of the particles. Once all of the powder is added, the bowl should be vibrated for about 10 seconds on a mechanical vibrator, or by tapping it on the countertop, to free up trapped air, which rises to the surface and out of the bowl (Fig. 9-4*C*).

Mixing

Mixing is initially accomplished by rotating the spatula in the material to help break up any remaining clumps and enhance the wetting of the powder (Fig. 9-4*D*). Then the material is vigorously mixed for 30 to 60 seconds by wiping the mix,

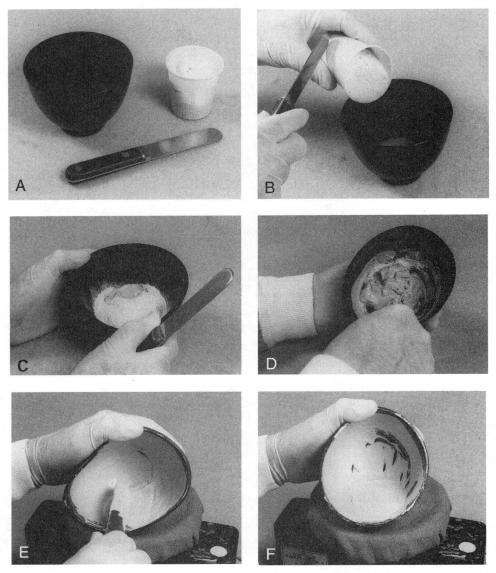

Figure 9–4 A. Stone and water dispensed for mixing. **B.** Stone being sifted into the water in a mixing bowl. **C.** Mixing bowl being vibrated to remove bubbles. **D.** Initial mixing of water and stone with a spatula. **E.** Stone mix being wiped against the side of the bowl as the bowl is mechanically vibrated. **F.** Glossy, creamy mix of stone.

keeping the spatula flat against the side of the bowl, to force the material against the side and thereby press the air bubbles out (Fig. 9-4*E*). After mixing, the material can again be vibrated or tapped to remove any remaining air bubbles. If one remembers that the presence of air bubbles, or **porosity**, in the mix produces holes on the surface of the object as well as reduces its strength, the rationale for mixing in this manner becomes clear. Mixing the gypsum mechanically in a vacuum-mixing device is also possible. Vacuum mixing is efficient for removing air bubbles and producing a denser product. The final mix will look glossy on its surface and have a smooth, creamy texture (Fig. 9-4*F*). If it appears watery or sandy and grainy, then an incorrect W/P ratio was used or mixing is incomplete.

Cleanup

After using the mix, the excess should be removed from the bowl with the spatula and discarded in the trash. The residual material can then be wiped from the bowl and spatula with a paper towel before washing both out with water in the sink, preferably one with a plaster trap.

■ *Setting Time*

The normal setting time for plaster and stone is 10 to 15 minutes. The working time, which refers to the length of time in which one can comfortably work with the material, is approximately 5 to 7 minutes, however. Once it reaches this point, which often is called the *initial set*, the gypsum begins to lose some of its glossy appearance and no longer flows. In this state, it will more than likely break up if manipulated. In contrast, the *final set* usually is determined by attempting to penetrate the surface of the mix with a weighted needle (usually a Gillmore needle weighing 1 pound). When the needle no longer penetrates the surface, the gypsum is set or hardened. The final set indicates that the material has reached a minimal state of hardness and abrasion resistance, but as the gypsum continues to dry over the next 24 hours, it will get harder and stronger. Therefore, care must be taken when handling a cast or other gypsum product until it is approximately 45 to 60 minutes old.

Several factors can affect the setting time of gypsum products; therefore, a brief description of the manner in which plaster (or stone) hardens is necessary to understand why the material behaves as it does. Plaster and stone dissolve in water. Gypsum also is soluble in water, but it dissolves only approximately one fourth as much as does plaster or stone. Once the plaster or stone particles contact water, they begin to dissolve. The hemihydrate enters into solution and reacts with the water to form the dihydrate. Because gypsum is less soluble than plaster or stone, the solution soon becomes saturated, and the dihydrate begins to precipitate throughout the mix as needle-like crystals of gypsum. The loss of hemihydrate from the solution by the formation of gypsum allows more hemihydrate to dissolve into solution. Soon, more dihydrate forms on the growing gypsum crystals, and the process continues to repeat itself.

The crystals get very long and needle-like and begin to impinge on one another (Fig. 9-5). This has two effects. First, it causes the needles to push one another out of the way, expanding the setting material. Second, as the needles interact, they begin to entangle with one another. Because each crystal is always supported by a neighboring crystal, it resists being moved, and thus the material is strengthened and hardened. Therefore, "setting" and "hardening" are synonymous. The setting time, then, is a measure of the extent to which the needles have grown and entangled with one another. *Is it not likely, then, that anything that affects the rate at which the crystals form or the number of crystals formed within the material will influence the setting time?*

Water-to-Powder Ratio

If one adds more water than is specified to the mixture of plaster or stone, what will be the effect on the setting time? Increasing the amount of water ensures that fewer gypsum crystals will be formed per unit volume of the mix. This increases

Figure 9–5 Photomicrograph showing the initial formation of gypsum crystals, with the growing gypsum needles impinging on one another.

the setting time by prolonging the time required for the crystals to grow enough to impinge on one another and produce strength. Conversely, reducing the W/P ratio causes a quickening of the setting reaction by increasing the number of crystals per unit volume. The danger here is that speeding the setting time also minimizes the working time, thus increasing the chance that one may not be finished using the mix before it becomes unworkable. Changing the W/P ratio by 0.1 can change the setting time by several minutes.

Gypsum Contaminants

What might you expect the effect to be of mixing plaster in a bowl that has not been completely cleaned of gypsum? The residual gypsum will serve as crystals on which to grow more gypsum, again increasing the number of crystals per unit volume. The result is a quickening of the setting time and a reduction in working time. In fact, a practical way to hasten the setting of plaster or stone would be to grind up some gypsum and place a pinch into a fresh mixture. ***What problems may arise if this is done before pouring a stone cast?***

> The most obvious problem would be the operator's unfamiliarity with the reduced working time, thus increasing the chances of producing a cast with many voids and defects.

Additives

Chemical agents are added to plaster or stone to alter the setting behavior, although the actual mechanism by which they work is not clearly defined. Potassium sulfate (K_2SO_4) is an example of a chemical that accelerates the setting of gypsum, presumably because it increases the rate at which the hemihydrate dissolves in water. In contrast, acetates or borates, such as boric oxide (borax), retard the set of gypsum products, possibly by "poisoning" the surface of newly formed crystals so that no more dihydrate can be formed on them. Therefore, in the small concentrations used by the manufacturers, these compounds can be added to subtly increase or decrease the setting rate to produce more useful plasters and stones.

Mixing Time

Prolonging the mixing time can disrupt the growing gypsum crystals, breaking each single crystal into two or more. The net effect is the production of more crystals in a unit volume and a faster-setting mix. This should not be a significant problem, however, if mixing is stopped once the material has gained a smooth, creamy consistency. It is of far greater concern to undermix the material.

Temperature

Most chemical reactions are accelerated when the temperature is raised. This is true to some extent for the setting of dental plaster or stone. Making a mix with warm water would likely hasten the setting time and reduce the working time by speeding the reaction. The effect is difficult to determine, however, because increasing the water temperature also increases the solubility of gypsum. The effect of this increased solubility is that it takes longer for the water to become saturated with gypsum, thus increasing the time required for gypsum to crystallize out of solution and solidify. Therefore, the two factors are in opposition, and it would be unwise to attempt to use water temperature as a way to alter the setting time for plaster or stone.

This discussion of factors affecting the setting rate for plaster and stone leads one to question what their effects are on other parameters, such as the expansion and mechanical properties of the final gypsum product. As mentioned, plaster and stone expand because the growing gypsum crystals impinge on one another, thrusting each other out of the way to some extent (Fig. 9-5). Therefore, the expansion must be related to how close together the crystals are or how many of them are found in a given volume. *From what we know about their differences in W/P ratio, what might we expect to be the difference in magnitude of setting expansion between plaster and stone?*

■ *Setting Expansion*

Generally, plaster materials expand more than stone expands. A mass of laboratory plaster will expand its volume by approximately 0.3% during setting. A similar mass of laboratory stone would expand only approximately 0.15%, or half as much as plaster. This seems to be the opposite of what we would expect based on our knowledge of these materials. If we increased the W/P ratio, we would expect to reduce the number of crystals in a unit volume. This would reduce the amount of interaction between the crystals and finally reduce the overall expansion. Therefore, plaster should have less expansion than stone, the opposite of what we find. The explanation can be found in the formulation of the materials. The accelerating and retarding additives used in laboratory plaster cause its expansion to be greater than that of stone, the opposite of what we predicted. *What would be the effect of the assistant raising or lowering the W/P ratio for a given composition of plaster or stone?*

Water-to-Powder Ratio

Increasing the amount of water used in the mix increases the space between growing crystals, thus slowing the setting rate and reducing expansion for the same reasons (i.e., fewer impinging crystals per unit volume). Therefore, the expansion of plaster can be reduced by increasing the W/P ratio.

If plaster were used as an impression material, it would be desirable for its expansion to be minimal to avoid distorting the impression. Obviously, it would be beneficial to have a plaster with a low setting expansion; however, increasing the W/P ratio would also cause the mix to be very fluid, possibly too fluid to be useful as an impression material because it would not stay in the tray. Therefore, it would be preferable to use additives, rather than W/P ratio changes, to alter the expansion. This is, in fact, how impression plasters are made. A similar concern arises when die stone is used to make accurate dies for fixed prosthetics. It is important to use a material with minimal dimensional change. Therefore, despite the very low W/P ratio used for die stones compared with laboratory stone, the expansion of die stone is slightly less (0.10%). Again, this is because of the presence of additives, which regulate setting as well as expansion.

Another significant consideration is the expansion of gypsum products and the effect of water. Briefly, the setting expansion of stone or plaster can be increased by allowing it to set while being submerged in water. This may seem contradictory at this point, but this phenomenon is treated later, when the use of gypsum as a binder for casting investments is discussed.

This discussion of the effects of various factors on the setting time and expansion of plaster and stone has failed to take notice of the effects on other important properties. The strength and hardness of gypsum products, although not as important as for restorative materials, are of significant interest. For example, if gypsum was extremely weak, it would crack and chip every time it was bumped against something. Imagine chipping the edges of teeth on a study model or a die. This is a problem in terms of the model's esthetics; more important, it severely limits the model's usefulness by eliminating areas of important information. Therefore, gypsum products must have a certain strength and hardness to resist breakage and abrasion during normal use. As one might expect, the differences in structure and W/P ratio between plaster, stone, and die stone affect their mechanical properties.

■ *Properties: Strength and Hardness*

In general, anything that affects the strength of gypsum materials also affects their hardness. One might expect that anything that alters the number of crystals formed in a given volume, or interferes with the formation of these crystals, will affect properties. As mentioned, it is the interaction and entanglement of crystals that give gypsum its strength. *Is it not then reasonable to assume that any factor that reduces the number of crystals in a unit volume will reduce the strength of the final gypsum product?*

In fact, this is precisely the case. An examination of the strength of gypsum formed from plaster (27.5 MPa or 4000 psi) and from stone (55 to 83 MPa or 8000 to 12,000 psi) reveals that stone is inherently stronger than plaster by a significant amount (two to three times). This is relatively easy to explain in light of the different amounts of water used to make each mix. Earlier in this chapter, it was suggested that to produce a workable mixture, it was necessary to mix 100 g of either plaster or stone with some quantity of water that exceeded the 18.6 mL required for the chemical reaction. What happens to the extra water when a gypsum cast sets? Initially, the water remains free in the cast. Water is not particularly strong. Filling a piece of gypsum with water does not add to its strength; it reduces it. Therefore, gypsum is initially much weaker because of the presence of the residual water. With time, the gypsum dries as the water evaporates, removing all of the residual water from the cast. This loss of water increases the strength of the cast. Often you will see the strength of gypsum cited as "wet" or "dry," where dry strength usually is two to three times greater than wet strength. Because gypsum fully sets within approximately 24 hours, the "dry" strength usually refers to a value taken at that time. The question then becomes ***What happens to the areas in the gypsum where the water used to be?***

When water evaporates, the space it leaves behind becomes occupied by air. Thus, any site in which water existed in the gypsum eventually becomes a porosity or air bubble (Fig. 9-6). An air bubble offers no resistance to force and, therefore, negatively influences the strength of the gypsum. There is a direct correlation between the amount of excess water used in the mix and the final degree of porosity. Both also are directly related to strength; this is the reason that plaster is weaker than stone, and stone is weaker than die stone. Increasing the W/P ratio for a given gypsum product reduces its strength and hardness, so it is important to use the recommended ratios. These have been established to optimize physical properties, setting time, and handling characteristics, such as the ability of the material to flow into an impression. The use of the gypsum product defines the properties and characteristics that are needed, and hence there are several types of plasters and stones.

■ *Types of Plasters and Stones*

The five types of gypsums, two plasters and three stones, are classified as American Dental Association (ADA) types I through V. They vary in their properties, and their handling characteristics are tailored for specific uses, as described in the following sections.

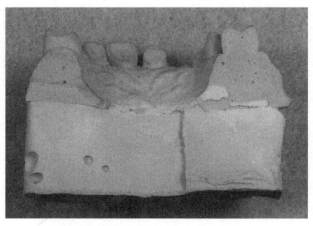

Figure 9–6 Porosity in a gypsum cast.

Type I: Impression Plaster

Type I plaster is used to make impressions of edentulous patients. Because it is hard and brittle and does not deform elastically, it cannot be removed from the under-cuts of teeth and, therefore, could not be used on dentulous patients. When placed in the oral cavity, this material has a relatively short setting time of approximately 4 to 5 minutes. This is important because a longer setting time would be more un-comfortable for the patient. Additives are introduced to produce the shorter setting time. Type I plaster has a relatively low expansion of 0.13%, in part because of the high W/P ratio of 0.6. The higher W/P ratio helps to ensure that the increase in temperature during the setting reaction will not be great enough to damage the mucosal tissues. The minimal expansion is important from the standpoint of accu-racy. The material is of minimal strength (27.5 MPa or 4000 psi), which is benefi-cial because when the impression is difficult to remove, it must be broken in the mouth and then "glued" together out of the mouth in the correct relationship.

Type II: Laboratory or Model Plaster

The requirements for model plaster are minimal because it is not used intraorally or for any precise operations. It is essentially the same material as plaster of Paris and is used to make study casts or to mount stone casts in the articulator or in the denture flask. It normally is mixed with a W/P ratio of 0.5 and, therefore, sets with a higher expansion (0.3%) than does type I plaster. This is of no clinical conse-quence, however. This plaster is stronger than type I plaster because of the lower W/P ratio, which results in less overall porosity when the material has dried.

A special type of plaster is referred to as orthodontic plaster. This plaster has properties similar to those of type II plaster but has a much faster setting rate. Or-thodontic plaster hardens within 2 to 3 minutes after mixing and is used to pro-duce rapid study casts to follow the progress of orthodontic treatment. The model provides a replica of the patient's mouth that can also be used to show the patient the progress of their treatment.

Type III: Laboratory Stone

Laboratory stone is the common stone used to make casts of impressions for the production of dentures and treatment planning. It is harder and stronger than type II plaster; hence, it is more durable. The greater strength is a result of the lower W/P ratio of 0.3. The expansion of this material is between 0.15 and 0.20%, which, because of the additives used in the formulation, is less than that of plas-ter. The dry strength of this stone is approximately 62 MPa (9000 psi).

Type IV: Die Stone

This high-strength (79 MPa or 11,500 psi), high-hardness, and low-expansion (0.08%) stone is used as a die material on which wax patterns of inlays or crowns are produced. The higher strength is a function of the low W/P ratio of 0.24 or less used for these materials.

Type V: High-Strength, High-Expansion Die Stone

This material is the most recent addition to the list of ADA gypsums. Its produc-tion is the result of a need for dies with increased expansion to compensate for the greater shrinkage that occurs in many of the newer, high-melting alloys used for dental castings. The setting expansion approaches 0.3% and is achieved by using a lower W/P ratio (0.18 to 0.22), which also results in a stronger gypsum product.

■ *Pouring and Trimming a Gypsum Cast*

The most common use of plaster or stone is to pour a model, cast, or die from an impression that has been appropriately disinfected. The procedure is not a difficult one but does require the operator to dispense, mix, and handle the material correctly to produce the optimum product. This is especially true when the material is used to make a die on which a wax pattern for a casting will be fabricated. The final restoration will not fit correctly if mistakes are made with any of the materials used during the process. The specific procedures for pouring a maxillary cast in stone, by using an alginate impression and then trimming the cast on a model trimmer, are described.

The surface of the impression should be dried of excess water. This can be done with compressed air for elastomeric impression materials or with an absorbent towel or tissue for hydrocolloid materials. The stone is then dispensed and mixed according to the procedures described previously, with care taken to vibrate excess bubbles from the mix. The impression tray is then held in one hand while a small amount of the stone is picked up on a spatula. A cement spatula works well because it is thin and limits the quantity of material that can be collected each time. But the spatula used to mix the plaster or stone can also be used with equal efficiency. The material is next dripped or wiped into one corner of the impression, in this case the last molar of the full arch (Fig. 9-7*A*). The impression is then gently vibrated to slowly move the mix into the adjacent teeth, essentially coating the impression with a layer of stone. Once no further movement occurs, a second small increment of stone is added and vibrated around while the impression is tilted to facilitate the movement of the mix (Fig. 9-7*B*). It is important not to vibrate the impression excessively, because this actually creates air bubbles in the material and on the surface of the cast. This process of adding increments of materials and vibrating is repeated until the entire surface of the impression is coated with stone and the teeth imprints are completely filled (Fig. 9-7*C*). Larger increments of stone then can be added to fill the impression completely up to the mucobuccal fold. This slow, careful process ensures that air bubbles will be displaced from the impression, producing a dense surface on the cast.

It is a good idea to place three or four small blebs of the mix onto the surface of the gypsum at this point (Fig. 9-7*D*). This produces a rough underside to enhance the retention between the stone poured into the impression and the base that will be made with a second mix of stone. The base gives bulk to the final cast and facilitates its handling during trimming. The impression tray is placed tray side down onto the table.

A second mix of stone is made, but with a lower W/P ratio (i.e., 0.26) to provide a heavier consistency, faster set, and increased strength. The second mix is dispensed onto a flat surface, such as a glass or plastic plate, and the sides are shaped with the plaster spatula into a square 0.75 inch in height. The poured impression (which should be past the initial set) can then be inverted onto this patty. (Note: If the cast has already set, it is recommended that it be soaked in water for 5 minutes to improve the adhesion to the base.) The tray is held steady while the sides of the patty are shaped with the spatula and smoothed to ensure that there is no gap between the two pours (Fig. 9-7*E*). Care should be taken not to "lock" the cast onto the tray by running the stone up too far. The material is then allowed

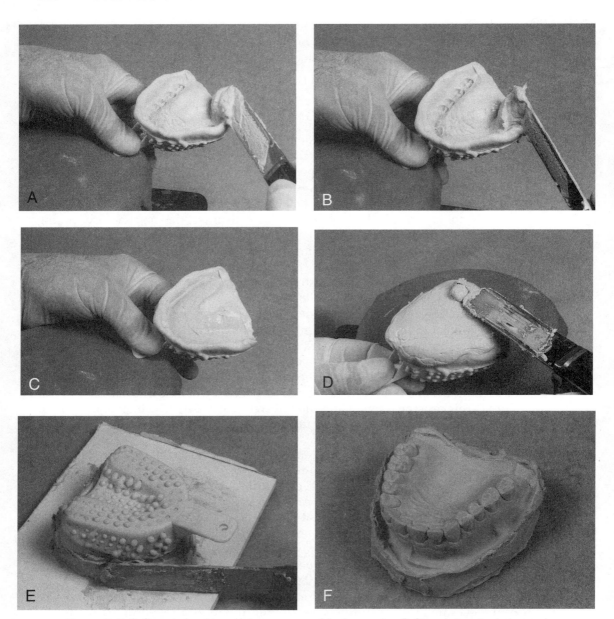

Figure 9–7 **A.** Stone being dripped into one corner of the impression. **B.** Stone being vibrated around the teeth imprints in the impression. **C.** Impression with all teeth imprints filled with stone. **D.** Placement of blebs on a surface of stone. **E.** Sides of a second pour being shaped with a spatula. **F.** Stone cast on removal from the impression.

to harden for at least 45 minutes to 1 hour before attempting to separate the cast from the impression. Because certain impression materials, such as the hydrocolloids, can dry out during this time, a damp towel should be placed over the cast during setting. This should maintain near 100% humidity and will not distort the impression before the stone has sufficiently hardened. Once the stone has set, excess stone can be trimmed from the cast with a utility knife. To remove the impression, the anterior portion is loosened first, by raising it slightly. The tray is then removed by pulling straight up. It is important not to rock the impression from side to side, to avoid breaking any portion of the cast (Fig. 9-7*F*). The cast is then ready to be trimmed on a model trimmer (Procedure Display 9-1).

Mixing Plaster or Stone

Equipment checklist
- Plaster, stone, or die stone powder
- Balance
- Water
- Graduated cylinder or measuring cup
- Rubber mixing bowl (usually green)
- Stiff steel plaster spatula

STEP 1: **Proportioning**
- Measure room temperature or cool water from faucet in graduated cylinder
- Weigh powder on balance in paper cup
- Add water to bowl
- Slowly sift powder into bowl, taking 30 to 60 seconds
- Vibrate or tap bowl on counter for 10 seconds to remove bubbles

STEP 2: **Mixing**
- Stir powder in water to wet particles for 10 to 20 seconds
- Mix vigorously for 60 seconds by wiping spatula with mix against side of bowl to press air bubbles out
- Vibrate or tap bowl on counter for 10 seconds to remove remaining bubbles, or use a vacuum-mixing device
- Visually inspect mix for glossy surface and smooth, creamy consistency

STEP 3: **Pouring cast**
- Drip small amount of stone into one of the molar areas of the impression and vibrate anteriorly into teeth imprints on mechanical vibrator
- Continue to add small amounts of stone in this manner until teeth imprints are full
- Place larger amounts of stone into impression until it is filled
- Place three small stone "blebs" on surface to aid retention with second pour
- Make second mix with W/P ratio of 0.26 and shape into square on plate or pad
- Invert impression filled with stone onto second mix and shape sides to fill in gaps completely (be careful not to lock tray into stone cast)
- Allow stone to set completely before removing impression (45 minutes)

STEP 4: **Cleanup**
- Remove bulk excess with spatula and discard in trash (note: if the material has hardened by this point, flex the bowl to break up the gypsum, and discard pieces in trash)
- Wipe insides of bowl with paper towel to remove residual mix
- Wipe spatula clean with paper towel
- Clean bowl and spatula in sink with plaster trap, using water only

The model trimmer contains a large, carborundum-coated disk that revolves at high speeds inside a cabinet (Fig. 9-8A). A model can be placed onto a table, the angle of which can be changed, and fed into the rotating disk under copious water spray to grind off material in a manner analogous to conventional sandpaper. The difference is that the disk is rotating at high speeds and can cause serious injury if the user does not pay close attention to the position of his or her hands at all times. Used properly, the model trimmer is a safe, efficient device that can be

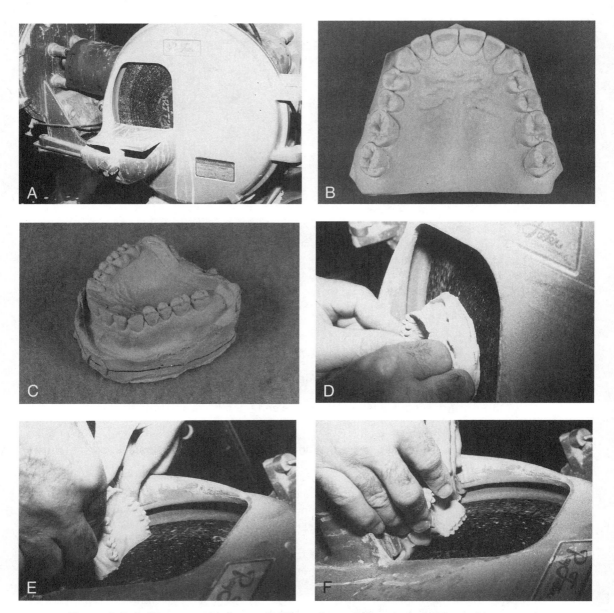

Figure 9–8 A. Gypsum model trimmer. **B.** Trimmed cast. **C.** Cast marked with pencil in preparation for grinding the base flat. **D.** Base of cast being trimmed. **E.** Back of cast being trimmed. **F.** Sides of cast being trimmed.

routinely used to enhance the appearance of gypsum casts. The final product should have a bottom that is parallel to the occlusal plane, should be symmetrical, include the anatomy of both the teeth and soft tissue, and be of sufficient bulk to provide structural stability (Fig. 9-8B). When both arches are being done, the assistant should ensure that the backs of both the upper and lower casts are even when in normal occlusion.

The cast is placed with the incisal edges resting on the table, and a line parallel to the table and 1 inch above the vestibule is scribed around it with a compass or Boley gauge (Fig. 9-8*C*). The base is then ground flat to this line by slowly feeding the base against the rotating disk of the trimmer, producing a cast with a base parallel to the occlusal plane (Fig. 9-8*D*). The posterior of the cast is then trimmed perpendicular to the midpalatal raphe by placing the flat base onto the table of the model trimmer and slowly feeding it in (Fig. 9-8*E*). With the base still resting on the table of the trimmer, the sides of the cast are ground parallel to a line running between the cuspid and the last molar on each side (Fig. 9-8*F*). The anterior portion of the cast is then trimmed at an angle from the cuspid to produce a peak in front of the midline. The heels of the cast are trimmed perpendicular to the sides of the cast. For a smooth, shiny finish, the cast can be soaked overnight in a special model soap and then dried; this also seals surface pores.

◼ *Disinfection of Stone Casts or Dies*

Disinfection of dental materials that have come in contact with oral fluids or tissues is an important consideration in the everyday practice of dentistry. An obvious situation presents with the handling of an impression. Although the impression itself should be disinfected before being handled further by the dental office staff or the laboratory technicians, whenever there is a question about whether this has been done, the stone cast or die also can be treated. The cast is disinfected by spraying the surface of the hardened gypsum with a sterilizing solution used in the office, such as an iodophor, glutaraldehyde, or phenol, and storing in a sealed plastic bag for 10 minutes. Although some differences have been observed, none of these solutions should significantly alter the accuracy, surface, or strength of the gypsum product. In addition, stone materials are available that contain disinfecting agents. These materials are essentially equivalent in accuracy and properties to conventional gypsum materials. Another option is to mix the stone with water containing a low concentration of the disinfectant. Although this has been shown to minimize viable microorganisms in a contaminated impression effectively, a full characterization of the properties and accuracy of stone mixed in this manner is not available. Therefore, this method should be used with caution. Autoclaving of the gypsum product is another possibility, but studies show that significant surface deformation, loss of strength, and dimensional change may occur when steam sterilization is used.

Summary

Plaster and stone are ceramic-type materials used in dentistry to produce models, dies, and investment materials. Plaster and stone powders are produced by heating gypsum, a mined mineral of hydrated calcium sulfate, under pressure to eliminate water. Stone is heated under pressure at high temperatures and is, therefore, denser than plaster. Plaster and stone powders are mixed with water and poured into impressions to produce gypsum dies and models. Because of its greater density, stone is mixed with less water than is plaster and, therefore, produces stronger and harder gypsum than does plaster, despite the fact that the chemical composition of both is the same. Therefore, stone is used for models and dies on which wax patterns of restorations are produced.

The setting of plaster and stone generates heat and is accompanied by expansion. The amount of expansion is controlled by chemical additives and the water-to-powder ratio; these variables also affect strength and setting rate. There are several different types of stones that vary in hardness and expansion and, therefore, are used for different applications. The hardest and most accurate is die stone. Like impression materials, gypsum products can and should be disinfected by approved techniques.

STUDY QUESTIONS AND PROBLEM SOLVING

1. **You are just filling the last teeth imprints for a stone model of a full-arch alginate impression and realize that the stone is beginning to thicken prematurely. Which of the following offer possible explanations for this unexpected occurrence?**
   a. You forgot to wash out the mixing bowl before beginning
   b. You did not measure and accidentally incorporated too much water into the mix
   c. The water you measured was 1 to 2° above room temperature
   d. You lost track of the time and overspatulated the mix
2. **You retrieve a die stone cast you poured from a quadrant polysulfide impression and are chagrined to find a complete cast containing numerous air bubbles on all of the teeth imprints. Which of the following are possible causes for the bubbles?**
   a. You used a surfactant on the impression before pouring the cast
   b. You failed to use a wiping motion during the mixing of the stone
   c. You vibrated the mix for 15 seconds before pouring the impression
   d. The stone was old and had been contaminated by moisture during storage
3. **The plaster study models you poured from alginate impressions have a much softer and less abrasion-resistant surface than normal. What might you have done to cause this problem?**
   a. You did not measure correctly, and mixed the plaster at a W/P ratio of 0.6
   b. You wet the impression with water and did not adequately dry it
   c. The plaster had been stored open and was contaminated by moisture
   d. You followed directions but mixed a type III stone instead of plaster
4. **You did not have time to clean out the plaster bowl after making a mix, and the material has hardened. The easiest way to remove the gypsum is to:**
   a. Soak the rubber bowl in water for a period of 24 hours
   b. Soak the rubber bowl in a detergent solution for 10 minutes
   c. Place the bowl on a vibrator to break up the gypsum
   d. Flex the bowl several times to break up the gypsum
5. **A cast crown fits the die well, but the dentist realizes that it is far too big for the tooth during try-in. What may have happened during the fabrication of the die to cause it to expand too much, producing this mismatch?**
   a. The water used to mix the die stone was taken from the cold tap only
   b. A new type V die stone was used, but a conventional gold alloy was cast
   c. The mix was not proportioned correctly, and a low W/P ratio was used
   d. The stone mix was overvibrated during the mixing procedure

6. The *most* likely reason for portions of teeth breaking off when a plaster or stone model is removed from an impression is:
   a. Use of an incorrect mixing technique
   b. Removing the cast from the impression too early
   c. Use of an incorrect W/P ratio during dispensing
   d. Waiting too long to remove the cast from the impression

SELECTED READINGS

Abdulla MA. Effect of frequency and amplitude of vibration on void formation in dies poured from polyvinylsiloxane impressions. Journal of Prosthetic Dentistry 80:490–494, 1998.
   This laboratory study showed that excessive vibration amplitude, especially at high frequency, produced more voids on the surface of stone casts poured from polyvinylsiloxane impression.

Brukl CE, McConnell RM, Norling BK, Collard SM. Influence of gauging water composition on dental stone expansion and setting time. Journal of Prosthetic Dentistry 51:218–223, 1984.
   This article evaluates the setting expansion and rate for stone mixed with various types of water, including one containing a slurry of gypsum particles, which proved to be an effective accelerator.

Cullen DR, Mikesell JW, Sandrik JL. Wettability of elastomeric impression materials and voids in gypsum casts. Journal of Prosthetic Dentistry 66:261–265, 1991.
   This article examines the wettability of various impression materials and its relation to voids produced in stone casts during pouring and shows that good wetting (low contact angles), which is achieved on certain hydrophilic impression materials and through the use of surfactants, produces casts with fewer voids.

Earnshaw R. Gypsum products. In: O'Brien WJ, ed. Dental Materials: Properties and Selection. Chicago: Quintessence Publishing, 1989;89–126.
   This excellent chapter describes the chemistry, manufacture, properties, and characteristics of gypsum products used in dentistry. It contains a detailed bibliography.

Mansfield SM, White JM. Antimicrobial effects from incorporation of disinfectants into gypsum casts. International Journal of Prosthodontics 4:180–185, 1991.
   This article describes a study in which dental stone that was mixed with water containing four different disinfectant solutions was effective in reducing viable bacteria intentionally placed into the impression.

Schneider RL. Hardening gypsum casts: An historical perspective. Quintessence of Dental Technology 9:186–187, 1985.
   This short article reviews many of the past attempts to increase the hardness and abrasion resistance of gypsum materials. The effect on setting expansion also is noted.

Stern MA, Johnson GH, Toolson LB. An evaluation of dental stones after repeated exposure to spray disinfectants: Part I: Abrasion and compressive strength. Journal of Prosthetic Dentistry 65:713–718, 1991.
   The repeated application of various disinfectant sprays is shown not to cause significant changes in the properties of type III or IV dental gypsums.

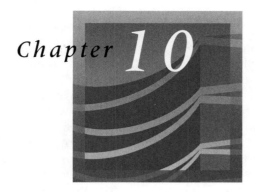
Provisional Restoratives

Objectives

- Identify the physical requirements for provisional restorative materials.
- List the components of zinc oxide eugenol provisional filling materials.
- Compare the strength and durability of zinc oxide eugenol to other cement-restorative materials.
- List the components of acrylic and bis-acryl provisional filling materials for crowns and bridges.
- Describe the procedure for making an acrylic or bis-acryl provisional restoration by the direct technique.
- Describe the procedure for making an acrylic or bis-acryl provisional restoration by the indirect technique.

■ *Uses of Provisional Restoratives in Dentistry*

Many dental procedures cannot be completed in a single appointment; often, laboratory work is required to complete a restoration. Other times, complications from an existing condition require a short-term treatment until a more permanent restoration can be designed. For example, there are times when the clinician needs to "buy time" to determine whether a wounded tooth will heal properly to allow a permanent restoration to be placed instead of proceeding directly with endodontic treatment. In either case, the patient and the dental team are faced with a prepared tooth without a restoration. In such cases, a provisional or temporary (note that the two terms are used synonymously) restoration must be placed over the preparation to prevent further insult by bacteria and their by-products. Although the filling may need to be sufficiently strong and durable to withstand occlusal forces, its length of service in the mouth usually is limited to a period of time measured in days or weeks. Therefore, high strength is not a requirement. In fact, high strength would be a significant drawback because it would greatly complicate the removal of the filling when the permanent restoration is placed. Of greater importance is the ability of the material to seal the tooth and prevent leakage, especially if it is to be left in place for more than a week or two, thus protecting the pulp. The provisional restoration also provides stability for the prepared tooth and the occlusion and enhances soft tissue health.

Another requirement for the provisional restoration of anterior teeth is some degree of esthetics. Although soft and ductile aluminum crowns often were used for the provisional restoration of posterior teeth, their use has been reduced by the development of self-curing and light-cured acrylics and composites, both of which are tooth colored. Clear, preformed polycarbonate crowns filled with tooth-colored acrylic or composite provide another esthetic alternative. Finally, and perhaps most importantly, the provisional restorative material must be easy and economical to prepare and place.

These requirements have led to the routine use of several materials as provisional restoratives. Reinforced **zinc oxide eugenol (ZOE)** cements and self-curing acrylics and composites are two of the most common examples. Light-curing technology also has expanded into this area of dentistry, and composite-type prosthetic resins often are used as temporaries. Light-cured composites have been developed as provisionals for inlay preparations. An interesting characteristic of some of these materials is that they first harden by self-curing to a semirigid state, remaining slightly rubbery. This facilitates its removal from the mouth and subsequent trimming of the excess material. The material is given a final light application to form the rigid final structure. Other provisionals never reach a completely rigid state, remaining hard but slightly resilient. The fact that it does not become completely rigid after curing facilitates its removal from the tooth at a later time. The compositions and characteristics of these materials are presented on the following pages. A protocol for the preparation and placement of an acrylic provisional also is presented.

■ *Types of Provisional Restoratives*

Zinc Oxide Eugenol

Zinc oxide powder can be mixed with eugenol liquid to produce a material used as a liner, base, provisional or permanent luting agent, impression material, endodontic sealer, periodontal dressing, and provisional restorative. The use of this material as a liner, base, and cement is described in Chapter 4, and its use as an impression material is described in Chapter 8. Its use as a provisional filling material is described in this chapter.

The composition of ZOE materials used for this large variety of applications is similar, except that the reinforced types are typically used as restoratives because they are more durable than the conventional material. These materials are based on powder-liquid (P/L) systems and are mixed like cements to a putty-like consistency. They are then packed into the prepared tooth, where they harden in a matter of minutes. They are generally considered to be nonirritating because eugenol has a neutral pH as well as an **obtundent**, or sedative, effect on pulpal tissue. In addition, ZOE efficiently seals cavities. This characteristic is probably due to the fact that it undergoes minimal overall dimensional change during setting and because it has some antibacterial properties.

ZOE restorative materials are usually P/L systems (Fig. 10-1). The powders basically are composed of zinc oxide (70% by weight). **Rosin** is added to reinforce the material and make it less brittle; rosin is a natural organic material available in powder form. In certain formulations, polymethylmethacrylate (PMMA) beads (approximately 20% by weight) are added to strengthen the restorative. These ZOE-PMMA materials are referred to as "polymer modified." Other ZOE materials used for cements are reinforced by the addition of approximately 30% by weight of hard aluminum oxide particles.

The liquid portion of the system is usually eugenol with the addition of a small amount of some other oil, such as olive oil. The liquid of the ZOE restoratives that contain aluminum oxide-reinforcing fillers contains approximately 65% ethoxybenzoic acid (EBA) and only approximately 35% eugenol. These materials are referred to as ZOE-EBA or, simply, EBA cements.

ZOE is mixed to a very thick consistency when used as a restorative. The powder and liquid are dispensed in the appropriate ratio onto a glass slab or an oil-impervious paper pad. Most of the powder is incorporated into the liquid within 30 seconds by using a cement spatula. Additional powder is introduced in stages until all of the powder has been incorporated and the mix becomes like a stiff putty.

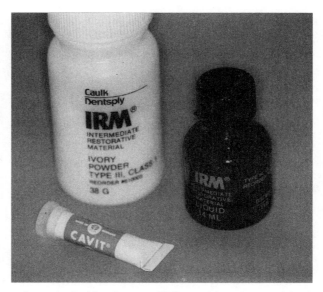

Figure 10–1 A powder-liquid and a paste ZOE material used as provisional restoratives.

In contrast to some of the restoratives, ZOE cements that are used to cement provisional restorations often are supplied as two-paste systems (Fig. 10-2). Equal lengths of the different-colored pastes are mixed on a pad to achieve a homogeneous color and relatively fluid consistency.

As described in Chapter 4, ZOE materials set by a chemical reaction. Therefore, their setting rate could be affected by temperature, although this usually is not a problem. The restorative has a long working time at ambient temperatures and sets rapidly once it is placed in the mouth. Moisture is a major factor contributing to the fast setting of ZOE materials in the mouth. The same effect could play a role during mixing if a glass slab is used that was not completely dried after cleaning, leading to a reduction in working time. Because it usually is not necessary to chill these materials to prolong working time, the humidity of the operatory may be the most important factor influencing the setting rate of the ZOE materials. *What other factor, which is in the hands of the assistant, may influence setting rate?*

> From previous discussions, it is known that mixing cements at high P/L ratios affects setting time. Thicker mixes set faster. Because it is desirable to achieve high P/L ratios to optimize the mechanical properties of the ZOE restorative, the assistant should always keep track of the time when mixing begins in order to ensure that the clinician has ample working time.

The properties of ZOE formulations vary. The unmodified versions are used for provisional cementation and are the weakest, having compressive strengths in the range of 2 to 20 MPa, depending on the P/L ratio used in the mix. The polymer-modified and alumina-reinforced ZOE-EBA formulations have compressive strengths of 40 to 60 MPa; the strengths of the reinforced ZOE materials are, however, still only 35 to 50% as high as those of the permanent cements that are also used as restoratives, such as glass ionomers. Therefore, the ZOE cements are indicated only as provisional filling materials. Clinical studies show that although ZOE provisional restorations are biologically acceptable and easily handled, they wear

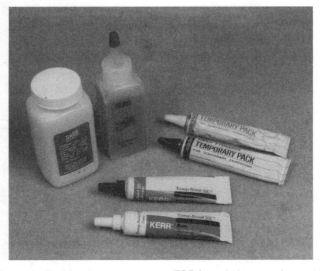

Figure 10–2 A powder-liquid and two paste-paste ZOE formulations used as provisional cements.

excessively. This limits their use to maximum periods of 1 year, which is perfectly acceptable for a provisional material.

Acrylic

Acrylics usually are used as provisional crown and bridge resins (Fig. 10-3). These materials have compositions similar to those of denture base or orthodontic resins. The powder generally is composed of small beads of PMMA polymer with small amounts of a peroxide initiator and oxide particles as pigments. The liquid is methyl methacrylate, which is used either alone or in conjunction with other methacrylate-type monomers, such as ethyl methacrylate. A small amount of amine activator is added to promote the polymerization reaction, as well as an inhibitor to provide shelf life and working time. Most of these acrylics are chemically cured materials, although light-activated composite denture base resin and tray resins also are used for constructing provisional restorations. The provisional acrylics are supplied in various shades to match a variety of tooth colors.

The powder and liquid are mixed to a creamy consistency in plastic cups according to the manufacturer's suggested P/L ratio. The restoration is produced by pouring the acrylic into a premade mold of the individual tooth or the several teeth involved in the bridge. The fabrication of a provisional crown and a provisional bridge is described later.

Similar to other acrylic materials, the liquid component of these provisional restoratives is highly volatile. Therefore, care should be taken immediately to replace the cap on the vial containing the liquid after its use. Also, the vapor can have an irritating smell, and exposure to it should be minimized.

Composites

Self-curing, light-curing, or dual-curing glass-reinforced resins are commonly used as provisional restoratives. These materials are based on urethane

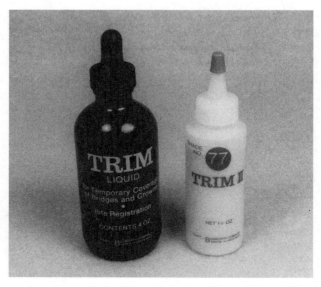

Figure 10–3 An acrylic resin powder-liquid formulation used for making provisional crown and bridge restorations.

dimethacrylate or bis-acryl resins and are similar to dental composite restoratives. They are usually supplied in tubes that fit within a gun cartridge, similar to many impression materials (Fig. 10-4). These materials are much more expensive but have several advantages over acrylic resins. The composite provisional materials generate less heat during polymerization and, therefore, are more compatible with oral tissues. In addition, they do not contain the same potentially irritating monomers found in acrylics.

Studies show evidence for discoloration, plaque adherence, and difficulties in handling that lead to marginal discrepancies with these composite provisionals. They are, however, physically strong and, when properly made, show good retention. As with the acrylic material, they can be used with a direct (in the mouth) or an indirect (on a cast) technique. These materials typically go through a doughy stage during setting. This allows them to be easily trimmed prior to final curing to produce a rigid structure. The material may cure on its own or be light cured, depending on the formulation.

Aluminum Crowns, Denture Resins, and Others

In addition to ZOE and acrylics, other materials are used as provisional restoratives. For example, certain provisional crowns are made of stainless steel or aluminum (Fig. 10-5). These thin metal crowns are stiff enough to bear occlusal forces when cemented onto a prepared tooth with a provisional cement, but they are also easy to cut and adjust to enhance their fit. One of their main drawbacks is their poor esthetic qualities.

For single-tooth preparations, such as inlays or onlays, light-cured denture resins also make useful provisionals (Fig. 10-6). These composite materials can be cured into undercuts in the tooth, eliminating the need for a cementation proce-

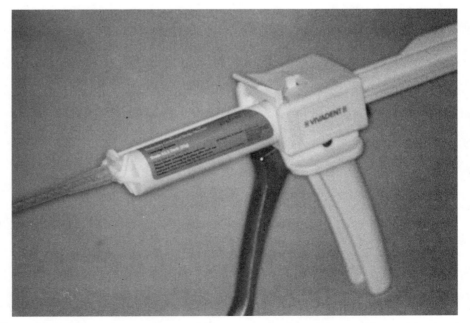

Figure 10–4 A bis-acryl composite material in a paste-paste formulation used for provisional restorations.

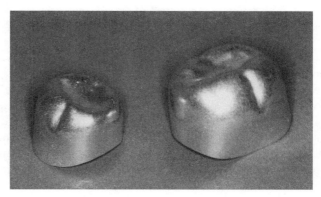

Figure 10–5 Aluminum provisional crowns.

dure. Often they are polymerized within a tooth that has been coated with a water-soluble lubricant. This enables them to be removed easily with an instrument and facilitates the cleaning of the cavity preparation. The provisional is then cemented into the tooth with a ZOE or noneugenol cement. The benefit of the latter procedure is that the cement fills up the gap created by the shrinking composite, thus minimizing leakage. When a cement is not used, leakage will occur and the tooth may be more sensitive during the interim period until a permanent restoration is placed.

A less rigid light-cured provisional filling material also exists (Fig. 10-6). This material is a cross between a composite and an impression material. It is of intermediate rigidity and is used frequently in preparations for composite or ceramic inlays (Fermit, Ivoclar). This composite-type material contains additives that keep it somewhat flexible after light-curing, similar to a very stiff putty impression material. The provisional material is cured in the preparation instead of being cemented in place. It undergoes minimal shrinkage during curing, so it "locks" into the tooth. It is easily removed because it does not bond to the tooth. Because of its flexibility, it is easily cut or pulled out of the preparation at the time of permanent restoration. Because it is not completely rigid, it is not recommended for large cavity preparations or bridges.

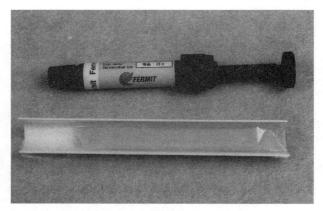

Figure 10–6 Two light-cured composite materials used for making provisional crown and bridge restorations, a semirigid formulation (*top*) and a rigid denture resin (*bottom*).

■ *Mixing and Placing an Acrylic Provisional Restorative*

Single-Tooth Provisional Restoration

When an acrylic provisional is made for a single crown, one customary direct technique involves the use of a clear plastic crown form made of polycarbonate polymer or celluloid (Fig. 10-7). These plastics are rigid and tough but can be easily cut by a blade or knife. The prepared tooth is first coated with a thin layer of petroleum jelly to keep the acrylic from sticking. At the same time, the surrounding tissue can be coated to avoid contact with the acrylic monomer. The appropriate crown form is then selected, and the provisional acrylic is mixed in a cup with a spatula until a creamy, fluid consistency is achieved. The acrylic is then poured into the plastic crown until it is approximately three-quarters full (Fig. 10-8). The filled crown is placed on the prepared tooth and held in place until the polymer begins to increase in viscosity and become doughy. The crown is then removed from the tooth and held for a few seconds before reseating. This process is continued until the acrylic hardens. ***What is the purpose of this "on-and-off" technique?***

As is discussed more fully in Chapter 12, when acrylic polymers harden, they emit heat. The heat could be significant enough to cause tissue damage or pain within the tooth. Studies have shown the temperature in the pulp chamber may exceed 50°C if the acrylic is allowed to set on the tooth the entire time. The "on-and-off" procedure allows for heat to be dissipated from the setting acrylic, but it ensures that the size of the provisional crown will be correct. In other words, the polymerization shrinkage that might cause the restoration to become too tight is minimized by continually repositioning the restorative on the tooth and forcing it to fit while it is still hardening.

After the acrylic has completely set, the clear plastic crown former is cut away from the acrylic with a scalpel. The crown is then trimmed with a blade and bur and refitted onto the tooth to ensure fit. Finally, it is cemented onto the tooth with a provisional cement. Either a ZOE or noneugenol cement is used when the permanent restoration is to be made from metal. A noneugenol cement would be chosen if the patient were known or suspected to be allergic to eugenol. If the permanent restoration is one that ultimately will be cemented to the tooth with a composite cement (e.g., a ceramic crown), then a noneugenol provisional cement also is more appropriate. Eugenol is difficult to clean completely from the tooth before final cementation, and it effectively inhibits the setting of composites. This is the same reason that ZOE bases cannot be used under composite restorations. If

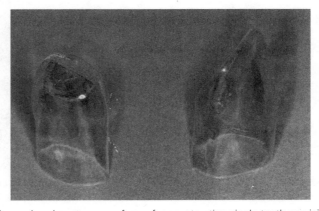

Figure 10–7 Clear polycarbonate crown forms for constructing single-tooth provisional restorations.

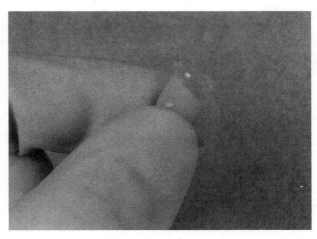

Figure 10–8 An acrylic provisional material mixed to a fluid consistency and poured into a plastic crown form to approximately three-quarters full.

a ZOE cement is used by mistake, a thorough pumicing of the prepared tooth before final cementation should be sufficient to eliminate the eugenol contaminants, but some concern remains because of the efficient manner in which eugenol penetrates into the tooth.

Another approach to making a direct provisional restoration of a single tooth is to make an impression of the prepared tooth, extending to at least one tooth on either side. The acrylic or composite provisional material is then placed into the impression and reseated in the mouth. The same "on-and-off" technique is used to minimize trauma caused by heat buildup. The provisional restoration is removed from the impression once it has set and is trimmed, adjusted, and finished prior to cementation onto the tooth.

Provisional Bridge

Provisional bridges can be constructed by a direct or indirect technique, with either a self-curing acrylic, composite, or light-cured composite denture resin used. Use of an acrylic will be described here. In either case, a study cast must be made of the patient's arch before cavity preparation. Typically, an alginate impression is made and the cast is poured in a fast-setting plaster. The missing dentition is then added to the model with either wax or a plastic denture tooth. A clear plastic shell or template is made on the model. This can be accomplished by softening the sheet over a flame and molding it onto the model or by using a vacuum-forming technique. For the latter, the model is placed onto the stage of the vacuum former (i.e., Omnivac), and the clear polypropylene or acetate plastic sheet is placed into the holder on the upper arm of the former (Fig. 10-9). The unit produces heat to soften the plastic sheet, which is then placed over the model. A vacuum is drawn from below the model, sucking the softened plastic down over the model, molding it tightly in all areas. The plastic is allowed to cool and harden and is then trimmed with scissors so that it extends to only one tooth on either side of the teeth to be prepared (Fig. 10-10). The excess is trimmed to ensure that the soft tissue will not be impinged on by the shell during seating of the provisional acrylic. The edges are smoothed with an acrylic trimming bur to avoid injuring the patient's mucosa or tongue. The teeth are then prepared and an impression is made. A plaster model is then made of the prepared teeth.

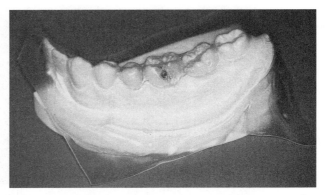

Figure 10–9 A clear plastic shell being formed on a plaster model in a vacuum former. The shell provides a template for the provisional bridge in the indirect technique.

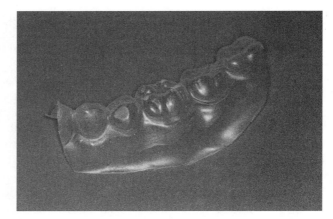

Figure 10–10 A trimmed plastic shell to be used for the indirect fabrication of a provisional bridge.

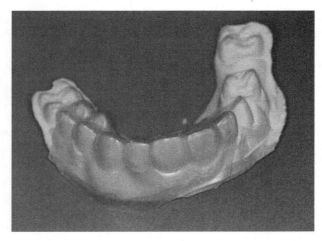

Figure 10–11 A plastic shell filled with acrylic after placing it onto a plaster model of teeth prepared for a bridge.

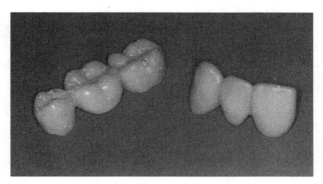

Figure 10–12 Finished acrylic provisional bridges.

For the indirect technique, a separating medium, such as petroleum jelly or liquid tinfoil substitute, is coated onto the plaster cast. The template is then filled approximately three-quarters full with the proper shade of an acrylic provisional material that has been mixed to a creamy consistency (Fig. 10-11). The pontic area is filled with an excess of acrylic to ensure complete filling. As an alternative to the acrylic pontic, a plastic denture tooth can be used as the pontic in the final provisional restoration. The acrylic becomes workable when it appears somewhat dull and begins to become doughy; it will have sufficient consistency or "body" to be shaped and remain where it is placed, while still possessing acceptable flow characteristics. It is then seated onto the cast and held in place with rubber bands until completely set. The setting for some materials can be hastened by placing the entire assembly in warm water at approximately 45°C. *Why isn't the "on-and-off" technique used here?*

After the acrylic has set, it is removed from the cast, and the shell is removed with a scalpel. The acrylic flash around the periphery of the provisional is removed with a separating disk and an acrylic finishing bur in a handpiece (Fig. 10-12). It is then polished and cemented in place with a ZOE or noneugenol provisional cement.

The procedure for the direct technique, in which the bridge is made in the mouth, is similar to that used for a single tooth with a polycarbonate crown form. First, the teeth and adjacent tissues should be coated with a lubricant. Once the acrylic has begun to set, it should be removed to avoid overheating the tissues during curing. The bridge can also be reinforced with fibers made from polyethylene or glass, as previously described (Chapter 7).

The light-cured material can be used in either technique and offers the advantage of allowing the removal of excess material before curing. In addition, repeated try-ins can be performed before curing to ensure proper seating and fit. The material is cured in a light-curing unit in the same manner as composite inlays and onlays.

Summary

Provisional restorative materials are used to occupy a cavity preparation until such time when a more durable and permanent restoration can be placed. Typical provisional materials in dentistry include ZOE cement, acrylic plastic, resin composite, and aluminum crowns. These materials are used for short durations and, therefore, have minimal requirements for strength and stability. ZOE is a relatively weak cement that can be used as a cementing agent or restorative for a single tooth. Acrylics are basically unreinforced, self-curing polymers that can be molded into crown and bridge temporaries. Self-cured and light-cured composites are also used routinely. These restorations can be made directly in the mouth or by an indirect technique on a model or die. Thin aluminum crowns can be shaped and fitted to a crown preparation but lack the structural rigidity needed for long-term use.

STUDY QUESTIONS AND PROBLEM SOLVING

1. An acid-etched composite would *not* make a good provisional restorative because it would:
   a. Have a poor marginal seal
   b. Not be strong enough
   c. Be too difficult to remove
   d. Set too slowly
2. Which of the following is *not* a component of a common ZOE provisional restorative?
   a. Eugenol liquid
   b. Rosin powder
   c. Zinc oxide particles
   d. Methyl methacrylate liquid
3. Which of the following is (are) a reason(s) that ZOE is not used as a permanent restorative material?
   a. It wears readily
   b. It has low strength
   c. It has poor biocompatibility
   d. It is difficult to use
4. The "on-and-off" technique is used when a direct acrylic provisional restoration is being made because the:
   a. Acrylic will never completely harden if left in the mouth
   b. Patient could be burned by the setting material
   c. The fit of the restoration is improved by repetitive removal
   d. Continuous squeezing removes air bubbles from the mix
5. Which of the following is *not* used in the procedure for preparing an indirect acrylic provisional restoration?
   a. A plaster model of the unprepared teeth
   b. An impression of the prepared teeth
   c. A plaster model of the prepared teeth
   d. An impression of the restored teeth
6. Composite materials offer several advantages over acrylics for provisional restorations, including:
   a. Less thermal production during setting
   b. Lower cost
   c. Significantly easier handling
   d. Less chemical irritation

SELECTED READINGS

Christensen GJ. Provisional restorations for fixed prosthodontics. Journal of the American Dental Association 127:249–252, 1996.
   This article provides a brief summary of the different types of provisional materials used specifically for fixed prosthodontic cases.

Duke ES. Provisional restorative materials: A technology update. Compendium of Continuing Education in Dentistry 20:497–500, 1999.

This article discusses the advantages of new composite provisional materials over previous acrylics.

Farah JW, Powers JM (eds). Temporization. Dental Advisor 9:1–8, 1992.

A review of the purpose, requirements, and techniques used for preparing provisional restorations is provided. This periodical compares current brands of materials and provides ratings and information on costs.

Gegauff AC. Provisional restorations. In: Rosenstiel SF, Land MF, Fujimoto J, eds. Contemporary Fixed Prosthodontics. St. Louis: CV Mosby, 1988;234–260.

This text contains a detailed chapter on the materials and techniques used to prepare various types of provisional restorations.

Hannon SM, Breault LG, Kim AC. The immediate provisional restoration: A review of clinical techniques. Quintessence International 29:163–169, 1998.

This article reviews numerous techniques for the immediate interim replacement of teeth and shows examples of the use of the patient's own extracted tooth in a denture, orthodontic wire stabilization of pontics in a bridge, and polyethylene fiber reinforcement as a periodontal splint.

Luthardt RG, Stobel M, Hinz M, Vollandt R. Clinical performance and periodontal outcome of temporary crowns and fixed partial dentures: A randomized clinical trial. Journal of Prosthetic Dentistry 83:32–39, 2000.

This article describes the results of a clinical study comparing four different composite provisional materials. The results show that the materials were all retained well and were sufficiently strong, but all collected plaque and were somewhat difficult to handle.

Schwartz R, Davis R, Mayhew R. The effect of a ZOE provisional cement on the bond strength of a resin luting cement. American Journal of Dentistry 3:28–30, 1990.

This article describes an experiment in which it is determined that bonding to enamel was not compromised by the previous application of a eugenol-containing material, as long as the tooth was pumiced and etched with phosphoric acid.

Small BW. Indirect provisional restorations. General Dentistry 47:140–142, 1999.

This article lists the requirements for provisional restorations and provides a step-by-step procedure for the indirect technique.

Wang RL, Moore BK, Goodacre CJ, Swartz ML, Andres CJ. A comparison of resins for fabricating provisional fixed restorations. International Journal of Prosthodontics 2:173–184, 1989.

This article compares four acrylic resins and two composite resin provisional restoratives in terms of hardness, fit, wear resistance, strength, roughness, and polishability. The results showed a variation among materials, with none being the best in all categories.

Chapter 11

Materials for Cast Restorations

Objectives

- Identify the different types of waxes used in dentistry and compare their properties and stability at room temperature.
- Compare the types and applications of the different die materials.
- Compare the composition and expansion characteristics of low-heat and high-heat investment materials.
- Explain the cause of the two types of expansion experienced by investment materials.
- Describe the sequence of procedures used to make a cast metal crown.
- Explain why investment materials must expand to produce accurate castings.
- Explain the rationale for vacuum mixing and vacuum investing.
- List the objectives behind the wax burnout procedure for the lost wax technique.
- Explain the purpose of using flux during the melting of metal in the casting process.
- List the factors that can influence the fit of a dental casting.

■ *Casting: The Basic Concept*

In dentistry, **casting** refers to the process of pouring a liquid material into a cavity in a mold to produce a restoration or appliance. The process is ancient, dating to approximately 2500 B.C., and in many respects has changed little over the course of time. Although casting is accomplished most often with metals, certain ceramics can be cast to produce restorations, and plastics can be cast to produce dentures. In this chapter, only metal casting is discussed, although the process for ceramics is similar.

The process by which inlays, onlays, crowns, bridges, and partial denture frameworks are made of gold or other metals is called the **lost wax casting technique**. The name derives from the fact that a wax pattern of a restoration is heated and vaporized and subsequently replaced by a metal. The process requires a high level of precision. Because many different types of materials are used in this process, strict attention to detail is required at every step to ensure success. Casting is an art form; jewelry is produced by using identical procedures. Many practitioners of the dental sciences use their training outside of dentistry and enjoy the hobby of jewelry making.

The entire casting process is described in detail in a later section of this chapter, after each of the materials has been discussed. It is instructive, however, to begin with a brief overview of the entire procedure. The dentist prepares a tooth for a restoration. An impression, or negative replica, is made of the prepared tooth. A temporary restoration is then placed, and the patient is sent home. A **die** material, usually a dental stone, is then poured into the impression to produce a positive replica of the prepared tooth. Next, a **wax pattern** is created on the die by adding melted wax; the wax pattern is essentially a restoration made from wax. The pattern is then **invested**, i.e., enclosed within a ceramic material that forms a mold around the pattern. The mold is then heated to high temperatures to melt and vaporize the wax, leaving behind an empty space or cavity within the ceramic investment. Next, a metal is melted and thrust into the investment by the centrifugal force produced by a casting machine. When the metal cools, it hardens to form the final restoration. The restoration is cleaned and polished and cemented into the prepared tooth at the patient's next appointment.

■ *Waxes*

Uses in Dentistry

Waxes find a great many uses in dentistry. They are used to make patterns for many types of cast restorations. They are used to attach or lute restorations together prior to soldering. Waxes can be used to make a registration of a patient's occlusion, although this is done less frequently today. They are used to simulate the gingiva and hold plastic or porcelain teeth during denture processing. They are also used by dental personnel during many other procedures performed both in and out of the mouth. They come in a variety of shapes and sizes (Fig. 11-1).

Types and Characteristics

Waxes are organic polymers made from molecules such as esters and alcohols. There are natural waxes, such as paraffin, carnauba, and beeswax, as well as syn-

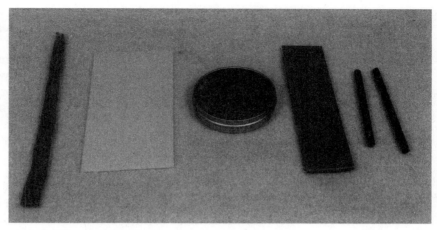

Figure 11–1 Different types of waxes, including wax ropes, baseplate wax, inlay wax, boxing wax, and sticky wax.

thetic ones. Most dental waxes are blends of different types. This is done to change the softening (or melting) range and hardness for a given application. For example, paraffin is soft and has a low melting range (approximately 50 to 70°C), whereas carnauba is much harder and melts over a higher temperature range (65 to 90°C). Mixtures of these two produce intermediate waxes. Waxes also contain other components, such as resins, oils, gums, and coloring agents, to optimize their handling and esthetic characteristics. Owing to their varied compositions, waxes have widely varying properties; they range from hard and brittle to soft and malleable. The waxes used in dentistry can be divided into several categories, including pattern waxes, processing waxes, and impression waxes. Each of these will be described briefly below.

Waxes have a variety of characteristics that limit their use to nonstructural applications in many dental procedures. They are essentially adjunct or temporary materials. Waxes are easily deformed under stress (i.e., they are weak), they flow and distort at low temperatures, and they have high coefficients of thermal expansion. During cooling, all waxes develop internal stress because of their low thermal conductivity and large amount of cooling shrinkage. In light of the manner in which waxes are used, this is an undesirable trait because it affects their dimensional stability. ***Can you think of an example in which the characteristics of waxes may influence a dental procedure?***

Consider the situation in which a wax is used to make a pattern for a cast inlay restoration. The wax is melted and then poured into the preparation on the die. As the wax cools to room temperature, it hardens and develops stresses within its internal structure. These stresses are produced because the outside surface of the wax cools and hardens before the inside surface does as a result of the insulating nature of the wax. Because it is on the outside, the outside surface is free to shrink and does so without restriction. As the internal part of the wax begins to cool, however, its shrinkage is restricted by the hardened wax shell that has formed on the outside. Therefore, the internal wax cannot move or flow to relieve the stress. This phenomenon leaves the completely hardened pattern in a state of internal stress. Any heating of the pattern at a later time (e.g., by a temperature change in its immediate vicinity) will cause the internal stress to be eliminated by flow of the wax, producing a distortion of the pattern. For this reason, it makes good sense to invest a wax pattern quickly before distortion can occur. Studies have verified poorer fit and accuracy of castings when patterns were stored for more than 24 hours before investing.

Another problem with wax is that it has only a minimal surface hardness and, therefore, can easily become deformed or scratched when touched with hard objects such as metal instruments. Even aggressive polishing can distort the surface of a wax pattern. This is significant because all flaws on the surface of a wax pattern eventually will be reproduced on the surface of the cast metal restoration. The dimensional instability and limited hardness always must be considered when working with waxes.

Pattern Waxes

These waxes are used to make inlays, onlays, crowns, and pontics (inlay wax), bridges and partial denture attachments (casting wax), and bases for setting denture teeth (baseplate wax).

There are two types of inlay pattern waxes. They differ in that one is meant to be softened and placed into the prepared tooth to form a "direct" pattern, which is then removed from the tooth and used to cast the restoration. The second type is for "indirect" patterns, which are made outside of the mouth by using an impression die technique, as mentioned in the synopsis of the casting procedure. As one would expect, a wax for a direct pattern would have to have a softening point higher than the normal oral temperatures of 34 to 37°C; otherwise, it would not hold its shape in the mouth or when removed from the tooth. Waxes for the indirect technique need only have softening points that are sufficiently higher than room temperature so that they will not distort under normal conditions in the laboratory.

Inlay pattern waxes are hard at room temperature, so their surfaces are not easily damaged during the preparation or smoothing of the wax pattern. These waxes usually are blue or purple in color. Casting pattern waxes most often are used in preparing partial denture frameworks and usually are supplied in sheets. They are relatively soft, compared with baseplate waxes. Denture teeth are set into baseplate waxes, which also are supplied in sheets, usually pink; however, they tend to be harder and more brittle than casting wax sheets. The baseplate usually is built up from layers of baseplate wax, which must be well heated so that the individual layers stick together. Because this wax will be tried into the mouth once the denture teeth have been set in one of the first stages of denture making, it must remain relatively hard and not easily distorted at oral temperatures.

Processing Waxes

Processing waxes are used in many dental procedures, such as bordering an impression tray (boxing or utility wax) and temporarily attaching objects for soldering (sticky and carding wax). Boxing and utility wax are soft and have low melting ranges. They often are colored red. Sticky wax is hard and must be heated with a flame to be melted. In the liquid state, it has good adhesive characteristics toward a variety of surfaces. It is usually black, brown, or yellow.

Impression Waxes

Impression waxes have been used for taking edentulous impressions; they also are used for bite registrations. Impression waxes must be deformable at oral temperatures to record the detail of the oral tissues. As waxes, however, they have minimal stability and largely have been replaced by elastomeric impression materials for these applications.

■ *Die Materials*

Uses in Dentistry

In dentistry, a **die** is a positive replica of a structure on which a wax restoration is prepared. The die can be of a single tooth or of several teeth. The die usually is prepared from an impression and, therefore, must be able to reproduce the fine detail that was initially recorded by the impression material. The die must also be stable over time and possess some minimal level of strength and hardness so that it will not distort, chip, or break during use.

Types and Characteristics

In Chapter 9, gypsum materials are discussed with respect to their use as model and die materials. As emphasized, the hardest dental stones are used in the fabrication of dies because they are the most resistant to chipping and abrasion. It also is stated that the setting expansion of gypsum could be minimized by adding certain chemicals, thus allowing them to produce accurate renditions of impressions. These characteristics, in conjunction with their low cost and ease of manipulation, make stone the most popular die material in dentistry (Fig. 11-2).

Stone dies can be plated with metal to make them harder and more stable. **Electroplating**, an electrochemical process, is used to place a thin layer of silver or copper metal directly into the impression. Stone is then poured into the plated impression. When the stone hardens and is removed from the impression, the metal shell remains attached to the stone, forming a plated die. The process requires special equipment and is complicated and time consuming. The major benefit is that it produces dies with hard metallic surfaces on which restorations may be finished with less concern over abrasion and destruction of the margins. Because of the water present within them, however, the technique cannot be used with hydrocolloid impression materials.

Stone can also be reinforced with a resin additive for the purpose of producing a die material with improved properties. A recent study has, however, shown little difference in the strength, brittleness, dimensional change, surface hardness, or abrasion resistance of the reinforced and the conventional gypsum dies.

Another die material that has been used in dentistry is epoxy polymer (Fig. 11-2). The material is supplied as two components, an epoxy resin and a hardener. The latter contains the amine catalyst, which can be toxic and should not be used in the mouth or allowed to contact the skin for any length of time. Although most

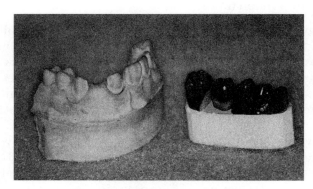

Figure 11–2 Stone and epoxy dies.

polymers undergo a large dimensional change during curing, die epoxies are formulated with relatively low shrinkage values. This usually is achieved by a slow curing reaction that builds up less shrinkage stress but causes the material to require up to several hours to harden fully. These materials are stronger, less brittle, and more abrasion resistant than is stone; they are not as accurate or as stable, however, because they still shrink during hardening. Because water inhibits their curing or polymerization reaction, they cannot be used with the hydrocolloid impression materials.

One other type of die that has emerged in recent years is a flexible material having a composition similar to that of polyvinylsiloxane impression material. In general, these very stiff but elastomeric die materials have not been shown to have better properties or surface characteristics than stone die materials have, and they cannot be used with polyvinylsiloxane impressions unless a separator is used. The problem is that the separator also contributes to inaccuracy and loss of surface detail in these materials.

■ *Investment Materials*

Uses in Dentistry

Investments are ceramic materials used as molds for casting molten metals or holding metal appliances in correct relation during soldering procedures. They are made from ceramics because they must be able to withstand the high temperatures associated with the casting process. In addition, they must not chemically react with the cast metal. Many investments have been developed in recent years as the casting of different types of metals, such as titanium and its alloys, and various ceramics have become more common. Because some of these other materials are cast at very high temperatures, investments that maintain their integrity at these elevated temperatures are necessary.

For the more common dental applications, three types of investments are used. One type is used for the casting of most gold alloys for full coverage. Another is used during the casting of the high-temperature alloys used in porcelain-fused-to-metal (PFM) restorations. The third is used for casting partial denture metals. Only the first two types of investments, known as gypsum-bonded and phosphate-bonded investments, are discussed in detail.

Types and Characteristics

Gypsum-Bonded Investments

Gypsum-bonded investments are composed of calcium sulfate hemihydrate (dental stone), which serves as the binder or matrix material and provides much of the strength of the investment. The investment also contains high concentrations of silica in the form of quartz or cristobalite. The silica serves as the **refractory**, the material that determines the temperature resistance and thermal expansion of the investment. Other additives include modifiers that control setting rate and expansion.

Gypsum investments are powders that are mixed with water in the same manner as discussed in Chapter 9 for plaster and stone. The materials are conveniently supplied in individual packages (Fig. 11-3). They also are supplied in bulk, but because the gypsum is **hygroscopic** (i.e., it absorbs water from the atmo-

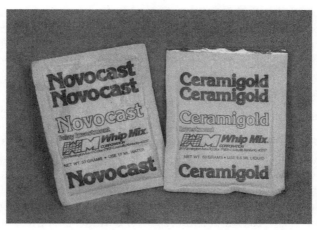

Figure 11–3 Gypsum-based (*left*) and phosphate-based (*right*) investment materials supplied in individual packages.

sphere), care must be taken to keep the powder dry at all times or it will begin to set.

As is discussed in the next section, casting involves the use of several materials that either expand or contract during the process. The overall goal of the casting procedure is to produce an accurate restoration; therefore, these expansions and contractions must be balanced. The use of an investment material that expands during setting and during heating to counteract the shrinkage of the cast metal during cooling is one example of how this is achieved. Because the bulk of the investment expansion can be attained through setting expansion or thermal (heating) expansion, gypsum investment material is manufactured in two different forms. One form is processed by the *thermal technique*, in which the bulk of the expansion takes place during the wax burnout procedure. The second is for the *hygroscopic technique*, in which most of the expansion of the investment occurs during setting in a water bath. The procedures for using these two materials are described later. In either case, the material usually is mixed in a vacuum to minimize the number of air bubbles incorporated.

Gypsum is thermally stable to temperatures approaching 730 to 750°C (1250 to 1300°F). The material begins to decompose when heated beyond that temperature. As discussed later, when it is heated to approximately 700°C, the expansion of a gypsum investment is maximized because the silica compound undergoes a physical change that creates an expansion. Therefore, there is always the danger of overheating a gypsum investment and causing some decomposition of the material during the expansion phase of the burnout procedure. When this happens, the casting becomes contaminated by the interaction between the decomposed investment and the molten metal. This problem can be avoided by paying strict attention to each step in the procedure; however, this characteristic limits gypsum-bonded investment materials to this temperature range.

As the technique of covering metal restorations with porcelain gained acceptance, it became obvious that metals with higher melting points were necessary to avoid distortion during the porcelain firing phase (see Chapter 7), which took place at temperatures near the melting point of many of the popular metals. Because these metals are melted at higher temperatures, they must cool over a greater temperature range after casting and, therefore, undergo greater thermal contractions than the common gold alloys used in all-metal crown and bridge restorations. The greater contraction necessitated an investment with greater expansion and one that would not interact with the metals at the higher casting temperatures. The phosphate-bonded investments were developed for this purpose. They are commonplace in dentistry today because of the many different types of metals used.

Phosphate-Bonded Investments

Phosphate-bonded investments contain the same silica refractory (i.e., quartz or cristobalite) present in the gypsum-bonded investments. The binder, however, is made from an acidic phosphate and magnesium oxide. The powdered investment is mixed with water or a special liquid containing small silica particles (Fig. 11-3). These materials set by a complicated, two-part reaction. One reaction begins after mixing, whereas the second reaction is induced by the heating process during wax burnout. This second reaction makes the investment extremely resistant to high temperatures and greatly improves its strength. The burnout procedure for the phosphate-bonded investment differs from that of the gypsum-bonded investment only in terms of the high-temperature step. The final heating step for phosphate investments takes place at 810°C (1400°F) for 30 to 60 minutes. Because the phosphate-bonded investment is much stronger than the gypsum-bonded one, it is much more difficult to break apart and remove from the casting.

The third common investment material is used for partial denture (cobalt-chromium) metals that melt at very high temperatures. These investments are silica bonded and set by a complex chemical reaction.

■ *The Lost Wax Casting Process*

Beginning with the creation of the impression of the prepared tooth and continuing until the final finishing, a multitude of factors influence the fit and marginal integrity of the cast restoration. Because the success of the entire process depends on the accuracy with which each step along the way is accomplished, the procedure is necessarily complex. A brief description of the process was given in the introduction to this chapter. In this section, a more detailed presentation of the technique for preparing a gold inlay is given in order to stress the importance of each event in the process, as well as to familiarize the student with the causes of ill-fitting and failed castings. Although many figures are included to assist the student in understanding the lost wax casting technique, fullest appreciation of the process is achieved by experiencing it in person.

The *first* step in the process requires an accurate recording (i.e., negative replica) of the surfaces to be restored. This is the role of the impression material. Dentistry is fortunate to have elastomeric materials that undergo minimal shrinkage (0.05%) and have the ability to reproduce and resolve features at the level of 1 μm. In other words, if one could scratch two lines 1 μm apart on a piece of glass and then take an impression of the glass surface, the two lines would appear as separate and distinct on the impression viewed under a microscope. As a frame of reference, the naked eye probably could see the two scratches as separate if they were 10 to 15 μm or more apart. Therefore, the naked eye of the dental worker is not capable of visualizing the detail that the impression material can reproduce. A poor impression guarantees a poor casting because the casting can only be as accurate as the initial impression. *Is it apparent why custom trays are used by many in the impression-making process?*

> Custom trays provide the best guarantee for an accurate impression, thus helping to ensure an accurate restoration.

The *second* step in the process is to produce a die (i.e., positive replica) on which a wax pattern will be fashioned. The die material is poured into the impression, with care taken to avoid bubble formation or distortion of the impression. Once hardened, it provides an accurate reproduction of the prepared tooth (Fig. 11-2). Note that some die materials, being made from gypsum, expand slightly (0.1%) during setting. This expansion offsets the shrinkage of the impression material, leaving the positive replica a bit oversized. In the final analysis, this will not be a problem. *Why won't it? (Consider what would happen if the casting were exactly the same size as the prepared tooth.)*

> Remember that the casting must be cemented into the tooth. If the casting fit the tooth exactly, there would be no room for the cement. The clinician would not be able to seat the casting without damaging the tooth.

The *third* step is to prepare a wax pattern on the die. The die is first coated with a thin film of separating solution or die lubricant so that the wax will not adhere to the die. Wax is then melted in a flame from a Bunsen burner or alcohol torch and added to the die in small increments. Each increment is allowed to cool to minimize shrinkage distortions, which may be produced within the wax if it is cooled too fast. The wax is built up to reproduce the anatomy of the tooth, and the pattern essentially becomes a wax model of the restoration (Fig. 11-4). It must be perfectly adapted to the die to ensure a good fit with tight junctions at the margins. As stated, the wax shrinks during cooling (0.2%) and, if cooled too fast, may distort at a later time. Therefore, the process must be handled with care and patience because the final casting will never be more accurate than the wax pattern. In spite of all these precautions, however, there will always be some internal stress within the pattern. Therefore, as mentioned, a wax pattern should not be subjected to temperature extremes that may cause stress relief and distortions in shape because this will result in a loss of accuracy in the final casting.

The *fourth* step in the process is the preparation of the wax pattern for invest-

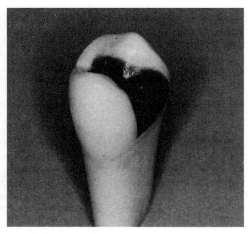

Figure 11–4 Two-surface inlay wax pattern on a stone die.

ing. The wax pattern will be enclosed in a hard investment material and will then be eliminated, leaving behind a cavity into which liquid metal can be poured. *If the wax pattern is surrounded by investment, how will the melted wax get out and the liquid metal get in?*

Obviously, the pattern must be invested with an opening to the outside that serves as a route for the removal of wax components and a channel through which liquid metal can flow in. This channel is called the **sprue**.

The sprue is fashioned on a base, called a *sprue former,* and the two suspend the wax pattern in the air before investing. After the wax pattern is created on the die, the sprue, a cylindrical piece of wax, is attached to it by slightly heating and pressing it onto the surface of the pattern. A waxing instrument is then used to add small amounts of wax at the attachment to secure the bond and produce a smooth surface (Fig. 11-5). The wax sprue (they also may be made of metal or plastic) is then attached to a cone-shaped rubber base (i.e., the sprue former; see Fig. 11-5). This attachment is also secured with additional wax. The sprue former is special in that it fits inside of a metal ring that will hold the investment material.

The *fifth* step in the process is called *investing.* A metallic ring, called the casting ring, is fitted into the rubber sprue former, encircling the wax pattern to a height of 10 mm or so above the edge of the pattern. The ring and sprue former provide a seal so investment material can be poured inside the ring to surround the wax pattern and sprue. Before this is done, the metal ring is lined with a moistened paper made from glass fibers. (Note: These liners once were made from asbestos, until asbestos fibers were proven to be carcinogenic and a major health hazard.) The purpose of this liner is to provide a cushion for the hardening investment material to expand into during the setting reaction. If the liner were not used, the investment could not expand outward because it would be completely constrained by the metal ring, which would push the investment back into the wax pattern. Because the investment, being made from gypsum, expands during setting by approximately 0.7%, if the outward expansion is inhibited, the gypsum will expand inward and press on the wax pattern. This would leave the cavity, formed when the wax is burned out, exactly the same size as the wax pattern. *Although this may seem desirable at this point, it will soon become apparent why the cavity must actually be increased in size to get an accurate casting.*

Therefore, the use of the soft ring liner with an expanding investment ensures

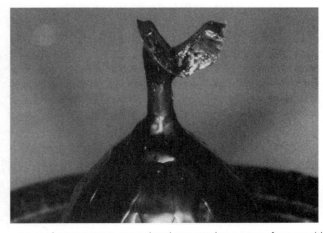

Figure 11–5 A wax pattern sprued and mounted to a sprue former with wax.

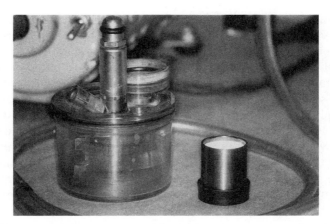

Figure 11–6 Vac-u-spat mixing apparatus and the lined casting ring mounted on the sprue former.

that the cavity will be larger than the wax pattern when the investment is completely set. The liner is moistened because a dry liner would absorb water from the investment and minimize the setting expansion. In recent years, ringless casting systems have been developed that do not require a ring liner or a metal ring. These systems utilize a flexible, resilient ring system to contain the investment material during its setting, which is removed prior to the burnout procedure. In either case, further expansion of the investment takes place during the high-temperature burnout procedure used to eliminate the wax. Thus, this investment technique is called the *high-heat investment technique.*

The investment powder is mixed with water in the correct proportions, usually under a vacuum to eliminate air bubbles. Special equipment, consisting of a plastic bowl with a plastic top containing a metal mixing blade, is used for this procedure (an example is the Vac-u-spat, Whip Mix Corp.; Fig. 11-6). The casting ring with the sprue former and wax pattern is attached to the top of the mixer. This allows the operator to flow the investment material directly into the open end of the casting ring, while the whole system remains under vacuum (Fig. 11-7).

Another common procedure is to disassemble the mixing container after the 15-second mixing procedure is complete and paint the investment onto the wax pattern with a paint brush. This is done to ensure that no air bubbles are trapped

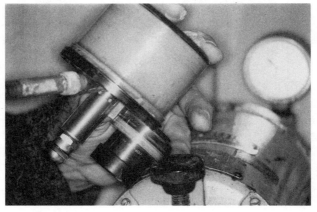

Figure 11–7 Casting ring attached to the Vac-u-spat and being filled while under vacuum in the Vac-u-vestor apparatus.

on the wax. The mixer is then reassembled, and the ring is completely filled under vacuum. Vacuum mixing and pouring is superior to hand mixing and pouring because most of the bubbles that may cling to the wax pattern are eliminated by the vacuum technique. One further way to eliminate bubbles is to brush a **surfactant**, a weak detergent solution, onto the wax pattern before investing. The surfactant improves the wetting of the hydrophilic investment onto the hydrophobic wax surface and minimizes bubble formation during investing.

Once the ring is completely invested, it is removed from the mixing device and allowed to harden on the countertop at room temperature for 45 minutes to 1 hour. If the burnout procedure will not be performed within 1 hour, the invested case should be stored in a humid environment to prevent the investment from drying and cracking. At this point, if one were to cut the casting ring in half from top to bottom, the cross section would appear as shown schematically in Figure 11-8.

In Chapter 9, it is stated that the use of a high water-to-powder ratio for mixing dental stone results in decreased setting expansion. Although this is true, additional water can actually be used to increase the setting expansion of gypsum investment materials. This apparent contradiction has to do with the effects of the surface tension of water on the expanding gypsum crystals. This subject is beyond the scope of this chapter, however, and the interested reader is directed to an excellent explanation of the effect in one of the textbooks appearing in the list of Selected Readings at the end of this chapter. It is enough to say that submerging the setting investment ring in a water bath will maximize the expansion of the investment material. This technique, called *hygroscopic expansion*, requires special equipment and produces a total setting expansion of 1.5%, more than twice the expansion produced by "air drying" the investment (0.7%).

The *sixth* step in the process is called *wax burnout*. The invested mold is heated to eliminate the wax and make room for the liquid metal. The following is a typ-

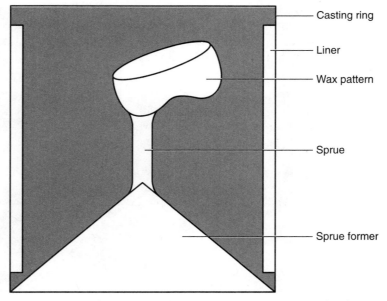

Figure 11–8 Cross section of a wax pattern invested in a casting ring.

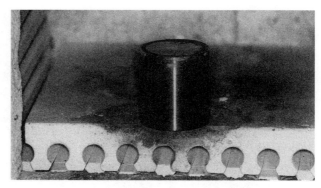

Figure 11–9 Casting ring in the casting oven during burnout. The sprue opening is pointed down.

ical procedure. The rubber sprue former is removed from the invested ring after the investment has hardened. The ring, which now contains the wax pattern and attached sprue completely surrounded by investment material, is then placed into an oven at 250°C (approximately 500°F) with the sprue end down, thus allowing the melted wax to flow out (Fig. 11-9). After 30 minutes, the wax will have been completely removed and vaporized. At this point, metal tongs are used to transfer the ring to an oven set at approximately 650°C (1200°F). The ring is placed with the sprue hole down so that no contaminants can fall into the hole. This slow heating process ensures that the investment material will not crack from excessive thermal shock, a problem for brittle materials. After 45 minutes at this elevated temperature, the ring is ready to be cast.

This high-temperature heating has two purposes, besides the removal of the wax. As the investment material is heated to 650°C, it undergoes a thermal expansion of 1.25%. Thus, the total expansion of the investment material in the high-heat technique is approximately 1.95% (setting = 0.7% + thermal = 1.25%). This creates a larger cavity for the metal to fill in the next step. For the hygroscopic technique, the mold also is heated, but to a lower temperature. This produces less thermal expansion, but the total expansion (2.05%) is slightly greater than that for the high-heat technique. The other important aspect of the heating is that it raises the temperature of the investment to a level closer to the temperature of the molten metal that will be cast into it. If the thermal shock produced by a very hot liquid metal hitting a very cold ceramic mold is too great, the mold may crack and cause a defective casting. Heating the investment to such a high temperature reduces the likelihood that this will happen.

The *seventh* step in the process is to melt and then cast or thrust the metal by centrifugal force through the sprue hole into the cavity within the investment. The machine used to accomplish this is called a centrifugal or "broken-arm" casting machine. It consists of a stage attached to an arm that has a counterweight at the other end and is supported in the middle by a rotating spindle (Fig. 11-10). The spindle is spring loaded and can be wound by hand (usually three to four full revolutions for gold metals). When the arm is released, it spins and throws the molten metal outward into the investment.

Metal, usually in the form of square "coupons" or "ingots" (each usually weighs 1 pennyweight), is placed onto a porcelain crucible on the stage of the casting machine and heated in the flame of a gas-air torch (Fig. 11-11). A proper flame has three visible cones. The middle, bluish-colored cone is the hottest and should

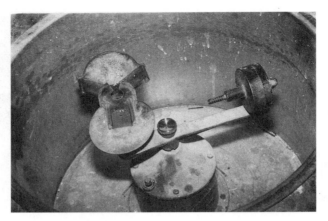

Figure 11–10 Broken-arm centrifugal casting machine.

be used to melt the metal most efficiently. Melting takes a minute or so and can be aided by the addition of a **flux** during the heating. Metals oxidize and form a "skin," or thickened outer surface; this is particularly apparent in a melting metal because the oxide skin keeps the surface together and inhibits the metal from flowing. This obviously would be detrimental to the casting process. The flux, which is a powder composed of borax and boric acid, reacts with the oxygen at the surface of the melting metal and removes the oxide skin, thus reducing the surface tension and allowing the metal to become very fluid (Fig. 11-12). At this stage, the metal takes on a shiny, mirror-like appearance and is extremely hot (approximately 1100°C or 2000°F). Higher temperatures can be achieved by mixing gas and oxygen, but they are not necessary for most non-PFM gold alloys. Certain high-melting-point metals are cast in special machines that heat the metal through an electrical process (i.e., induction heating) rather than by an open flame.

Immediately after the metal is melted, the invested ring is retrieved from the nearby oven with metal tongs and placed into a metal cradle directly behind the crucible holding the molten metal (Fig. 11-13). The crucible has a hole in it, and

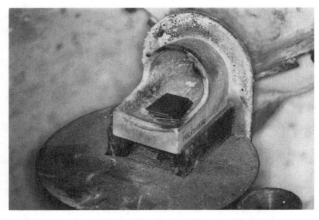

Figure 11–11 Metal coupons just before being heated in a crucible on the stage of the casting machine.

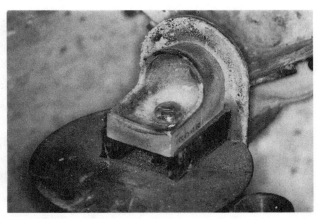

Figure 11–12 Melted metal appears shiny after flux has been added to enhance flow.

when the casting arm is released and begins to spin, the metal is thrown through the hole and directly through the sprue hole into the cavity in the investment material. Because the metal will cool quickly, two things are important. First, the torch flame must remain directed at the metal until the casting arm is released, so that the metal does not cool down and decrease in fluidity. Second, the casting arm must provide enough rotational force to fill the cavity quickly before the metal freezes in the thin sprue region.

Once the casting machine stops spinning, the hot metal ring is removed from the cradle with tongs and placed onto a heat-resistant block to cool. When the exposed metal surface becomes a dull red color, the ring is quickly placed into a container of cold water. This process, called **quenching**, usually causes the investment material to crack, and this can facilitate its removal from the surface of the casting. After 10 seconds, the casting is sufficiently cool to be retrieved from the water (Fig. 11-14). The sprue is then removed from the restoration by using an abrasive disk mounted in a handpiece. The surface of the casting may be cleaned in an acidic solution (**pickling**) before being finished and fitted onto the die (Fig. 11-15).

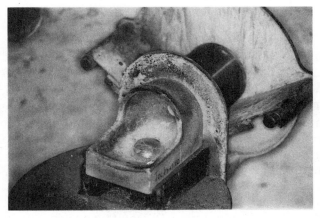

Figure 11–13 Casting machine with the casting ring placed onto the stage directly behind the crucible, just before casting.

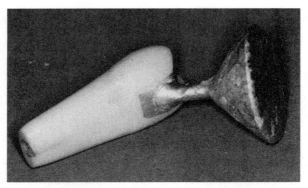

Figure 11–14 The fit on the die of the cast inlay while it is still attached to the sprue and metal button.

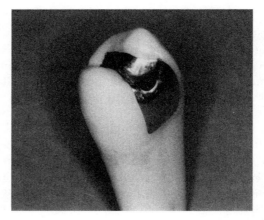

Figure 11–15 Polished casting as it fits on the die.

Because the metal must cool to room temperature from a very high temperature, a significant thermal contraction occurs, resulting in a shrinkage of the casting of approximately 1.4 to 1.5%. This shrinkage is offset by the expansion of the investment, producing a casting with good fit characteristics when each step of the procedure is performed properly.

Summary

Many materials are used during the process of manufacturing a dental casting. These materials are not usually used intraorally. Natural and synthetic waxes are used for many applications, including the formation of patterns for restorations and setting teeth for dentures. Die materials are made from either gypsum or polymer resins, such as epoxy, and they serve as an accurate representation of the prepared tissue on which the wax pattern is fashioned. Investment materials are used to encase the wax pattern; they eventually provide a mold within which liquid metal or ceramic can be poured to produce the actual cast restoration. Different types of investment materials are used for different metals because high casting temperatures require phosphate- or silica-based investments instead of the gypsum-based investments commonly used for gold alloys with lower melting points.

The lost wax casting process is the most common procedure for making cast dental restorations. The procedure involves many steps in which the dimensional changes of the various materials are accounted for to produce restorations with acceptable fit.

STUDY QUESTIONS AND PROBLEM SOLVING

1. **Which of the following waxes is hardest at room temperature?**
   a. Baseplate
   b. Boxing
   c. Inlay pattern
   d. Impression

2. **In contrast to low-heat investments, high-heat investments:**
   a. Cannot be heated beyond 750°C
   b. Are used for PFM alloys
   c. Undergo greater expansion
   d. Are made with gypsum

3. **Dimensional changes that affect the accuracy of a cast dental crown include:**
   a. Setting expansion of the investment material
   b. Shrinkage of the wax pattern during cooling
   c. Shrinkage of the metal during burnout
   d. Expansion of the impression material during setting

4. **The number of bubbles in an investment material can be reduced by:**
   a. Investing the pattern under water
   b. Mixing the investment under vacuum
   c. Using a higher water-to-powder ratio
   d. Using a lower water-to-powder ratio

5. **Flux is added to the casting metal during melting to:**
   a. Minimize oxidation of the metal
   b. Enhance the esthetics of the metal
   c. Increase the stiffness of the metal
   d. Enhance the fluidity of the metal

6. **Which of the following is *not* a likely cause of an inaccurate or unacceptable cast crown?**
   a. Vibrating the casting ring during investing
   b. Quenching the casting ring 1 minute after casting
   c. Underheating the casting metal during melting
   d. Rapidly heating the investment during burnout

7. **Which of the following is *not* a rationale for the wax burnout procedure?**
   a. Increase the density of the investment material
   b. Expand the investment material
   c. Vaporize the wax pattern from the mold
   d. Increase the temperature of the investment

8. **Mixing a die stone with a higher water-to-powder ratio than normal will result in a die that:**
   a. Is oversized because of excessive expansion
   b. Is less resistant to abrasion and chipping
   c. Has a significantly slower setting rate
   d. Has a lower density after hardening

9. **An epoxy die has the following characteristics, compared with a stone die:**
   a. Greater strength
   b. Greater setting expansion
   c. Lower abrasion resistance
   d. Less brittleness

SELECTED READINGS

Chew CL, Land MF, Thomas CC, Norman RD. Investment strength as a function of time and temperature. Journal of Dentistry 27:297–302, 1999.
   This article describes the results of a study in which the strength of phosphate-bonded investments at high temperatures is verified to be greater than that of gypsum-bonded investments.

Diwan R, Talic Y, Omar N, Sadig W. The effect of storage time of removable partial denture wax pattern on the accuracy of fit of the cast framework. Journal of Prosthetic Dentistry 77:375–381, 1997.
   This study showed the importance of time after wax pattern production on the accuracy of cast partial denture frameworks.

Diwan R, Talic Y, Omar N, Sadig W. Pattern waxes and inaccuracies in fixed and removable partial denture castings. Journal of Prosthetic Dentistry 77:553–555, 1997.
   The types of dental waxes that are used to make castings for prosthodontics are reviewed in this article. Many of the important properties of the waxes that need to be considered to make accurate castings are discussed.

Duke P, Moore BK, Haug SP, Andres CJ. Study of the physical properties of type IV gypsum, resin-containing, and epoxy die materials. Journal of Prosthetic Dentistry 83:466–473, 2000.
   This study compared the properties of resin-modified and conventional type IV gypsum die materials and showed that they had equivalent properties, such as hardness, strength, abrasion resistance, dimensional change, and detail reproduction. It also showed that epoxy die materials exhibited the best properties but that the setting shrinkage was a concern in terms of accuracy.

Gerrow JD, Price RB. Comparison of the surface detail reproduction of flexible die material systems. Journal of Prosthetic Dentistry 80:485–489, 1998.
   This study compares the characteristics of several flexible, polyvinylsiloxane die materials with a type IV stone die. Only one of the flexible dies showed any improvement over stone, and most were incompatible with many popular impression materials.

Morey EF. Dimensional accuracy of small gold alloy castings. Part 1: A brief history and the behavior of inlay waxes. Australian Dental Journal 36:302–309, 1991.
   This article is the first in a four-part series addressing the lost wax casting process. This first article provides a short history of the discovery and development of the technique and reviews the literature pertaining to dimensional changes in wax that may lead to inaccurate castings.

O'Brien WJ. Dental Materials: Properties and Selection. Chicago: Quintessence Publishing, 1989.
   This text provides a concise explanation of the casting process.

Phillips RW. Skinner's Science of Dental Materials. 9th ed. Philadelphia: WB Saunders, 1991.
   This excellent text contains several chapters dealing with the lost wax casting process. The chapters contain detailed descriptions of the procedures, as well as complete explanations of the causes of many types of casting failures.

Polymers for Prosthetics

Objectives

- Identify the steps in addition and condensation polymerization and describe the different methods available to begin the reaction.
- Explain how the size of a polymer affects its strength, stiffness, and dimensional stability.
- Explain the effect of cross-linking agents and plasticizers on the structure and hardness of a polymer.
- List the components in the powder and liquid of both heat-cured and cold-cured dental acrylics for dentures, appliances, and custom trays.
- List the different types of formulations of denture base plastics and explain the way(s) in which they are an improvement over conventional acrylic.
- Describe the stages during the setting of dental acrylic in terms of the physical and chemical changes occurring.
- Explain the physical and compositional differences between denture bases, liners, and tissue conditioners.
- Describe the general procedure for the production of a heat-cured denture.
- Explain the effect of improper heating, cooling, and pressure application on the strength, fit, and esthetics of a heat-cured denture.
- Describe the procedure for constructing a cold-cured acrylic custom tray.

The use of polymers was made possible by Charles Goodyear's discovery of vulcanized rubber in approximately 1840. Fifteen or twenty years after that discovery, the material was introduced as a denture base, under the names Ebonite or Vulcanite, to be used with porcelain teeth. These remained the principal denture base materials for 75 years, despite the fact that they had poor esthetics, tasted bad, and became foul smelling. In about 1868, a printer by the name of John Hyatt discovered the first plastic molding material, celluloid, by dissolving nitrocellulose (a cotton derivative) under pressure. His goal was to make a synthetic substitute for ivory billiard balls. Celluloid was tough and somewhat flexible and had better esthetics than vulcanized rubber, but it too tasted bad and smelled foul. It also was difficult to process and was not particularly stable. In about 1909, Dr. Leo Bakeland discovered phenol-formaldehyde resins while trying to make an artificial shellac. This material, which became known as Bakelite, was tried as a denture base but was not dimensionally stable in the mouth. It was later modified to produce a better, more acceptable material, but by that time another discovery had been made. In the 1930s, Dr. Walter Wright and the Vernon brothers working at the Rohm and Haas Company in Philadelphia developed polymethylmethacrylate (PMMA), a hard plastic. Although other materials were used for dental prosthetics, none could come close to PMMA, and by the 1940s, 90 to 95% of all dentures were made from this acrylic polymer.

■ Polymeric Materials: The Basics

Definitions and Uses in Dentistry

A **polymer** is a long-chain organic molecule. It is produced by the reaction of many smaller molecules called **monomers,** or mers. When many identical, small molecules chemically react, adding together like beads on a string, they produce a long chain of many mers, or a polymer. If the reaction occurs between two different but compatible monomers, the polymeric product is called a **copolymer.** The ability to add many different types of monomers together to make copolymers gives the polymer chemist a tremendous ability to "tailor-make" molecules for specific applications. For example, a patient who cannot tolerate a hard denture base made from PMMA requires a softer liner to be placed on the tissue surface of the denture. There are many rubber-like polymers compatible with the PMMA, but they would be too flexible and have limited durability for dentures. A copolymer can be produced, however, by having the molecules that produce the hard denture base react with the rubbery material, resulting in a liner with properties intermediate between the two, i.e., not too soft or too hard. This type of technology is used throughout all forms of the industry to produce ideal properties as well as to reduce costs for certain materials. Because many types of small molecules can be reacted to form polymers the possibilities are almost limitless.

Polymers of different types are used in dentistry as denture bases and artificial teeth, denture liners or tissue conditioners, composite restoratives and pit and fissure sealants, impression materials, custom trays for impressions, temporary restoratives, mouthguards, maxillofacial prostheses, space maintainers, veneers, cements, and adhesives. They can be processed in the laboratory, in the office, or in the oral cavity, and they can be produced with nearly ideal esthetics.

Chemistry of Polymerization

Monomers react to form polymers by a chemical reaction called **polymerization**. This can occur in several ways, depending on the composition of the monomers. The most common polymerization reaction for polymers used in dentistry is *addition polymerization*. The reaction is as the name implies; monomers are added one after the other to make the long polymer chain. This distinguishes it from the other common type of polymerization known as *condensation*. In condensation, a small molecular by-product is produced by the union of each monomer. A typical example is the way amino acids join together to produce proteins, with the condensation of a water molecule as a by-product. Bakelite was also a condensation polymer. Most of this discussion of the chemistry of polymers concentrates on addition reaction materials because they are dominant in dentistry.

Addition Polymerization

Addition reactions usually involve monomers containing carbon-carbon double bonds ($C=C$). The $C=C$ bond is of high energy and is relatively unstable, so it reacts rather easily with other molecules. In general, monomers with these groups will not react quickly on their own, but their interactions with one another can be enhanced under the appropriate conditions. This usually requires a special molecule called an **initiator**, since it initiates the reaction. Some means to activate the initiator is also necessary. The **activator** can be light, heat, or a chemical, and all are used in dentistry. The first step in the polymerization is to break down or activate the initiator and cause it to initiate the reaction by joining with a monomer and making it reactive (Display 12-1). When the monomer is attacked by the initiator, the carbon-carbon double bond splits, leaving the molecule with a carbon-carbon single bond and a free, unpaired electron. This electron is often called a **free radical**, which explains why the addition reaction is often called free-radical polymerization. This radical is very reactive and quickly bumps into and reacts with a nearby monomer. These two join, splitting the $C=C$ on the second monomer and transferring the free electron to it from the first monomer. Thus far, two monomers have reacted and begun to form the polymer chain. This type of reaction begins at many sites throughout the mixture of monomers, so there are numerous polymer chains forming simultaneously. This **propagation** stage continues with many more monomers being added at a rapid rate. Finally, as fewer monomers remain and the viscosity of the mixture increases, the reaction enters the final stage where it stops, or *terminates*, by the combination of the

DISPLAY 12–1

Steps in the Free-Radical Polymerization Reaction

$$I^* + M \rightarrow I-M^*$$
a. Initiation
$$I-M^* + M \rightarrow I-M-M^*$$
b. Propagation
$$I-(M)_n-M^* + I-(M)_m-M^* \rightarrow I-(M)_n-M-M-(M)_m-I$$
n and m > 1
c. Termination

I, initiator; *, a free radical; M, monomer; n and m, integers.

remaining free radicals. Because of the rapid rate of reaction and the fast increase in viscosity, however, some monomers remain unreacted and become trapped within the polymer. These unreacted **residual monomers** may alter the properties and stability of the final polymer and, therefore, are of significance.

Two more important points should be made about the addition reaction. First, every time a $C=C$ bond is broken, heat is evolved. As one might expect, this heat accelerates the chemical reaction. It also can pose a problem, which is discussed later. *Try to predict what effect a large amount of heat buildup within the polymer may have on the dimensional accuracy of a polymer component.* Second, as each monomer reacts, the entire mass of polymers shrinks. This follows from the fact that two molecules held together by a primary chemical bond, such as a covalent $C—C$ linkage, occupy less total volume than they did when they were next to one another in the liquid state and interacting through secondary bonds. Therefore, there is an overall shrinkage of polymers based on this type of reaction. This shrinkage may have a significant effect on polymers used as dental restoratives or prosthetic devices. An intensive effort is underway to develop polymers for dentistry that do not shrink during polymerization.

Some of these materials are made from monomers that polymerize by a mechanism called *ring-opening* polymerization. Simply stated, a molecular ring of atoms at the reactive end of the molecule is forced to open up during the polymerization reaction. Because of the ring opening, two reacting molecules actually elongate and increase their volume at the same time that the total volume is decreased by the formation of a covalent bond. The goal is for the two-dimensional changes to offset one another, with a net result of no actual change in volume (i.e., no shrinkage). Dental composites based on ring-opening monomers are currently being developed. The ring-opening reaction also is used for polyether impression materials and some epoxies used as die materials.

Condensation Polymerization

Another type of polymerization is called condensation polymerization. In this process, it is common for a small molecule, such as water or alcohol, to be released as a by-product of the reaction between the two monomer units. One dental example is the reaction that forms polysulfide rubber impression materials. In this case, the reaction between the —SH groups produces water as a by-product during the reaction to form the final polymer (Display 12-2). Polymers that form by this mechanism are seldom used in dentistry because the reactions tend to be too slow and do not produce polymers of suitable length within an adequate time. Polymer chain length is important because this characteristic influences properties.

Polymer Size and Its Effects

In general, the strength, stiffness, and stability of a given polymer are increased the longer the individual polymer chains are. This is because of the nature of the

DISPLAY 12–2

Condensation Polymerization Reaction

$$(X)_n—OH + (Y)_m—H \rightarrow (X)_n—(Y)_m + H_2O$$
$$n \text{ and } m > 1$$

interactions between the chains. In Chapter 2, it was noted that secondary bonding was responsible for holding a polymeric material together. This might lead one to believe that most polymers would be weak, unstable, and easily pulled apart; tremendous frictional forces between the polymer chains keep them from slipping past one another, however, thus giving the polymer strength by making it difficult to pull it apart or change its shape. These interactions are called *entanglements*. They are analogous to making a loop in a piece of thread and holding both ends in one's left hand, and then looping a second thread through the first and holding both ends of it in the right hand (Fig. 12-1). It is difficult to pull the threads apart because to do so would mean breaking the center portions where they interact. In the case of the polymer, breaking the chain would mean breaking the strong covalent bonds. These entanglements, therefore, provide much strength and stability. Polymers with longer chains have a greater opportunity to become entangled and are, therefore, stronger than polymers with shorter chains. This concept is easy to understand for anyone who has ever tried to unravel a long strand of tangled Christmas lights.

The length of the molecules or chains in a polymer is usually described in one of two ways: as the average molecular weight of each chain or as the **degree of polymerization** (DP). The latter relates to the average number of monomers that reacted to make each chain. In any case, as the average molecular weight or the DP increases, the strength, stiffness, solubility resistance, and dimensional stability of the polymer increase. A third way to describe the extent to which the polymerization reaction has taken place would be to count the percentage of $C=C$ bonds that disappear during the reaction. This can be done with infrared spectroscopic techniques and provides a value for the **degree of conversion** (DC) of the polymer system. Because the polymerization reaction also is referred to as a curing reaction, "DC" is synonymous with **degree of cure**. This is an important method for expressing the extent of the polymerization reaction in cross-linked network polymers such as dental composites, adhesives, bis-acryl provisionals, and pit and fissure sealants.

Polymer Structure and Its Effects

The discussion to this point has been confined to polymers that are **linear** in nature. In other words, there are no primary chemical bonds between the individual chains; if they could be separated, they could be placed onto the table and oriented in straight lines lying next to one another. The internal structure that results from

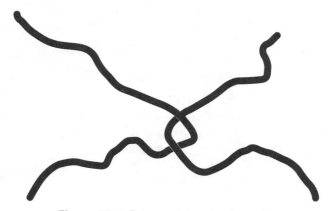

Figure 12–1 Polymer chain entanglements.

the formation of linear polymers used in dentistry is **amorphous**, having no identifiable order (Fig. 12-2*A*). Some monomers, however, have two functional C=C groups per molecule instead of only one. These monomers are called difunctional because they may react with two other monomers, forming actual chemical bonds to link together two individual polymer chains (Fig. 12-2*B*). These **cross-linkages** create a **network** structure that makes these polymers stable and resistant to many solvents. The polymer appears similar to a spider web on a microscopic scale. The individual chains can no longer be separated, and the polymer becomes a single, giant molecule in an amorphous arrangement. A monomer with two C=C groups can be added in small quantities to a linear polymer such as PMMA so that the polymer cross-links and forms a network with increased stability. This is done for most denture base materials.

Properties of Polymers

Another important factor affecting the properties of a polymer is the structure of the monomers themselves. Certain monomers are very stiff and produce rigid, glass-like polymers because they make it difficult to bend the main polymer chain

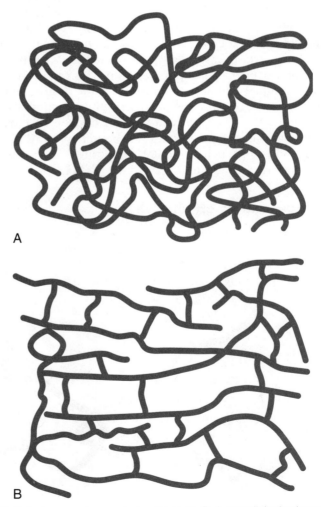

Figure 12–2 **A.** An amorphous polymer structure. **B.** A cross-linked polymer structure.

or "backbone." Other polymers contain flexible linkages such as those in impression materials, which cause their polymers to be rubbery. Another factor that affects the polymer is the nature of the side groups on the polymer chains. When the molecules have large, bulky side groups, they tend to push the polymer chains apart and reduce the number and effectiveness of the entanglements between chains (Fig. 12-3). The overall effect is to make the polymer more flexible and rubber-like. The process is called **plasticizing** because the polymer becomes more moldable (i.e., plastic) and less rigid. If the side groups are small, the chains stay closer together and are less mobile; thus, the plasticizing effect is less and the polymers are harder. The plasticizing effect can be predicted by an evaluation of the properties of the polymer at different temperatures. When subjected to elevated temperatures, some polymers undergo a softening before they melt or decompose. These polymers are called **thermoplastic** because they are transformed from a rigid, glassy material into a more plastic, moldable material when their temperature is raised beyond a certain point. The critical temperature is called the **glass transition temperature**, and it is determined by the structure of the monomers and the presence or absence of plasticizers. Some practical aspects of this phenomenon are discussed later.

A polymer can be plasticized by adding small molecules that do not chemically interact with the polymer but simply reside within its folds and bends (Fig. 12-4). The effect of these plasticizers is to push the chains apart and reduce entanglements, thus softening the polymer. The difference between this softening method and that produced by the bulky side groups, however, is that these molecules are unattached and will eventually diffuse out of the polymer. *What is the effect of this diffusion?*

The polymer chains can then move closer and improve their interactions, causing the material to harden (Fig. 12–4). When this occurs in certain denture liners, irritation of the patient's gums can result.

Because polymers routinely absorb water and lose components demonstrates that they are not as stable as most metals or ceramics. In addition, they do not possess the same level of mechanical properties or abrasion resistance as metals or ceramics. Thus, their usefulness is limited. Their esthetic possibilities as soft tissue replacement materials, however, are unequaled. In addition, their ability to

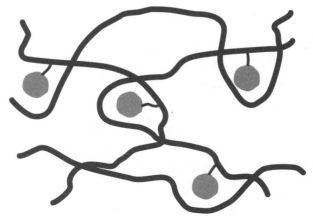

Figure 12–3 Effect of a bulky side group on plasticizing the polymer.

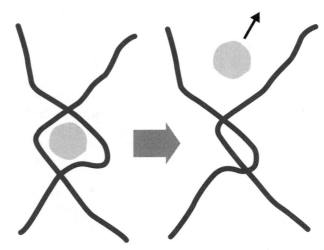

Figure 12–4 A plasticizing molecule diffusing out from a polymer entanglement.

reproduce hard dental tissues is exceeded only by ceramics. Polymers are good thermal and electrical insulators, but their high thermal expansion coefficient poses a potential problem in maintaining sealed margins. Perhaps the biggest drawback for polymers used in restorative dentistry is the volumetric contraction that accompanies polymerization. This problem was discussed in detail for composites in Chapters 5 and 6.

■ *Prosthetic Resins*

The composition and the characteristics of the polymeric materials used to make denture bases and liners are presented here in some detail. The factors under the control of the dental team that influence the properties of these materials are also addressed. Subsequently, polymeric materials used in other dental applications are introduced.

Denture Base Materials

Types of Denture Base Polymers

The most common denture base polymer is dental acrylic, or PMMA. This dental resin has essentially the same composition as commercial Plexiglas but is pigmented and processed differently. The conventional versions are cured or hardened by the application of heat. There are similar formulations, however, that are cured by a self-curing reaction or by the application of microwave energy.

Conventional Heat-Cured Polymethylmethacrylate

Conventional heat-cured PMMA is supplied as a powder and liquid. The powder can be supplied in bulk but usually is dispensed in individual packets (Fig. 12-5). The liquid is supplied in a brown glass jar with a measuring cylinder. The powder contains a copolymer of PMMA in the form of spheres or beads to which the benzoyl peroxide initiator is added. Coloring pigments and fibers often are added for improved esthetics. The polymer is polymerized by the manufacturer to a very high molecular weight. The liquid is methyl methacrylate (MMA) monomer with

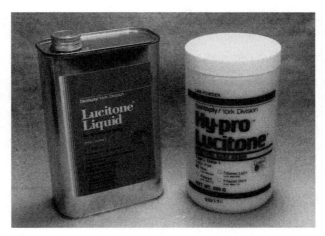

Figure 12–5 Bulk packaging of the liquid and powder of a commercial denture base resin.

a cross-linking agent (usually 5 to 15% ethylene glycol dimethacrylate) and a small amount of inhibitor (hydroquinone) to avoid premature polymerization and enhance shelf life. The cross-linking molecules are added to reduce the likelihood that small surface cracks will form in the denture when it is allowed to dry. These small cracks are called **craze** cracks and are produced by stresses created during the drying.

MMA is a flammable liquid of low viscosity, like water. It is extremely volatile and boils at approximately 100°C. When it polymerizes, it shrinks approximately 21% by volume. It can be a physical irritant to the skin, producing an itching feeling, and is a known allergen. A correctly heat-processed denture base could have as little as 0.3% to as much as 2% residual MMA monomer. The high temperature at which conventional dentures are processed ensures a thorough, although not complete, polymerization. The high-temperature processing also leads to a greater dimensional change, however, resulting in a shrinkage of approximately 0.4% across the molar region.

Cold-Cured Polymethylmethacrylate (Pour Resin)

Cold-cured, or self-curing, PMMA often is referred to as "pour resin" because it is poured into a processing mold made of agar hydrocolloid to form a denture base. The composition of this material is the same as the heat-cured version, with two differences: 1) the powder contains beads of polymer that have a lower molecular weight than those of the heat-cured material; and 2) the liquid contains a chemical activator (an amine molecule) to start the reaction. Denture bases made from these resins are processed quickly at room temperature. They have more residual monomer (1 to 4%) but a lower dimensional change (0.2%) than dentures produced by heat processing.

High-Impact-Resistant Acrylic

This denture base resin is similar to the heat-cured material and is processed the same way, but it has a much higher impact strength. It is more expensive than the conventional material but is less likely to be accidentally broken if dropped by the patient. These resins are produced by substituting the PMMA in the powder with a copolymer. The copolymer is made with a rubbery monomer that causes the material to behave as if it contained an internal shock absorber. In addition, there often is no cross-linker used in the liquid. The materials have high-impact resistance, low crazing, and fit in a way comparable with that of the conventional materials.

Injection-Molded Polymers

Injection-molded polymers are usually made of nylon or polycarbonate. The material is supplied as a gel in the form of a patty that must be heated and injected into a mold. The equipment for processing these polymers is more expensive than that for processing conventional denture resins. In addition, the craze resistance of these materials is not equivalent to that of the conventional acrylic. These polymers have high impact resistance, however, and do not contain MMA monomer, so they may be used for patients who are allergic to MMA.

Rapid Heat-Polymerized Polymers

The denture base resins used with rapid heat-polymerized polymers are the same as those used with conventional material, except that they contain an altered initiator system. The initiator allows them to be processed in boiling water for 20 minutes, which is a much faster processing than that used in the conventional heat-curing method. A problem with these dentures is that areas of the base thicker than approximately 6 mm have a high level of porosity. As a point of reference, a correctly processed conventional acrylic should have little porosity up to a thickness of almost 20 mm. The short duration of the heating also leaves a higher level of residual monomer, three to seven times greater than that of conventionally heat-cured denture base.

Microwave-Polymerized Polymers

The resins used with microwave-polymerized polymers have the same composition as those used with conventional material and are processed in a microwave. Their properties are optimal when a special liquid is substituted for the normal monomer liquid. Although the denture base cures well in the special polycarbonate (instead of metal) flask with the normal monomer liquid, it shows a higher level of porosity than dentures processed with the special liquid. The properties and the accuracy of these materials have been shown to be as good as or better than those of the conventional heat-cured material, and the processing time is much shorter (4 to 5 minutes).

Light-Activated Polymer

Light-activated polymer is a composite, consisting of a paste of urethane dimethacrylate monomer with fillers. It is used as a denture base resin, as a repair material for prosthodontics, and as a custom tray material. It, like the composite inlays discussed in Chapter 7, is processed in a light-curing unit. Some studies have shown that the properties of these denture polymers are slightly lower than those of the conventional PMMA materials and produce slightly rougher surfaces that seem to stain more readily. One study, however, showed their fit to be better than that of conventional heat-cured material, although not quite equivalent to cold-cured or microwave-processed dentures.

Fiber-Reinforced Polymer

Glass, carbon/graphite, aramid, and ultrahigh-molecular-weight polyethylene have been used as fiber-reinforcing agents for PMMA removable and fixed prosthetic appliances. Metal wire also has been used, although, like graphite, metal has minimal esthetic qualities. The premise behind fiber reinforcement is that the fibers are stronger than the matrix polymer, thus their inclusion strengthens the composite structure. The reinforcing agent can be in the form of unidirectional, straight fibers or multidirectional weaves. Their main purpose in denture acrylics is to reduce the chance of fracture and accidental breakage.

Mixing and Handling of Polymethylmethacrylate Resins: Processing Variables

The use of acrylic materials in dentistry was made possible by the development of the dough technique. As mentioned, the curing of MMA is accompanied by a nearly 21% reduction in volume. The shrinkage can be reduced by reducing the amount of monomer. This can be accomplished by substituting a powder containing previously polymerized material of the same composition (i.e., PMMA) for some of the liquid. Suppose one needed four parts of liquid monomer to produce an object. If three parts of powder were substituted for three parts of the liquid, the shrinkage would be only approximately one fourth as much as it normally would be, because only one part of monomer was used. For MMA, this would effectively reduce the shrinkage from 21% by volume to approximately 5% by volume (approximately 1.7% in any direction). The material also would be easier to handle because the mixed powder and liquid form a doughy mass that can be manipulated. The only concern is achieving good bonding between the newly formed polymer and the preexisting PMMA beads. This is ensured by the fact that the outer surface of the PMMA polymer beads can be dissolved in the MMA monomer, facilitating a bond between the two.

The powder and liquid are mixed in the correct proportions, which are obtained either by weighing and measuring or by using prepackaged materials. A series of physical changes then takes place before polymerization is initiated. The important factor is that sufficient monomer be used to wet the beads completely but that an excess be avoided because this increases shrinkage and reduces accuracy. When the powder is incorporated into the liquid, the mixture is initially somewhat "sandy" (Fig. 12-6A). Within a minute or so, the monomer begins to diffuse into the polymer beads, causing them to swell. Some of the lower-molecular-weight polymers begin to dissolve from the surface of the beads into the monomer at this point, and the mass becomes very sticky and fibrous. This is often called the "stringy" stage (Fig. 12-6B). Within another minute (approximately 3 to 4 minutes total), the material becomes less glossy on its surface and no longer sticks to the fingers; it can be kneaded like a bread dough (Fig. 12-6C). This "dough" stage is produced by the continued diffusion of the monomer into the beads and the movement of polymer from the beads into the monomer, increasing the viscosity of the mixture. This stage lasts for about 2 minutes and is the appropriate time to work with either a heat-cured or a cold-cured acrylic. As the monomer continues to penetrate completely through to the center of the beads, the mass will become much like a rubber. It no longer retains its shape but instead springs back. A cold-cured material begins to polymerize at this point, hardening within 8 to 10 minutes. The heat-cured material does not harden until sufficiently heated.

The polymerization reaction is accompanied by evolution of a significant amount of heat, caused by the breaking of $C=C$ bonds throughout the mass. Therefore, even a cold-cured material heats up during hardening, and care should be taken not to burn oneself or the patient when using these materials. The evolution of heat has a significant effect on the dimensional stability of the denture material. Because free shrinkage of the material is restrained by the casts and

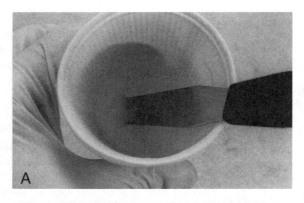

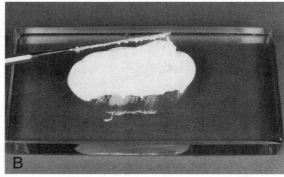

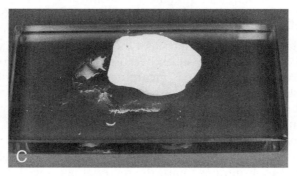

Figure 12–6 A. The "sandy" stage after mixing acrylic monomer and powder. **B.** The "stringy" stage for a mix of acrylic monomer and powder. **C.** The "doughy" stage for a mix of acrylic monomer and powder.

molds during processing, stress is built up within the acrylic in a way analogous to the stress built up within one's arm muscles as they push against a solid, immovable object. In addition, because the material may reach a temperature of 75 to 80°C when cold-cured and a temperature of well over 100°C when heat-cured, further shrinkage accompanies the cooling process. This sets up additional internal stresses. The magnitude of the stress, and thus the overall distortion during stress relief after the denture base is removed from the cast, depends on the maximum temperature and cooling rate. Higher temperatures create more internal stress and greater distortion. Thus, although heat-processed dentures are clinically acceptable, they may not have the same dimensional accuracy as cold-cured dentures. Also, after processing the denture has to be allowed to cool slowly. This allows the residual stresses to relax, so when the denture is removed from the cast, there is less distortion, or "pulling in," which can make a maxillary denture fit

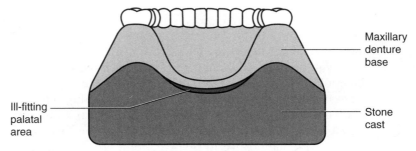

Figure 12–7 Distortion of a denture on a cast as a result of shrinkage.

poorly in the palatal area (Fig. 12-7). During the process of making a custom tray, similar shrinkage and contraction stresses will be present within the tray. ***What is the clinical significance of this?***

> If the tray is used too soon after it is processed, the impression may distort as the tray changes dimension, leading to an inaccurate replication of the tissues. It usually is a good idea to make the tray the day before it is needed.

The rate and duration of heating also are important factors influencing the esthetic qualities and properties of the denture base. Rapid heating causes the internal temperature of the acrylic to rise quickly to a high level. Because the monomer boils at approximately 100°C, it may do so during the processing if the temperature within some portion of the mass exceeds this level. Monomer boiling creates small bubbles in the denture, particularly in the thicker regions where the temperature rises the most because of the insulating nature of the acrylic (Fig. 12-8). Therefore, a slow rate of heating is preferred; it is difficult to heat an acrylic too long. In contrast, reducing the processing time can be deleterious because it results in an incomplete polymerization, leaving more residual monomer and producing a weaker polymer.

The last consideration with respect to acrylic processing is the application of pressure. Pressure forces out air bubbles created during mixing and manipulation, improves the adaptation of the denture base around the teeth, and squeezes out some pores generated during curing. In addition, the application of insufficient pressure to a heat-cured denture increases the vertical height of the base, thus reducing the fit within the mouth.

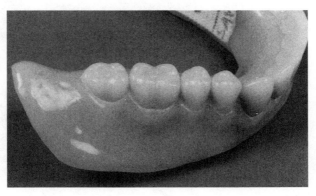

Figure 12–8 Small bubbles in a denture, caused by a processing error.

Physical and Mechanical Properties

The most significant properties of a denture base are those relating to durability and dimensional stability. Generally, the strength and stiffness of a denture resin are adequate unless the denture is processed with very thin areas, specifically at the midline. This may cause it to break in service during chewing or by squeezing the mandibular denture too tightly during cleaning (Fig. 12-9). The acrylics have relatively low abrasion resistance; this problem usually is encountered only during cleaning, however, and the patient can be instructed to use soft-bristled brushes. The main concerns revolve around the low impact strength and poor fatigue resistance of these materials. The greatest cause of fractured dentures is accidental breakage as a result of being dropped. The reinforced materials are superior in this respect, but not ideal. The physical properties of denture base materials also are generally adequate. Their esthetic qualities are very good. They have sufficient thermal stability because the glass transition temperature of most denture base materials is about 100°C. Warping is a potential problem, however, if the denture is cleaned in very hot water or if high temperatures are generated on their surfaces during polishing. This may be partly the result of their poor thermal conductivity (see Chapter 2). The insulating nature of the denture base creates another problem in that the temperature of hot and cold foods is not transferred as readily to the underlying tissues. This causes the denture to feel somewhat unnatural. Of greater concern is the risk of burns when the patient fails to realize how hot or cold the ingested food or beverage is until the soft tissues in the throat are contacted.

The dimensional stability of most denture base resins is adequate. Although every denture undergoes some contraction, it is believed that the magnitude is well tolerated by the patient's tissues. Also, the shrinkage is offset to some extent by the expansion that occurs as a result of water uptake, which can be as much as 2% by weight of the denture. Most of this water uptake occurs quickly, although it can continue for several weeks. Therefore, it often is recommended to soak the denture for 24 hours or more before giving it to the patient; this aids in equilibrating the dimensions of the denture, improving its fit, and limiting the amount of change that will take place over time. The soaking is beneficial in another way: During immersion, residual monomers, which could be a source of irritation to the patient, are dissolved out from the denture. Most of the monomer is removed within 24 hours.

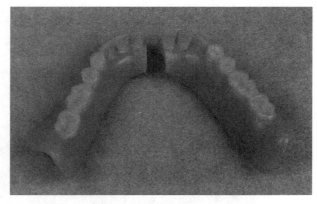

Figure 12–9 A denture broken in service.

The effect of chemicals on dentures warrants some discussion. These polymers have fairly good resistance to most of the acids and bases they encounter. Common cleansers and detergents do not adversely affect them. Cleaning a denture containing a soft liner with an effervescent cleanser or a brush, however, can have deleterious effects on the lining material. It is recommended that dentures with soft liners be rinsed after each meal and cleaned by soaking for 20 minutes in an alkaline (i.e., nonacidic) hypochlorite solution every evening. Alcohol can cause acrylic dentures to craze because of its drying effect, but the length of contact time usually is not long enough to be of concern. Similarly, other organic solvents that would severely damage the surface of a denture do not routinely come into contact with them. A significant problem does arise with the use of denture cleansers containing chlorine, specifically for partial dentures constructed from a chromium-containing alloy. These solutions cause a severe tarnish and surface discoloration and may actually attack the metal by corrosion processes.

The last consideration is the biologic characteristics of these materials. The potential irritating effect of the monomer and its allergenic effect have already been mentioned. In addition, working with the highly volatile monomer places dental personnel at risk for toxic exposure. The most common symptom of exposure is a mild headache; other ill effects, however, have been shown in studies in which MMA monomer was administered to animals for long periods of time at very high doses. Therefore, the operator should take care not to breathe excessive amounts of the monomer vapor. Exposure can be minimized easily by using the material in a room with adequate ventilation. Finally, the denture base itself provides a site for the growth of organisms present in the oral cavity. This can lead to simple discoloration and staining of the surface and to mucosal irritation if the organisms attach to the underside of the base. Soaking the denture in a solution containing nystatin or chlorhexidine has been shown to be effective in inhibiting the growth of *Candida albicans* for several days. Various ways have been studied to treat the surfaces of the base to inhibit the adhesion of microorganisms. They are effective, but usually for only a few months duration.

Denture Liners and Conditioners

Denture liners are used to cover the tissue-bearing aspect of a denture to improve its fit or to improve its comfort for patients who cannot tolerate the hard dental acrylic on their mucosa. Patients with thin ridges are ideal candidates because they lack supporting structures for the denture. Denture liners are resilient materials, but they are not spongy. They are made from acrylics, silicones (similar to but of a different formulation than those used for bathroom caulking), or newer polymers based on a fluoroelastomer. They differ from one another in composition, adhesiveness to the denture base, rate of staining and fouling, and appearance.

Acrylic-based **soft liners** can be heat cured or cold cured. Heat-cured liners generally are considered permanent and are processed along with the denture base. These materials are copolymers containing ethyl methacrylate and plasticizers. Because they are methacrylates and similar to the denture acrylics, they adhere well to the denture base. They have the feel of a stiff rubber material and may become somewhat hardened over time because of the loss of some of the plasticizing molecules. They have a glass transition temperature slightly below room temperature, which causes them to be resilient at oral temperatures but be "rock hard" when placed in ice water. The practical significance of this is that a technician can place the denture in ice water and make the liner hard, which facilitates the polishing process because a hard material is easier to polish than a soft one. Because of their limited durability, the service life of a soft liner usually is about 1 to 3 years, although at least one study has shown success with silicone soft liners for up to 9 years.

Silicone rubbers of both the heat-cured and cold-cured (temporary) type have been used as denture liners. These polydimethylsiloxane materials are somewhat similar to the addition silicone impression materials. They have a vastly different formulation than the denture base; therefore, adhesion between the two is limited. They must be applied with an adhesive, but peeling from the denture base remains a problem. These materials also leach or dissolve out plasticizers over time and have poor tear strength. In addition, they tend to allow the growth of microorganisms that are difficult to remove and foul the liner.

Another type of soft liner is based on a polyphosphazine fluoropolymer. It has a very low glass transition temperature, which makes it softer than the acrylic type but also makes it more difficult to polish. It cannot be placed in ice water to facilitate polishing. The surface of this polymer seems to roughen with time, resulting in the formation of pits, and causes increased friction with the patient's mucosa. The problem may be great enough to produce mucosal irritations, often referred to as "rug burns." In contrast to the acrylic type but similar to the silicones, its surface stains from the growth of microorganisms that are difficult to remove.

A more temporary form of liner is available for patients whose mucosa is so irritated that they cannot wear their dentures; although they want to wear the prosthesis, the gums need time to heal. A **tissue conditioner** is the appropriate material in these cases. These materials are based on polymethylmethacrylate polymers loaded with plasticizers, such as alcohol, to increase softness. They are mixed as powder-liquid systems, but no polymerization reaction occurs. Instead, they are poured onto the tissue surface of a denture and pressed against the tissue to form an impression by a physical gelation (like Jell-O) between the polymer in the powder and the plasticizers in the liquid. Because of the alcohol, the patient may experience a slight stinging with application, but no lasting adverse affects are noted. There also is no concern over heat generation because these materials do not polymerize. The soft conditioner occupies the space between the irritated tissue and the hard denture base, acting as a shock absorber. The material is temporary, lasting only a week or so, because the plasticizers leach out and cause the conditioner to harden in the mouth. The goal is for the tissues to be sufficiently healed by that time to enable the patient to wear the denture again.

Other Resin Systems

Polymers are used in numerous other applications in dentistry, many of which have been discussed, such as the application of polymers as mouthguards, pit and fissure sealants, composite restoratives, provisional restorations, impression materials, and cements. PMMA polymers are also used for many other applications. They are used to repair cracked or broken dentures or appliances. They are ideally suited for this application because of the identical chemical characteristics, which facilitate good adhesion between the components. Appliances for maintaining distance between teeth also are produced from cold-cured orthodontic resin. This resin is essentially the same material as that used in a cold-cured denture base. Often a metallic orthodontic appliance is produced by alternating applications of polymer powder and resin liquid, the so-called "salt and pepper" technique, to build up the bulk of an appliance and enclose the wire framework. This technique is more appropriate than trying to mold a dough when thin, uniform layers are desired. The same material is used to produce an occlusal splint for a patient with temporomandibular joint dysfunction. Acrylic splints can be heat processed like a denture or can be made from cold-cured acrylic. Light-cured materials have been used for these applications because of their ease of fabrication.

Another application of a hard polymer is in the manufacture of denture teeth. These usually are made from highly cross-linked PMMA. Composite materials may also be used and are expected to have improved wear resistance. The natural appearance is produced by building the tooth up with successive layers of different-colored resins. The advantages of plastic teeth over porcelain are an improved adhesion to the denture base, a lack of the clicking sound caused by porcelain-to-porcelain contact, and the ability to use them in partial dentures opposed by natural teeth. Porcelain is detrimental to the opposing dentition because it wears down the natural teeth. In contrast, the plastic teeth wear in preference to the natural dentition, conserving tooth structure. Plastic teeth are also relatively easy to replace and are polishable.

A further application for the soft polymers is in the reconstruction of facial tissues in oral and maxillofacial prostheses. This is perhaps the most dramatic use of dental polymers and makes the greatest demand on their esthetic capacities. Common materials for these applications are silicone and polyurethane polymers. The most significant drawbacks to these materials are their limited durability and color stability, which limit their service life to 1 to 3 years. In addition, stabilization on the head often is difficult and may involve attachment to the facial bones with dental implants.

■ *Production of a Heat-Processed Denture*

A common technique for the fabrication of a heat-processed acrylic denture is briefly reviewed to familiarize the student with the basic procedures involved. The denture is processed through the application of heat and pressure in a brass flask to produce a well-cured denture base with minimal porosity. Wax, plaster, and stone are used at various stages of the procedure in conjunction with the dental acrylic.

The denture teeth are initially set into a denture base made of wax placed onto the cast of the edentulous arch (Fig. 12-10A). The wax keeps the teeth in their correct relation and is ultimately replaced by the denture base resin. The waxed-up denture is placed into a brass flask and invested with plaster up to but not including the wax. This stabilizes the cast in the flask. A separating agent, such as a tinfoil substitute, is coated onto this "first pour" of plaster to keep it from sticking to the "second pour." A second mix of plaster is then poured in to cover the denture teeth completely (Fig. 12-10B). The top of the flask is assembled before the gypsum hardens. After 45 minutes, the invested flask is placed into boiling water for 4 to 5 minutes to soften the wax (Fig. 12-10C). The flask can then be taken apart. The softened wax is removed in one piece, leaving the teeth held in plaster in the upper part of the flask (Fig. 12-10D). The mold is then washed with hot water to remove all traces of the wax. If the flask were put back together at this point, there would be a space between the original cast and the invested teeth where the acrylic denture base belongs.

The mold is then painted with a separating medium to ease removal of the processed acrylic. The denture base resin is mixed in a jar according to the manufacturer's directions and then sealed to allow it to "dough" without monomer evaporation. This keeps the surface from becoming dry. When the mix reaches the dough

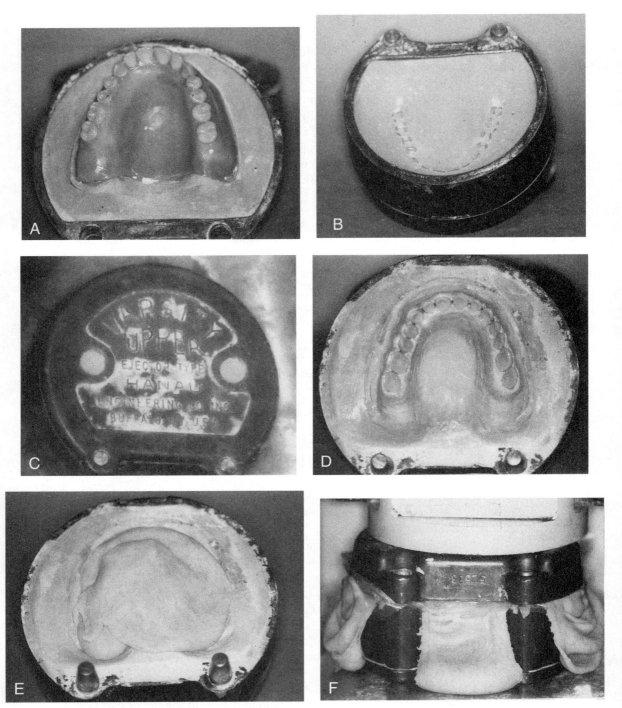

Figure 12–10 A. Denture teeth in a wax base. **B.** Denture wax-up invested in a flask with plaster. **C.** Assembled flask placed in water to soften wax. **D.** Invested denture in a flask after wax has been removed. **E.** Doughy acrylic being placed into a flask. **F.** Doughy acrylic being placed under pressure to squeeze out excess. *(Continues on next page.)*

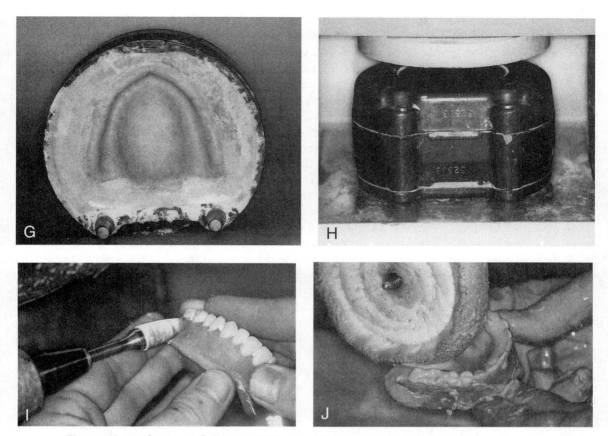

Figure 12–10 *Continued.* **G.** Disassembled flask after first pressure application. **H.** Flask placed under pressure in a vise. **I.** Denture being trimmed. **J.** Denture being polished.

stage, it is removed from the jar and placed into the flask (Fig. 12-10*E*). A piece of cellophane is placed onto the acrylic, and the flask is reassembled and gently pressed together to compress the acrylic (Fig. 12-10*F*). The flask is reopened, excess acrylic is removed (Fig. 12-10*G*), and the process is repeated several times to provide an appropriate amount of acrylic and ensure that sufficient pressure is applied to eliminate voids. Finally, the flask is pressurized in a press and left for an hour or two (Fig. 12-10*H*). This allows the monomer to diffuse completely into the polymer beads and ensures that a good bond will form between the two during heat curing.

The denture is then placed into a water bath and cured by using either of two methods. The first procedure involves heat processing at 75°C for 8 hours or more (overnight is convenient). The second method is quicker and includes a 1.5- to 2-hour soak in the 75°C bath followed by 30 minutes at 100°C (boiling water). An important factor is that the heat should be generated slowly. Rapid heating raises the internal temperature of the denture above 100°C, especially in the thicker regions, and causes uncured monomer to boil and produce porosity in the denture. A second consideration is that a sufficient temperature be achieved for a sufficient period of time to maximize the cure of the polymer. If the denture is undercured, its strength and hardness are reduced, and it will be left with a high concentration of residual monomer. This monomer may be a source of irritation to the patient.

After curing is complete, the flask is allowed to cool slowly to room temperature. It is important not to remove the denture from the flask until it has completely cooled. As the denture cools, a dimensional change occurs. The change in the denture base resin is greater than that occurring in the plaster because the acrylic has a higher coefficient of thermal expansion. Because the gypsum somewhat restricts the acrylic from shrinking, stress is built up within the denture. Over time, this stress will be relieved. If most of it is relieved while the denture is in the flask, there will be little distortion in the base on removal. It would be impractical to wait until all of the stress is relieved, so there is always some shrinkage, usually in the range of 0.2 to 0.4%. This amount of shrinkage appears to be well tolerated by the patient. If the denture is removed from the flask too soon, however, the dimensional change will be greater and the fit will be poorer.

The denture is removed by disassembling the flask and breaking out the gypsum; this is one of the benefits of the limited strengths of gypsum products. The denture is then trimmed with an acrylic bur (Fig. 12-10*I*) and polished on a lathe with a rag wheel (Fig. 12-10*J*). The technician takes care not to generate too much heat, which could warp the denture. The polished denture is stored in water before being delivered to the patient. This has two benefits. The first is the extraction of unreacted monomer. There usually is 0.2 to 0.5% unreacted monomer in a properly processed heat-cured denture and 1 to 3% unreacted monomer in a cold-cured denture. Most of this monomer can be extracted by soaking the denture in water for 24 hours. The second benefit of the soaking is to allow the denture to take up water and expand. With time, the denture continues to equilibrate with water and expand in the patient's mouth, perhaps continuing to change for the first 1 to 2 months. Water uptake is most rapid within the early time periods, however, and this soaking enhances the fit and comfort for the patient. The denture should be placed into a sterilizing solution for 10 to 15 minutes and then rinsed well just before delivery to the patient.

■ *Construction of an Acrylic Custom Tray*

Dental acrylics are also routinely used to make custom impression trays. The most accurate impressions are produced when there is a uniform layer of impression material between the teeth and the tray holding the impression. Excess or inadequate impression material in some area of a stock tray may lead to differences in the strain produced in the impression during removal and negatively affect accuracy. It is common to use a two-part impression system with stock trays, the so-called putty-wash system, as discussed in Chapter 8. The most accurate impressions, however, can be made by producing a **custom tray** for the specific case. These trays can be made with a cold-cured acrylic similar to that used in the denture base or repair resins. The only difference is that these materials contain ground glass fillers to thicken them and help keep the material in place before setting. It is also common to use certain composites for making a custom tray (see Fig. 10-6). Though these materials are more expensive, they are more convenient and quicker to use because they do not require mixing and can be light cured.

Acrylic custom tray resins are cold-cured powder-liquid systems that harden within 5 to 7 minutes from the start of mixing. Because of the exothermic nature of the curing reaction, the tray is made on a gypsum study cast of the patient's teeth instead of in the mouth. A relatively large mass of material is used in this procedure, and enough heat is generated to produce temperatures of 70 to 80°C at the surface, sufficient to burn the oral mucosa. Remember that the same concern applies when direct acrylic temporaries are made, and they must be removed from the mouth before being completely set.

The tray should be made at least several hours and, ideally, 1 day before it is needed. The tray continues to change dimension for up to 24 hours after hardening because the curing reaction continues and internal stresses are relaxed. If the tray were used immediately, the continual dimensional change accompanying the cure might distort the elastic impression material.

The greatest benefit of the custom tray is the accuracy attainable in the impression from the uniform layer of material. To ensure that a uniform space will be present for the impression, the study cast must be covered with a spacer that mimics the desired thickness of impression material. The spacer usually is made from two thin sheets of baseplate wax placed over all areas to be recorded on the cast. The wax should extend beyond the gingival margin by approximately 4 mm on the buccal and lingual mucosa.

Once the wax has been adapted to the cast, it is necessary to take a wax spatula or utility knife and cut out small areas or "stops" (approximately 3 × 3 mm) of the wax on a cuspal region of a noncritical tooth in both the anterior and the posterior region of the quadrant (Fig. 12-11A). A thin layer of petroleum jelly is then coated onto the exposed gypsum. When the acrylic is placed onto the cast, it will flow into the "stops" and contact the gypsum. The lubricant ensures that the

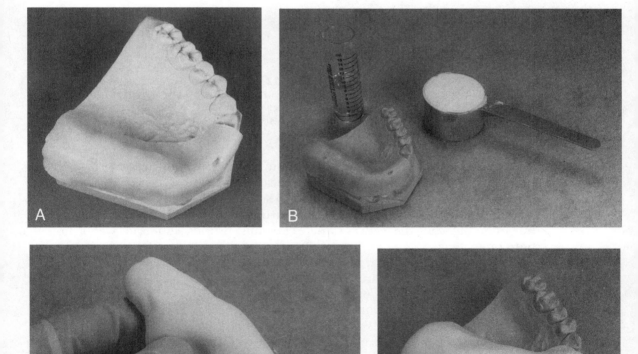

Figure 12–11 A. Cast with baseplate wax placed over the appropriate quadrant and "stops" cut into the appropriate areas. **B.** Powder and liquid dispensed for the mixing of the acrylic to prepare the custom tray. **C.** Doughy mass being shaped for placement on a cast. **D.** Placement of doughy mass on the waxed areas of a cast. *(Continues on next page.)*

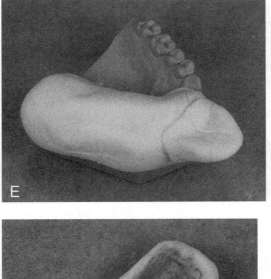

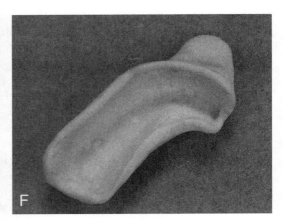

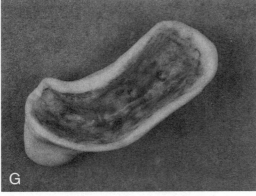

Figure 12–11 *Continued.* **E.** Formation of a handle for the custom tray. **F.** Custom tray after removal from the cast. **G.** Finished custom tray with adhesive for impression material.

acrylic does not stick to the cast during curing. The "stops" provide a mechanism to stop the custom tray from being seated against the teeth when the impression is made. Otherwise, it would be possible to squeeze nearly all of the impression material out from between the teeth and the tray. The "stops" prevent the custom tray from contacting the teeth anywhere else, thus ensuring a uniform layer of impression material.

The powder and liquid tray materials are dispensed into a wax cup or glass jar according to the manufacturer's instructions (Procedure Display 12-1). A ratio of 2.5 g of powder to 1 mL liquid is common (Fig. 12-11*B*). Usually, the powder is added to the liquid. A cement spatula or wooden tongue blade is used in a stirring motion for 30 to 60 seconds to mix the ingredients, with care taken to wet all of the powder with the liquid monomer to produce a homogeneous material.

The acrylic will advance through the usual stages. It is very fluid during the initial mixing and becomes thicker and very sticky as the monomer is taken up by the polymer beads in the powder. Within 2 to 3 minutes, the material becomes doughy and easily manipulated by hand without sticking to the fingers. If the material is used before it reaches the dough stage, it will be too fluid and will not stay in place. Conversely, if the operator waits too long to form the tray, the material will begin to get rubbery and cannot be shaped correctly on the cast. The working time should last for 2 to 3 minutes.

Gloves can be worn to manipulate the acrylic, but it often is easier to manipulate the material if the operator coats his or her hands with a very thin layer of petroleum jelly before handling the material. The acrylic is removed from the mix-

PROCEDURE DISPLAY 12-1

Making an Acrylic Custom Tray

Equipment checklist
❏ Powder–liquid tray acrylic with appropriate dispensers
❏ Wax cup or glass jar
❏ Steel cement spatula or wooden tongue blade
❏ Gypsum casts
❏ Baseplate wax
❏ Utility knife
❏ Petroleum–type jelly lubricant
❏ Heat source (warm water or Bunsen burner)

STEP 1: **Proportioning**
❏ Dispense liquid according to manufacturer's directions, using the measure pro-vided (alternatively, measure appropriate volume, using the graduated cylinder)
❏ Dispense powder according to manufacturer's directions, using the scoop device provided (alternatively, measure appropriate mass, using a balance)

STEP 2: **Mixing**
❏ Dispense liquid into cup or jar, followed by powder
❏ Mix vigorously 30 to 60 seconds, ensure that all powder is wet by monomer
❏ Let stand for 1 to 2 minutes until material becomes doughy—test for "nonsticki-ness" with finger

STEP 3: **Making a custom tray**
❏ Shape the doughy acrylic into a cigar-shaped mass
❏ Gently place the acrylic over the waxed region of the cast and press down to mold it, but do not let it extend beyond the wax
❏ Form a small amount of leftover dough into a handle and attach it to the front of the tray (squirt a small amount of monomer onto the region to which the handle will attach to facilitate adhesion)

STEP 4: **Cleanup**
❏ Remove excess acrylic from jar and spatula before set
❏ Remove hardened acrylic from jar and spatula by soaking in water for several hours

ing container and formed into a cigar-shaped mass long enough to overhang the areas to be recorded by several millimeters (Fig. 12-11*C*). The cigar-shaped mass is then gently placed onto the waxed regions of the cast and molded down to but not beyond the wax (Fig. 12-11*D*). If the acrylic is extended beyond the wax, it may stick to the cast and become difficult to remove. It is important that a uniform layer of acrylic be placed throughout and that no area is thinned too much. The material should not be manipulated excessively because this often introduces folds that result in a rough and unesthetic tray.

A small amount of material while still doughy can be formed into a handle on the most anterior portion of the tray. The handle should be oriented parallel to or at an angle slightly upward from the cast to ensure that it can easily be gripped when the tray is being placed into or removed from the patient's mouth (Fig. 12-11*E*). If the handle is oriented downward or is allowed to sag during setting, it will impinge on the patient's lips. A handle also can be formed from a small piece of excess acrylic. First, a small amount of monomer liquid is squirted onto the tray to improve the bond between tray and handle. Then the piece of acrylic is squeezed between the thumb and forefinger and flattened against the monomer-wetted area to make the handle. At this time, excess acrylic should be removed from the glass jar and steel spatula. Soaking these implements in water for several hours will release the plastic if it has been allowed to harden.

After the tray has hardened and is cooled sufficiently to be handled, it is removed from the cast and the wax spacer pulled from the interior (Fig. 12-11*F*). Any rough areas on the surface, especially on the borders, can be trimmed with an acrylic bur and polished smooth. Before use, the tray must be coated with the adhesive recommended for the specific impression material to be used (Fig. 12-11*G*). The adhesive should be brushed on and allowed to dry to ensure an adequate bond and avoid the impression being left on the teeth during removal of the tray from the patient. If an adhesive is unavailable, small holes can be drilled into the tray with a bur to provide retention sites for the impression.

Summary

Polymers are a class of material made from natural or synthetic molecules strung together like beads on a string to produce very long, complex structures. The reaction of the molecules, called monomers, to produce polymers is called polymerization and can take place in a number of ways. The most common polymerization reaction used in dental polymers is called addition, or free-radical, polymerization. It can be initiated by chemicals (self-curing composites), light energy (light-cured composites), or heat (denture base acrylic resins). The number of monomers linked during the reaction influences the size, strength, stability, and biocompatibility of the polymer; therefore, it is desirable to maximize this reaction. As a class of materials, polymers have only minimal strength and stability but have optimum esthetic qualities. They are used to a great extent in prosthetic dentistry to produce full and partial dentures. By correctly altering composition, polymers can be produced in a rigid or flexible state.

Rigid polymethylmethacrylate (acrylic) resin provides sufficient structural integrity to be used as a denture base, whereas the reaction of the methyl methacrylate monomer with other monomers can produce a much softer, resilient polymer to line the underside of a denture for improved fit and comfort for some patients. The rigid acrylic can also be used to produce a custom-made tray for carrying an impression material into a patient's mouth to maximize accuracy.

STUDY QUESTIONS AND PROBLEM SOLVING

1. **Polymerization in which water or alcohol by-products are produced during the reaction is called:**
   a. Addition
   b. Condensation
   c. Ring-opening
   d. Cross-linking

2. **Which of the following does not represent a mode of activation commonly used to cause polymerization of dental polymers within the oral cavity?**
   a. Heat
   b. Light
   c. Chemical
   d. Microwave

3. **Denture acrylics contain cross-linking agents, mainly to improve their:**
   a. Internal color
   b. Tissue compatibility
   c. Surface hardness
   d. Craze resistance

4. **The hardness of denture base acrylic plastic is:**
   a. Greater than that of glass
   b. Greater than that of enamel
   c. Less than that of metals
   d. Less than that of gingival tissue

5. **Tissue conditioners are temporary materials because they:**
   a. Are too expensive for permanent use
   b. Are not color stable over time
   c. Harden over time in the mouth
   d. Are always irritating to the gums

6. **You inspect a denture that has been returned from the laboratory for presentation to a patient that afternoon and notice a large number of bubbles, but only in the thickest areas. You suspect that the bubbles were caused by:**
   a. Heating the denture to less than 75°C during processing
   b. Heating the denture rapidly during the early stage of processing
   c. An inadequate application of pressure during packing
   d. Mixing with too low of a monomer-to-powder ratio

7. **You have just made a custom tray for a quadrant impression. When you try the tray back on the stone cast, you notice that it seats all of the way down and is very tight. What is causing this problem?**
   a. You forgot to make cutouts in the wax for stops
   b. You manipulated the acrylic beyond the dough stage
   c. This is normal because of the shrinkage of the acrylic
   d. You mixed the acrylic with too high a powder-to-liquid ratio

SELECTED READINGS

Bafile M, Graser GN, Myers ML, Li EKH. Porosity of denture resin cured by microwave energy. Journal of Prosthetic Dentistry 66:269–274, 1991.

The porosity is measured in heat-cured and microwave-cured dentures and found to be the same as long as the special liquid is used for the microwaved material.

Braden M, Wright PS, Parker S. Soft lining materials—a review. European Journal of Restorative Dentistry 3:163–174, 1995.

This article provides a review of the composition and characteristics of the different types of polymer materials used as soft liners for denture applications. Results from clinical studies of permanent and temporary soft liners are discussed.

Eichold WA, Woelfel JB. Denture base acrylic resins: Friend or foe? Compendium of Continuing Education in Dentistry 11:720–725, 1990.

This article reviews the advantages and disadvantages of denture base acrylics and discusses certain properties and the attempts that have been made to improve them.

Jagger DC, Harrison A. Complete dentures—the soft option. An update for general dental practice. British Dental Journal 182:313–317, 1997.

This article provides information concerning the use, indications, and maintenance of permanent and temporary soft lining materials for dentures.

Mack PJ. Denture soft linings: Materials available. Australian Dental Journal 34:517–521, 1989.

This article reviews the history of development and composition of the various soft lining materials available for dentures. The advantages and disadvantages of the various materials are discussed.

Phoenix RD. Denture base materials. Dental Clinics of North America 40:113–120, 1996.

This article presents a review of the materials, both historical and contemporary, that have been used in the fabrication of dentures.

Qudah S, Harrison A, Huggett R. Soft lining materials in prosthetic dentistry: A review. International Journal of Prosthodontics 3:477–483, 1990.

This review article describes the composition and properties of the various soft lining materials available. It also includes a brief history of the development of soft liners, a list of their deficiencies, and a summary of their indications for use.

Rudd KD. Processing complete dentures. Dental Clinics of North America 40:121–145, 1996.

This article describes the technique for fabricating and processing acrylic dentures.

Takamata T, Setcos JC. Resin denture bases: Review of accuracy and methods of polymerization. International Journal of Prosthodontics 2:555–562, 1989.

This article reviews the methods used to polymerize various denture base resins and their effect on fit. It also discusses the many different methods that have been used to evaluate accuracy.

Vallitu PK. A review of fiber-reinforced denture base resins. Journal of Prosthodontics 5:270–276, 1996.

A summary of the use of fiber reinforcement for denture base resins is presented. The article describes the types of fibers that have been used, as well as the results of studies investigating the potential for reinforcement of PMMA with fibers.

Chapter 13

Metal Alloys for Orthodontics, Prosthodontics, and Pediatric Dentistry

Uses of Metal Alloys in Dentistry

Types of Alloys
  Stainless Steels
  Cobalt-Chromium Alloys
  Pure Titanium and Titanium Alloys
  Nickel-Chromium Alloys

Properties of Alloys
  Alloys for Orthodontic Wires
  Alloys for Prosthodontics

Biocompatibility

Summary

Objectives

- Describe the uses of base metals in dentistry.
- Explain what is responsible for the corrosion resistance of each of the alloys used in orthodontics and prosthodontics.
- Compare the composition of the four major types of alloys used to make orthodontic wires.
- Compare the properties of the four major types of alloys used to make orthodontic wires.
- Compare the composition of nickel-chromium and cobalt-chromium prosthetic alloys.
- Compare the properties of nickel-chromium and cobalt-chromium alloys to those of gold alloys.
- Describe concerns over the biocompatibility of certain types of alloys used in dentistry.
- Explain pitting corrosion and identify alloys that may be susceptible to it.

Uses of Metal Alloys in Dentistry

Non-noble metals are used frequently in dentistry for a variety of applications. These **base metals** are used in the instruments to clean teeth, prepare teeth for restorations, and place restorations. They are used in crowns for single-tooth restorations and as frameworks for appliances such as bridges, partial dentures, and retainers. They are used as wires and brackets for moving and repositioning teeth. They also are used in implants. The high strength and durability of certain base metals makes them the logical choice for many of these applications. Specific important qualities include ductility (the ability to be bent and shaped without breaking) and stiffness (the ability to resist being elastically deformed). Many types of metals are available, but some are not suitable for dentistry because they do not possess adequate corrosion characteristics or acceptable biocompatibility. Through many years of testing, specific metals and alloys have been developed for dentistry and medicine on the basis of their ability to resist corrosion in biologic fluids. This is important from a structural standpoint because a corroding metal may deteriorate and become more prone to fracture. Of greater importance, however, are the biologic consequences of the products of corrosion because these may be swallowed or absorbed by oral tissues after they dissolve from the metal appliance or instrument.

Many of the noble metals and alloys used in dentistry are discussed in previous chapters. The purpose of this chapter is to acquaint the reader with the composition and characteristics of some of the other metals used in the profession.

Types of Alloys

Noble metals are used infrequently in orthodontics and pediatrics. Years ago, gold wires were used in orthodontics to straighten teeth; because of cost and the short-term nature of their use, however, these materials have mostly been replaced by more economical and better-suited base metals. Because of its reasonable cost and ease of handling, stainless steel is the most popular metal used in orthodontics and pediatrics. Other alloys, based on cobalt, nickel, and titanium, are also used extensively in these fields and in prosthodontics.

Stainless Steels

Uses

Crowns made of stainless steel are used in pediatric dentistry to repair severely damaged primary teeth or when rampant caries is present (Fig. 13-1). Stainless steel also is used to make bands, brackets, and wires for orthodontics. Steel wires often are soldered onto steel bands or crowns to maintain space (space maintainers) until the primary molars erupt, and they are embedded in acrylic orthodontic retainers to stabilize them on the teeth (Fig. 13-2). Extraoral uses of stainless steel include prophylactic instruments, cavity preparation instruments, instruments such as amalgam condensers and carriers that are used to place fillings, pliers for bending orthodontic appliances, burs and bur shanks, orthodontic headgear, and instrument trays.

Composition

Steel is a base metal alloy of iron with a small amount of carbon. Although pure iron is comparatively soft, the addition of a fraction of 1% of carbon causes iron

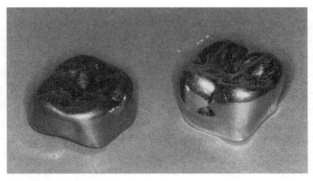

Figure 13–1 Stainless steel crowns used in pediatric dentistry.

to become very hard. The term "cast iron" is reserved for alloys of iron that contain more than about 2.5% carbon. These alloys are very hard, but too brittle to be useful in dentistry. The typical steel used in dentistry is called **stainless steel**. There are several types of stainless steel, but what is important to remember is that it is the chromium in steel that makes it "stainless," i.e., resistant to tarnish and corrosion. Stainless steel generally contains more than 12% chromium. Chromium is very reactive toward oxygen. When an alloy containing sufficient chromium is exposed to air, it quickly forms an oxide film that serves as a **passivating**, or protective, coating. The coating is extremely thin and transparent. It cannot be seen by the naked eye, but it provides protection from corrosion for the metal it covers.

Everyone has seen chrome-plated bumpers on cars. These are simply ordinary steel bumpers that have been treated with chromium to form a coating that does not corrode and stays shiny until it chips or cracks off. The chromium oxide on stainless steel is more durable than a chromium-plated bumper because the chromium is added directly to the stainless steel metal and forms a tightly bonded oxide layer on the surface. When scratched, the surface oxide usually can reform to protect the underlying metal. This protective layer does not form as easily in a solution containing chloride ions, however. ***Could this be a problem in the oral environment?***

Because saliva and body fluids contain high levels of chloride ion as a result of the presence of sodium chloride, stainless steel surfaces can be corroded in the

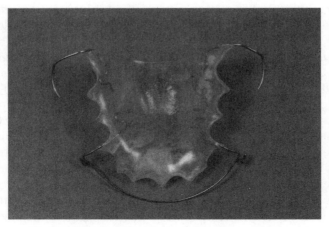

Figure 13–2 Stainless steel wire/acrylic space retainer.

body or in the mouth when they are scratched or nicked. Because repassivation does not readily occur, the corrosion can be accelerated in the area of the scratch, producing a small but deep pit.

This process is called **pitting corrosion**. Although pitting corrosion has caused some concern over the use of stainless steels, it is rarely a problem in orthodontics or pediatric dentistry, in which the service life of a given restoration or appliance is limited to a few years. Should extensive pitting corrosion occur in a thin section of an appliance, however, it may be sufficient to weaken the metal to the point of failure by fracture.

The type of stainless steel most commonly used in dentistry has the following approximate composition: 69% iron (Fe), 18% chromium (Cr), 8% nickel (Ni), 5% molybdenum (Mo), and 0.2% carbon (C). The nickel is present to stabilize a specific alloy structure, and molybdenum is added to cause further hardening. A similar type of stainless steel with slightly less carbon is used in orthopaedics for plates, screws, rods, and articulating surfaces for joint replacements. Therefore, the specific alloy is often referred to as surgical stainless steel.

Two common stainless steels are used for permanent crowns for pediatric patients. One has a composition similar to that described above (i.e., 70% Fe, 18% Cr, 11% Ni, and 0.1% C). The other is a nickel-based alloy containing 76% Ni, 16% Cr, 8% Fe, and 0.05% C. Both are corrosion resistant by virtue of their high chromium content.

Cobalt-Chromium Alloys

Uses

Base metal alloys made of cobalt (Co) and chromium (Cr) are used in both orthodontics and prosthetic dentistry. Some wires for straightening teeth are made from Co-Cr metal alloys. The other common dental use of Co-Cr alloy is as a framework for partial dentures or as the upper palatal portion of a full denture.

Composition

The common Co-Cr alloy used in dentistry has the approximate composition of 60% Co, 25% Cr, 10% Ni, 5% Mo, and 0.3% C. Cobalt and nickel are similar and are used almost interchangeably in alloys. Both produce a hard alloy, but the nickel slightly enhances ductility (i.e., percent elongation). As in stainless steels, molybdenum is added to harden and strengthen Co-Cr alloys. The concentration of carbon is important. Only small additions are acceptable because greater amounts cause the alloy to become extremely brittle, making it more difficult to bend during adjustments and leaving it more prone to accidental fracture. *What would be the purpose of the high concentration of chromium in these alloys?*

As expected, the chromium imparts corrosion resistance. As with stainless steel, however, environments with high concentrations of chloride ions enhance the possibility of pitting corrosion in these alloys. In addition, a high-chlorine environment may discolor or tarnish an appliance made from Co-Cr alloy. Although this is not a significant problem within the oral cavity, discoloration may occur when certain denture cleansers are used to clean partial frameworks made from this metal. Therefore, a partial denture should not be cleaned in commercial denture cleansers or in common at-home cleansers containing sodium hypochlorite [bleach (Clorox)]. An alternative solution for partial denture cleansing can be made as follows: 1 teaspoon sodium perborate tooth powder, 1 teaspoon dishwashing liquid (or powder), and half a glass of water.

Pure Titanium and Titanium Alloys

Uses

Titanium has become a metal commonly used in dentistry, in large part because of the demonstrated biocompatibility of the pure metal and its alloys. Wires made from titanium alloys are used in orthodontics. Pure titanium and titanium alloys are used as implant materials for patients needing single-tooth restorations or partial or complete dentures. The instruments used to place these implants are also made from titanium. Because of its tremendous reactivity with oxygen, titanium is a difficult metal to cast. Casting of titanium requires special furnaces for melting the metal under inert gas conditions, in which oxygen is excluded. The metal causes an acceptable and predictable response when placed in contact with epithelial tissues and, therefore, is ideal for many types of prosthetic appliances and restorations.

Composition

Titanium (Ti), like gold, is used in essentially its pure form as a dental implant material. The implant metal contains only trace amounts (i.e., less than 1%) of oxygen, carbon, and nitrogen, but the introduction of these elements must be carefully controlled or the metal becomes brittle. Thus, production of titanium implants is a sensitive procedure. An alloy of titanium containing approximately 6% aluminum (Al) and 4% vanadium (V) is also used successfully as an implant material.

Several types of titanium alloys are used to make orthodontic wires. One has a composition of 55% Ni and 45% Ti. Certain compositions of these Ni-Ti alloys are highly elastic (superelastic); they can be severely deformed without losing their elasticity. Often, small amounts of specific alloying elements, such as copper, are added to impart superelastic properties to Ni-Ti orthodontic wires at oral temperatures. They are ideal for the rapid but painless movement of severely misaligned teeth. It has become more common to use these wires during the initial stages of orthodontic therapy, in which large tooth movements using low levels of applied force are required.

Specific formulations of Ni-Ti alloys have a special **shape memory** effect. A wire made from this alloy can be bent into a certain shape at some temperature that exceeds its "critical temperature." Subsequently, the wire can be reshaped at a temperature below its critical point. On reheating the wire to a temperature above the critical temperature range, the wire will automatically "remember" its original shape and try to recover it. If it is free to do so, it will spontaneously deform to change back to its original shape. If its movement is restrained, for example, by the teeth, it will exert a force as it attempts to return to its original shape. Although these "shape memory" alloys are used in orthodontics because of their tremendous elasticity, the shape memory effect itself has not yet been commercialized. Dental researchers, however, envision many applications in which these special properties may be useful in anchoring restorations or moving tissue slowly.

Another type of titanium alloy used in orthodontics is called β-titanium (β-Ti). The approximate composition of this alloy is 79% Ti and 11% Mo, with further additions of zinc (Zn) and tin (Sn). The molybdenum is added to stabilize the desirable structure of the titanium crystals (i.e., the "β" structure), which makes the metal easier to bend and shape.

The corrosion resistance and the biocompatibility of titanium and its alloys are the result of its tremendous reactivity with oxygen. Titanium oxides rapidly form

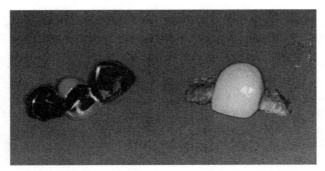

Figure 13–3 Lingual and facial views of a resin-bonded bridge.

on the surface of either the pure metal or its alloys and serve to passivate it to an even greater extent than the chromium oxide on stainless steel and Co-Cr alloys. After rupture or scratching, the invisible titanium oxide film immediately reforms in any environment containing oxygen. Therefore, titanium and its alloys are less susceptible to pitting corrosion than are chromium-containing alloys.

Nickel-Chromium Alloys

Uses

Nickel-chromium (Ni-Cr) alloys are used mainly as substrates for porcelain-fused-to-metal (PFM) restorations. These base metal alloys are much less expensive than noble metal alloys, although they also are more difficult to cast into restorations and to adjust for fit. The other common use of these alloys is in resin-bonded bridges. The conventional bridge requires the clinician to grind crown preparations on the teeth "abutting" or adjacent to the space to be filled. Resin-bonded bridges do not use crowns as **abutments** but instead require a minimal preparation of the lingual portion of the adjacent teeth. The prepared enamel on these abutment teeth is then acid-etched and bonded to the wings or extensions of the bridge by using a composite cement (Fig. 13-3). The pontic is a PFM tooth.

Composition

The approximate composition of Ni-Cr alloys is 80% Ni and 15% Cr; they also contain some aluminum and manganese. Beryllium (Be) is added to some of the alloys to make them easier to cast and to enhance their ability to be bonded with porcelain and composite cements. Because exposure to beryllium dust may be harmful, however, many alternative alloys without beryllium have been developed. Concerns over beryllium dust are warranted only during grinding procedures in which the element may be present in the debris generated. Laboratory personnel can essentially eliminate their risk of exposure by grinding these alloys in well-ventilated areas while wearing protective masks. The beryllium does not pose a concern for other dental personnel or patients.

The excellent corrosion resistance of these alloys is a function of their high chromium content. Therefore, they have similar characteristics to stainless steel and Co-Cr alloys.

■ *Properties of Alloys*

The discussion of the properties of the alloys described above is most conveniently divided into two sections. The first section will cover the alloys used as arch wires in pediatrics and orthodontics. The second section will cover the alloys used in prosthodontics.

Alloys for Orthodontic Wires

Stainless steel, Co-Cr, β-titanium, and Ni-Ti are the alloys commonly used for orthodontic wires. The properties of each type of alloy vary, as do the properties of the different compositions within each alloy. For example, there are several types of Co-Cr wires that differ in their stiffness. These wires are designed for different applications or for use at different stages during the treatment of a given patient. The manufacturer produces these different wires from the same alloy composition by giving them different heat treatments to alter their elastic limit and **working range**. The working range of an orthodontic wire is essentially equivalent to its maximum flexibility (see Chapter 2). A wire with a greater working range can move teeth greater distances than one with a lower working range before needing a "tightening" or adjustment. In addition, wires come in different sizes and shapes, providing different capacities for tooth movement from the same type of alloy. The selection of a particular type of wire depends on its properties as they relate to the requirements of the specific case, as well as the cost and handling characteristics of the different wires. Wires can be sterilized and reused several times, but this practice is not common.

The properties of alloys for orthodontic wires are compared in Table 13-1. The table lists the important characteristics of elastic limit (how much elastic deformation can take place before the wire is permanently deformed), elastic modulus (how difficult is it to bend the wire), resilience (how much energy is stored in the wire that can be used to move the teeth), working range (how much tooth movement can be accomplished before the wire must be repositioned), ductility (how much can the wire be shaped before it breaks), and cost. Note that the titanium wires have a lower elastic modulus and a greater working range than the steel or Co-Cr wires. This makes them better suited for the large tooth deflections necessary early in the orthodontic treatment of patients with badly misaligned teeth. This is especially true for the regular and superelastic types of Ni-Ti wires. Although these wires cost more than the chromium wires, the cost has been reduced in recent years, thus imposing fewer limitations on their use. A more significant problem with the wires is their low ductility. Owing to their tremendous elasticity, they are difficult or impossible to form into shapes such as loops and springs (Fig. 13-4). Although it is possible to bend them severely, they return back to their

TABLE 13–1. Comparison of the Properties of Alloys Used in Orthodontic Wires

	Stainless Steel	Co-Cr	β-Ti	Ni-Ti
Elastic limit (MPa)	1300	1100	900	400
Elastic modulus (GPa) stiffness	180 (high)	185 (high)	72 (medium)	41 (low)
Relative resilence (stored energy)	Low	Low	Medium	High
Relative working range (maximum flexibility)	Low	Low	Medium	High
Relative ductility (formability)	High	Medium	Medium	Low
Relative cost	Low	Low	Medium	High

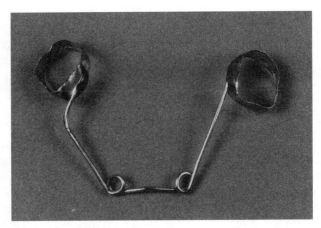

Figure 13-4 An orthodontic wire containing a loop structure.

original shape on removal of the force, with no permanent deformation. Wires made from the β-titanium alloy offer much better formability but do not have the extensive working range of the wires made from the Ni-Ti alloys. In addition, β-titanium wires experience more friction during sliding through steel brackets, thus slowing the rate of tooth movement.

The key concept in tooth movement is that it must occur slowly and, ideally, with low force applications to move teeth effectively with little pain or injury. The brackets and wires are placed to apply force to the teeth. As the teeth move, the force decreases, and the ability of the wire to move the teeth further declines, thus requiring an adjustment. The "wire tightening" that occurs at routine intervals in orthodontic cases is actually an adjustment of the position or replacement of an existing wire to continue to apply low-level forces in the appropriate directions and to the required extent as dictated by the particular demands of each case at each time period. The use of wires of different properties and variable sizes and shapes for a single composition provides a wide selection of choices for the orthodontist to accomplish this task. For example, at the same amount of applied force, certain alloys can produce much greater tooth movement than others (Fig. 13-5).

One other characteristic of orthodontic wires that is of importance to clinicians is the ease with which they can be joined to other structures, such as steel bands. It is common to **weld** or **solder** pieces of wires to bands or to other wires during the construction of an orthodontic appliance (Fig. 13-6). Welding refers to the joining of two metals and, in its purest sense in dentistry, requires no intermediate agent, such as another piece of metal. β-Titanium is the only orthodontic wire material truly capable of being welded. Two wires made of β-titanium can be joined by heating them where they are in contact. A fusion takes place through metallic bonding. Stainless steel can be welded to stainless steel, but the joints are not very strong and must be reinforced with solder, usually made from silver. The same is true of Co-Cr alloys. Ni-Ti wires cannot be welded or soldered and can be joined together only by mechanically squeezing or "crimping" them, which causes them to bond.

Alloys for Prosthodontics

The properties of the alloys used in prosthodontics are usually compared with those of the gold alloys they have replaced (Table 13-2). Although the properties

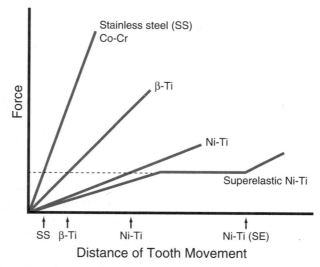

Figure 13–5 Plot of force versus tooth movement for different orthodontic alloys, showing the greater amount of movement possible for the superelastic Ni-Ti alloy than for the Ni-Ti, β-titanium, and stainless steel or Co-Cr alloys.

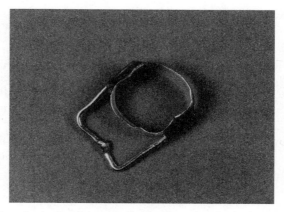

Figure 13–6 An orthodontic wire welded/soldered to a band to make a space-maintaining appliance.

TABLE 13–2. **Comparison of the Properties of Alloys Used in Prosthodontics**

	Gold Alloy	**Ni-Cr**	**Co-Cr**
Density (g/cm³)	15	8	8
Melting temperature (°C)	1000	1200	1300
Hardness (kg/mm²) (compared with enamel)	150–220 (softer)	350 (similar)	380 (harder)
Elastic modulus (GPa) (stiffness)	100	200	210
Relative cost	High	Low	Low

of each of the alloys are acceptable for these applications, there are specific differences between them.

The weight of a large dental appliance can become a significant factor for the comfort of a patient. For example, consider a denture made with a metallic base for greater strength. Because the density of the two base metal alloys is only half as much as that of the comparable gold alloy, the same denture made from the base metal alloys will weigh much less than that made from the gold alloy. This may help to keep the maxillary denture in place in the mouth. In addition, the elastic modulus of the two base metal alloys is nearly twice as great as that of the gold alloy, meaning that the base metals are significantly stiffer. The combination of low density and high stiffness of the base metals allows for the fabrication of a thinner appliance than would be possible with gold, thus reducing bulkiness and enhancing comfort without compromising stability.

Note that the hardness of the gold alloy is less than that of enamel, whereas that of the two base metal alloys is equivalent or greater (Table 13-2). This characteristic ensures that a prosthesis or appliance made from these alloys, such as a bridge covering the lower posterior teeth on one side of a patient's mouth, will not be easily scratched or abraded. The base metals, however, may produce more damage to opposing teeth than would the gold alloy. Usually, this is not a problem, but excessive wear of the opposing teeth may be a consideration for a patient who **bruxes** or grinds his or her teeth excessively. In addition, the high hardness of base metals makes grinding of components for fit adjustments much more difficult and time consuming for the laboratory technician. Also, the high elastic modulus makes chairside bending of partial denture clasps made from the Co-Cr alloy more difficult than it is for clasps made with gold alloys.

The greater difficulty in handling the base metals becomes most apparent when one examines the melting point of the different alloys. The Co-Cr metals are the most difficult to cast, requiring special casting machines to reach the high temperatures necessary for melting the metal. Ni-Cr alloys may be melted with torches with a mixture of gas and oxygen (instead of the gas-air torch described in Chapter 11) and are, therefore, less difficult to cast than Co-Cr alloys. The gold alloys, however, are much easier to cast than is either of the base metals. A major benefit of the two base metals, however, is their low cost, and this was the predominant driving force behind their development.

■ *Biocompatibility*

All of the alloys described in this chapter are considered to be compatible with the body in that they do not cause toxic reactions. Their biocompatibility is based on their corrosion resistance. Although every alloy releases ions into solution to some extent, the corrosion process is very slow for these metals, and the release of ions is often considered to be a negligible hazard. Some specific questions have arisen, however. As mentioned, beryllium is a carcinogen, and care must be taken that its dust is not inhaled. An acceptable level of beryllium dust to which a person may be exposed in a normal 8-hour-day, 5-day workweek is 2 $\mu g/m^3$ of air. Note that this is less than 5% of the safety level for occupational exposure to mercury vapor (50 $\mu g/m^3$). Beryllium poses no health risk to a patient wearing an appliance containing the metal. Nickel may present a greater hazard.

Nickel allergy is common. It is estimated that 9 to 10% of women in the United States are allergic to nickel. The initial sensitization to the metal most likely originates from wearing costume jewelry and pierced earrings. Only 1 to 2% of the male population appears to be allergic to nickel. Side effects caused by dental materials, most often allergic reactions, are most prevalent in orthodontics. This seems to be directly related to the wide use of nickel-containing stainless steel appliances in this dental specialty. Although allergic reactions are more difficult to produce in the oral cavity than on the skin, the wearing of headgear and other extraoral stainless steel appliances can provoke allergic reactions on the face and lips in people who are allergic to the metals. Of greater concern, perhaps, is the question of whether nickel causes tumors. Although there is no proof of the carcinogenic potential of nickel-containing dental appliances, studies have suggested that nickel may be of concern, and authorities in certain countries have seriously considered the safety of these alloys for continued use in dentistry. No restrictions have been imposed on the use of nickel in dental alloys in the United States.

Summary

A variety of metal alloys (mixtures of metals) are used in dental specialties. In general, these alloys are very strong and stiff, have excellent tarnish and corrosion resistance, and are biocompatible. Stainless steels, alloys of Co-Cr, and titanium and its alloys are commonly used in orthodontic wires and appliances. The steels and Co-Cr alloys are more rigid, stronger, and more easily shaped than titanium and its alloys, but they are not as elastic as titanium. Therefore, certain Ni-Ti alloys are commonly used where large tooth deflections are needed in the initial stages of orthodontic therapy. Co-Cr and Ni-Cr alloys are commonly used in prosthodontics to make, respectively, removable partial dentures and fixed bridges with porcelain facings. The high strength and melting temperature of the alloys make them well suited for these applications. In addition, the high chromium content imparts corrosion resistance. Stainless steels and Ni-Cr alloys are also used to make thin crowns that can be shaped and trimmed for pediatric dental applications.

STUDY QUESTIONS AND PROBLEM SOLVING

1. **The excellent corrosion resistance of the base metal alloys used in restorations can be attributed to which of the following:**
   a. The formation of a protective oxide film
   b. Painting the surface with varnish as a final step
   c. The presence of sufficient chromium within the metal
   d. Their extremely smooth surfaces
2. **Which of the following elements is (are) *not* found in any common type of orthodontic wire?**
   a. Iron
   b. Molybdenum
   c. Mercury
   d. Copper
3. **The large working range of orthodontic wires made from which alloy allows the most tooth movement with the fewest adjustments:**
   a. Nickel-titanium
   b. Stainless steel

c. β-Titanium

d. Cobalt-chromium

4. **A patient comes into the office showing extensive tooth wear on the upper left side of her mouth, which opposes a long-span, all-metal bridge. Although it is difficult to be certain, you suspect that the bridge is made of a:**

a. Nickel-titanium

b. Nickel-chromium alloy

c. High-copper amalgam alloy

d. Gold-silver-copper alloy

5. **If a patient cannot wear common pierced earrings because of an allergic reaction, which alloy would *not* be a good choice for her porcelain-fused-to-metal crown?**

a. 90% gold, 10% palladium

b. 80% nickel, 20% chromium

c. 50% gold, 50% platinum

d. 70% palladium, 30% silver

SELECTED READINGS

Brantley WA. Orthodontic wires. In: O'Brien WJ, ed. Dental Materials: Properties and Selection. Chicago: Quintessence Publishing, 1989;381–395.

This textbook chapter describes the composition and properties of orthodontic wires. An explanation of the clinical significance of the important properties of orthodontic wire alloys is presented.

Hensten-Pettersen A, Jacobsen N. Toxic effects of dental materials. International Dental Journal 41:265–273, 1991.

The toxic potential of dental materials is reviewed in this article. The authors conclude that there are frequent reactions to metals used in orthodontic appliances but that reactions to other dental metals are rare.

Kapila S, Sachdeva R. Mechanical properties and clinical applications of orthodontic wires. American Journal of Orthodontics and Dentofacial Orthopedics 96:100–109, 1989.

This study reviews the compositions, properties, and uses of the metals used to make orthodontic wires. It contains a section on the optimal clinical applications of orthodontic wires.

Kusy RP. Materials and appliances in orthodontics: Brackets, arch wires, and friction. Current Opinion in Dentistry 1:634–644, 1991.

This article reviews the materials used for orthodontic brackets and arch wires and discusses in depth the factors that determine the friction generated between them during tooth movement.

Kusy RP. A review of contemporary archwires: Their properties and characteristics. Angle Orthodontics 67:197–207, 1997.

This review article provides an update on the different alloys used for orthodontic wires and compares and contrasts their mechanical characteristics.

Wolfaardt JF, Peters E. The base metal alloy question in removable partial dentures: A review of the literature and a survey of alloys in use in Alberta. Canadian Dental Association Journal 58:146–151, 1992.

This article describes the historical background behind the use of base metals in prosthodontics and compares the composition of currently used alloys. An extensive review of the literature concerned with the biocompatibility of these alloys, particularly the effects of nickel, also is presented.

Chapter *14*

Abrasion and Polishing

Objectives

- Identify the goals of finishing and polishing of dental restorations and tooth structure.
- Define abrasion, finishing, and polishing and explain how they differ.
- Identify the factors that affect the rate and efficiency of abrasion in dentistry.
- Explain the Moh's scale and use it to make relative comparisons between the abrasives and substrates found in dentistry.
- Explain the rationale for the components of dental prophylaxis pastes and dentifrices.
- Identify the abrasives used and the typical procedure to be followed to finish and polish dental composites.
- Identify the abrasives used and the typical procedure to be followed to finish and polish dental amalgams.
- Identify the abrasives used and the typical procedure to be followed to finish and polish dental casting alloys.
- Identify the abrasives used and the typical procedure to be followed to finish and polish dental ceramics and porcelains.
- Identify the abrasives used and the typical procedure to be followed to finish and polish dental acrylics.

DISPLAY 14-1

> ### *Potential Benefits of Smooth Dental Restorations*
>
> - Minimal irritation of soft and hard tissues
> - Simulates natural tooth surface esthetics
> - Less likely to trap food debris and plaque
> - Reduced potential for corrosion
> - More hygienic

The goals of finishing and polishing of dental restorations and appliances are fairly obvious. For example, material must be ground from both the tissue-bearing surfaces, such as the tooth or gingiva, as well as the occlusal surfaces to make the restoration fit and maintain correct occlusal relationships. Because most of the materials used as permanent restoratives cannot be cut with hand instruments because of their hardness, a rotary handpiece is used for most of these contouring applications. Another obvious goal of finishing is to produce a smooth surface on a restoration. A restoration with a smooth surface has several benefits; it simulates natural tissue and is not irritating (Display 14-1). A rough or irregular surface can be irritating to the tongue and may become annoying to the patient. A rough surface at a gingival margin may be of even greater consequence because it may irritate the gingiva and cause it to become inflamed. A second benefit of a smooth surface is that it appears more natural and esthetically pleasing. A third benefit derived from the production of a smooth surface on a restoration is that it is less likely to trap food debris and plaque, compared with a surface containing deep grooves and scratches. Again, this can be especially important for restorations with subgingival margins.

In any event, the end result of finishing and polishing is to produce a more hygienic restoration or appliance. One final benefit of finishing and polishing relates to metallic restorations. Because corrosion is enhanced on rough and irregular surfaces, polishing is expected to reduce intraoral corrosion of metal restorations.

■ *Definitions and Theory of Finishing*

Abrasion can be defined as the wearing away or removal of material by the act of rubbing, cutting, or scraping. The object that does the abrading is called the **abrasive.** Finishing and polishing are two abrasive procedures commonly used in dentistry. **Finishing** refers to the process by which a restoration or appliance is contoured to remove excess material and produce a reasonably smooth surface. **Polishing** follows finishing and refers to the final removal of material from a restoration or appliance, resulting in the production of a very smooth, highly reflective surface that does not contain scratches. The polished surface most resembles the natural surfaces in the oral cavity. Therefore, finishing and polishing are both wear processes, but they differ in intent and degree. The object of finishing is to make a restoration that is acceptable in fit, occlusion, and contour while achieving reasonable surface quality through the removal of large quantities of material by abrasion. The object of polishing is to produce a final smoothing of the surface with a minimal removal of material, thus causing no further change in contour.

The theory behind finishing and polishing is to use a series of hard objects, or abrasives, to remove material from a softer object, such that the surface scratches produced by each abrasive are sequentially replaced with ones of smaller and smaller dimension. Therefore, any factor that either improves or impedes the efficiency of producing scratches and "gouging" the surface material is important to the overall process. *Anyone who has ever sanded a piece of wood can probably think of several variables that influence the efficiency of the abrasion process. What are some of them?*

■ Factors Affecting Finishing

In dentistry, finishing is accomplished with abrasives made from metals, oxides, and diamonds. Some of the abrasives are particulate in nature, whereas others are burs with a precise cutting pattern, similar to those found in ordinary drill bits and files. Although the nature of the cutting instrument is determined by the manufacturer, the manner in which it is used is solely the responsibility of the clinician. Therefore, the characteristics of the finishing instrument and the manner in which it is manipulated are important factors determining the rate and efficiency of cutting. Other factors that affect cutting efficiency include the hardness of the abrasive and the object to be cut (i.e., the substrate), the size and shape of the abrasive, the speed at which the abrasive moves, the pressure applied to the abrasive, and the use of appropriate lubricants.

Hardness

An important consideration in cutting is the difference between the hardness of the abrasive and the hardness of the substrate. To demonstrate this point, consider the following example. Glass is very hard, yet it can be cut by a diamond. Diamond is the hardest material known; therefore, it can be used to cut virtually anything, since everything else is at least a little softer than diamond. As discussed in Chapter 2, hardness is a measure of a material's ability to resist indentation. Several hardness scales exist to compare materials. There is, however, an alternative scale—the Moh's scale—which ranks materials in terms of their ability to resist being scratched. The Moh's scale is applicable to the study of abrasion because abrasion is essentially equivalent to scratching. The relative ranking of various materials and abrasives on the Moh's scale is given in Table 14-1.

Diamond has the maximum Moh's rating of 10. Silicon carbide, another abrasive material commonly used in dentistry and other fields, is close to diamond, with a Moh's value of 9 to 10. When one compares these materials with glass, which has a Moh's rating of 5 to 6, it is easy to understand why diamond and silicon carbide easily cut and scratch glass. The greater the difference in hardness between the abrasive and the substrate, the more rapid and efficient the cutting and abrasion. Tooth enamel has a Moh's rating of 5 to 6. As expected, dentin is softer and easier to cut than enamel and has a rating of 3 to 4. It is instructive to keep these values in mind as the different types of abrasives are discussed in this chapter.

TABLE 14–1. **Relative Ranking of Abrasion Resistance for Materials Using the Moh's Scale**

Material	Moh's Value	Material	Moh's Value
Diamond	10	**Composite**	**5–7**
Silicon carbide	9–10	**Enamel**	**5–6**
Emery	9–10	**Glass**	**5–6**
Tungsten carbide	9–10	**Chromium metals**	**5–6**
Aluminum oxide	9	Rouge	5–6
Zirconium silicate	7–7.5	**Amalgam**	**4–5**
Cuttle	7	**Gold alloys**	**3–4**
Quartz	7	**Dentin**	**3–4**
Tin oxide	6–7	Chalk	3
Porcelain	**6–7**	Gypsum	2
Garnet	6.5–7	**Acrylic**	**2–3**
Tripoli	6–7	Talc	1
Pumice	6		

Shape

Common sense can be used to predict which is more abrasive, a spherical object or one with an irregular shape and sharp edges. The irregular object has a tendency to dig into a surface instead of roll across it. Therefore, its cutting efficiency is enhanced by having numerous sharp edges. The blade of a kitchen knife has two edges. The sharpened one is much more effective for cutting into an object than the blunt edge. Consider an abrasive as being like a knife; the sharper the abrasive, the more effective it is as a cutting instrument. With repeated use, however, the knife loses sharpness and no longer cuts as well as it did when it was new. The same happens to the abrasives in a dental bur or stone. Some cutting instruments, such as knives, can be resharpened to enhance their cutting efficiency. Most instruments, such as burs and stones, however, cannot be sharpened and simply are disposed of when they become dull or clogged with cutting debris (Fig. 14-1).

Size

In general, under the same conditions, larger particles abrade a surface more rapidly than smaller ones because the former plough deeper grooves or cuts into the surface. Not surprisingly, the roughness of the ground or finished surface is directly related to the size of the abrasive particles. Particles usually are classified by their size in micrometers (μm), with coarse being 100 μm or more, medium being 10 to 100 μm, and fine being 0 to 10 μm. Abrasives of all sizes are used in dentistry. The procedure for finishing and polishing involves a sequential reduction in the size of the abrasive particles. By so doing, the scratches left in the surface by the previous abrasive are removed and replaced by smaller and shallower scratches from the current abrasive. Eventually, the abrasive is so small that the scratches are no longer visible.

Although abrasives made with smaller particles are usually less effective abraders than those made with larger particles, the cutting efficiency of a smaller-particle abrasive can be increased by increasing the applied force. This can be undesirable in some instances. Therefore, it is important to monitor pressure during the finishing procedure, even with fine abrasives.

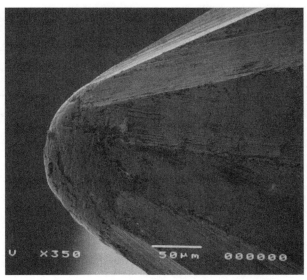

Figure 14–1 Scanning electron micrograph showing the point of a cutting bur that has been used and become dulled by cutting.

Pressure

Use of a greater force during finishing causes a more rapid removal of material by forcing the abrasive to cut deeper into the surface. Care must be taken, however, when using pressure application to regulate finishing, because greater pressures also create additional heat and raise the temperature within the substrate. The higher temperatures can lead to distortion or physical changes within the appliance or restoration. This is especially true for acrylics and amalgams. For example, high temperatures created during the polishing of amalgam may cause discomfort for the patient because of the transmission of the heat to vital tissues through the thermally conductive amalgam. One laboratory study showed temperature increases of 15 to 20°C in the pulp chamber when amalgams were polished without water coolant.

Possibly the greatest concern with the use of pressure to enhance cutting efficiency is the danger of overabrading the substrate. This often is a problem at the margin, where the restorative material may not be as hard as the enamel and becomes abraded away more quickly. This can lead to overcontouring of the restoration (Fig. 14-2). Overcontouring can negatively influence occlusion as well as the adaptation of critical margins.

Speed

The speed of abrasion also influences the cutting efficiency. Faster speeds result in faster cutting rates, and the clinician must take more care to keep the cutting instrument under control. This situation is similar to that discussed for pressure. Higher speeds create greater temperatures and a greater danger of overcutting the object.

Lubrication

The abrasive instrument transfers its energy into removal of material. There is extra energy that does not get used up, however, but instead is transferred to the sur-

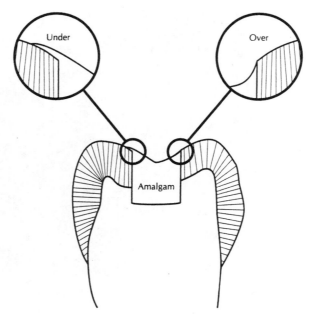

Figure 14–2 An overcontoured margin produced on a restoration as a result of using excessive pressure during finishing.

face in the form of heat. Because there are several factors that can create unwanted heat at the site of finishing, it is of interest to understand how to minimize heat buildup. One method is to flood the site with a lubricant that carries the heat away from the surface. In tool and die machining, oils often are used, but they cannot be used in the mouth. Water, conversely, poses no problems and is the most common lubricant used in dentistry. When excessive heat builds up under a cutting instrument, the instrument loses efficiency. Lubricants, therefore, act to lessen this problem. In addition to having a cooling effect, a lubricant such as water facilitates the movement of the cutting edge into the surface and carries away debris that would otherwise clog the cutting edge. Both the cooling and the removal of debris by the lubricant enhance the efficiency of the abrasion process and are integral to successful finishing of dental restorations. It should also be noted that the use of a lubricant can obscure the cutting surfaces, making it difficult to visualize it, especially at the margins. There are times when a final finish may be carefully conducted dry to avoid this problem.

■ *Instruments Used in Cutting and Abrading*

Numerous types of abrasive materials are used in dentistry to remove material or finish surfaces. Given the compositions of the many types of materials used in the field, it is clear that many types of abrasives are needed. The abrasives are supplied as powders, pastes, particles bonded to steel shanks or paper disks for use in the handpiece, and particles bonded to paper strips for use by hand. Other cutting instruments work like conventional drill bits or files in that they contain parallel cutting edges, or flutes.

The composition of the different materials and their specific uses are discussed in the next section; the materials are presented in the order of most abrasive to least abrasive. The most abrasive materials include diamonds, carbides, emery, and aluminum oxides (alumina), which are used to cut tooth structure and produce gross and fine finishing of restoratives. The less abrasive materials are cuttle, tin oxide, pumice, rouge, and the like, which are used primarily in final polishing or for the finishing of soft materials such as acrylic. ***How is it that diamonds and alumina, which are so hard, can be used as final polishing agents?***

Composition of Abrasives

Diamond

Diamond is composed of carbon. It is the hardest substance (10 on the Moh's scale) and, therefore, makes an efficient abrasive because it does not wear down or lose sharpness as easily as do other abrasives. Diamond chips of various sizes, either natural or synthetic, usually are bonded to metal shanks to be used in the handpiece (Figs. 14-3 and 14-4). Very fine diamond chips also can be mixed with glycerin and water to produce a polishing paste. Diamonds frequently are used to cut tooth structure for crown and bridge and for finishing composites. Diamond finishers usually are used with water to avoid excessive heat buildup and clogging of the particles by the abrasion debris, both of which reduce cutting efficiency.

Carbides

Included among the carbides are abrasives such as *silicon carbide* (SiC), boron carbide (B_4C), and tungsten carbide (WC). These abrasives have a Moh's value higher than 9. Silicon and boron carbide finishing instruments usually are supplied as particles pressed with a binder into disks or wheels for use on a handpiece. They also are attached to steel shanks as burs or stones (Fig. 14-3); for example, green stones contain silicon carbide. Tungsten carbide burs usually are used to cut tooth structure; they look like drills in that they have many flutes (Fig. 14-3). Gross reduction of material is accomplished with a bur with few flutes (i.e., 6 to 8), whereas smoother surfaces are produced with burs containing 12 or more flutes. These burs usually are used in a high-speed handpiece for cutting cavities or finishing composite restorations.

Emery

Emery is composed mainly of a natural form of an oxide of aluminum and is often called *corundum*. It looks like sand. This commonly used abrasive is familiar to ev-

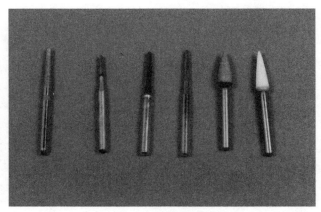

Figure 14–3 Various dental cutting instruments (*left* to *right*): diamond, 6-fluted carbide bur, 12- and 30-fluted carbide burs, green stone, and white stone.

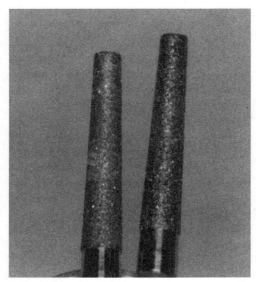

Figure 14–4 Diamond cutting instruments. The one on the left has been used and is partially clogged with debris.

eryone who has filed his or her fingernails with an "emery board." Emery has a Moh's value higher than 9. Emery particles usually are bonded to paper strips or disks to make finishing instruments. Emery is commonly used to make arbor bands, which attach to a dental lathe and are used to grind off rough areas and contour acrylic appliances and custom trays (Fig. 14-5).

Aluminum Oxide

Aluminum oxide refers to a specific composition (Al_2O_3) of an extremely abrasive material that has a Moh's value of 9. It has generally replaced emery as an abrasive material and is used in similar applications. Aluminum oxide usually is produced as particles bonded to paper disks and strips (reddish brown in color) or impregnated into rubber wheels and points. Aluminum oxide is the abrasive used in white stones (Fig. 14-3). Very fine particles of aluminum oxide (and diamond) can be mixed into a paste and used to produce smooth polished surfaces on many types of restorations, such as acrylics and composites (Fig. 14-6).

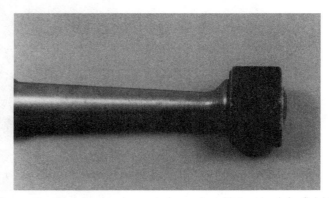

Figure 14–5 Emery abrasive arbor band mounted on a dental lathe chuck for finishing an acrylic appliance.

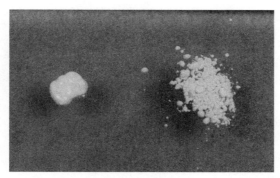

Figure 14–6 Aluminum oxide polishing paste and tin oxide polishing powder.

Zirconium Silicate

Zirconium silicate is a natural mineral (i.e., zircon) that is used as a polishing agent in strips and disks, as well as in **prophylactic pastes**. It has a Moh's value of 7 to 7.5 and is, therefore, not as effective as diamonds, carbides, or aluminum oxides in cutting hard substances.

Cuttle

Cuttle is a fine-particle form of quartz, or sand. Its composition is that of silicon dioxide (SiO_2). Originally, this material was produced from the bones of certain fishes. Cuttle, however, now refers to quartz particles with a Moh's value of 7. The particles are attached to paper disks. These beige-colored disks are used in the handpiece to finish gold alloys, acrylics, and composites.

Tin Oxide

Tin oxide (SnO_2) has a Moh's value of 6 to 7, making it less abrasive than quartz (sand). It is used as a polishing agent for metallic restorations, especially amalgams. It is supplied in the form of a powder or paste, the latter of which is produced by mixing the powder with water, glycerine, or alcohol (Fig. 14-6). It also produces an excellent polish of enamel.

Garnet

Garnet has a Moh's value similar to that of tin oxide (6.5 to 7.5). This mined mineral is composed of oxides of silicon, iron, and aluminum. It is reddish in color and, similar to cuttle and aluminum oxide, is used on disks. Owing to its low hardness compared with that of many other abrasives, it is used mainly for the polishing of acrylic appliances but could also be used for composites.

Tripoli

Tripoli is another polishing agent used commonly for alloys of gold. The main component of this mined material is a form of silicon dioxide that is less abrasive than quartz; thus, its Moh's value is 6 to 7, or slightly less than that of cuttle. The material is usually supplied in a bar that is applied to a rag wheel and mounted in a dental lathe or handpiece (Fig. 14-7).

Pumice

Pumice is a natural glass that is rich in silica (SiO_2) and is produced from volcanoes. This abrasive is used in the laboratory to polish acrylics, and it is added to pro-

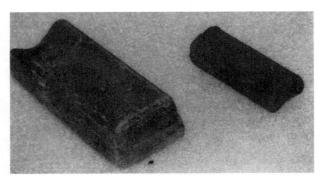

Figure 14–7 Bars of tripoli and rouge for polishing dental alloys, with use of a rag wheel mounted on a dental lathe.

phylactic pastes to polish teeth. It is commonly used also as a material to remove dried skin (as in a "pumice stone"). It has a Moh's value of 6.

Rouge

Rouge is used in facial makeup because of its reddish color, but it also is used as a polishing agent in dentistry. It is iron oxide (Fe_2O_3). Iron oxide has a Moh's value of 5 to 6. Although it is normally a powder, it can be formed into a block or cake and used on a rag wheel in a dental lathe or in a handpiece to polish gold alloys (Fig. 14-7). It adheres relatively well to skin, which explains its use in cosmetics. It is this quality that also makes handling it a messy proposition.

Chalk

Chalk is *calcium carbonate* ($CaCO_3$). This material has a very low Moh's value of 3, which makes it only mildly abrasive. It was commonly used in prophylactic pastes. At one time, it was used in many dentifrices but has since been replaced by other materials.

Prophylaxis Pastes, Dentifrices, and Denture Cleansers

Prophylaxis Pastes

Prophylaxis pastes must remove surface stains but must not produce damage or extensive roughening of the underlying tooth structure. Therefore, they usually contain only moderately abrasive materials, such as pumice. Silicon dioxide and zirconium silicate, however, are also used in these pastes, which are applied to the teeth through a rubber cup on a slow-speed handpiece. *How can a material as abrasive as zirconium silicate be used in a prophylaxis paste?*

> Remember that even a very harsh abrasive produces only minimal removal of a hard substrate when it is used in a very fine particle size.

The benefit of having an aggressive abrasive is that difficult stains can be removed more easily. Because of the particle sizes used, little damage is done to the tooth, and smooth surfaces are maintained. The abrasives in these pastes can abrade certain dental materials, such as composites and acrylics, however. Therefore, care should be taken during routine cleanings to avoid excessive polishing of such restoratives, which could alter anatomy and leave surfaces in a roughened condition.

Dentifrices

Dentifrices (toothpaste) are used to clean teeth and promote oral hygiene. Although much oral debris can be removed by the bristles of a toothbrush, the nylon fibers themselves, being plastic, are not very abrasive. Therefore, **pellicle** (the organic coating that forms on surfaces in the mouth) and stains must be removed by some more abrasive agent. Typical abrasives used in dentifrices include calcium pyrophosphate, dibasic calcium phosphate dihydrate, tricalcium phosphate, hydrated alumina, hydrated silica, and sodium metaphosphate. The use of a dentifrice with a stiff toothbrush can enhance the abrasion of the teeth by exerting more force on the abrasives as they move across the enamel, thus increasing their cutting efficiency. Although this is helpful in removing stains, it can be harmful in that it may lead to excessive removal of enamel (Fig. 14-8). Therefore, softer-bristled brushes usually are recommended.

In addition to the abrasive, dentifrices contain water, humectants such as glycerine to keep the paste from drying out, a detergent such as sodium lauryl sulfate to help the dentifrice clean the teeth by improving the wetting on enamel, a binder such as carboxymethylcellulose to keep the solid and liquid components of the paste from separating, coloring agents such as food dyes, flavoring agents such as specific oils and extracts, and a fluoride compound for caries protection.

Denture Cleansers

Deposits collect on dentures as a result of normal use. These deposits can be unesthetic and may cause the denture to be foul smelling or irritating. Removal of surface stains and debris from a denture can be accomplished with a soft-bristled toothbrush and toothpaste or another type of abrasive powder (i.e., calcium carbonate). There also are solutions in which the denture can be soaked. These solutions rely on chemical means to remove the stains and deposits and may contain sodium perborate (i.e., Efferdent, Warner-Lambert) or hypochlorites (Mersene, Colgate-Palmolive). Other solutions contain alkaline peroxide or dilute acids, such as phosphoric acid. Any of these solutions may be effective for full-arch dentures. As mentioned, however, partial dentures should not be soaked in acidic solutions or those containing chlorine (such as the hypochlorites) because the metal may become tarnished.

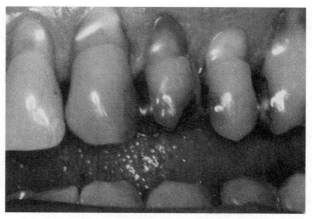

Figure 14–8 Erosions of the cervical region of the anterior and posterior teeth.

■ *Finishing Procedures*

Composites

Composites are a mixture of relatively soft polymers (having a Moh's hardness similar to acrylic) and very hard, abrasive filler particles (having a Moh's hardness of 5 to 8). The overall hardness of a specific composite depends on its composition but is in the range of 5 to 7 on the Moh's scale. For some formulations, this is higher than the hardness of enamel, and such composites actually pose a clinical problem in that they tend to wear down opposing dentition, which leads to improper occlusal relationships. The procedure for finishing composites has changed as formulations with "softer" fillers of smaller size have been developed. There are many different ways to produce a smooth surface on composites. Although the material continues to strengthen with age, most of the hardening occurs within the initial few minutes after curing, so composites are finished within minutes of hardening. There is evidence that the marginal integrity and surface properties of the material may be improved by delaying finishing, but this is not practical. Therefore, many clinicians recommend a final light activation of the finished composite surface to improve the properties.

The initial contouring of a composite can be performed with either carbide burs or diamonds rotating in a high-speed handpiece (Fig. 14-9). Only light pressure should be applied to avoid overcontouring the composite. There is some debate over the use of water spray during the procedure because although water acts as a coolant to minimize heat buildup, it makes it difficult to observe the margins clearly because of the esthetic nature of the material. When the tooth and restoration are the same color, it is difficult to identify a margin that is submerged in water containing finishing debris. Studies have shown that equivalent smoothness and surface hardness can be obtained on composites polished wet or dry. Nevertheless, water usually is recommended, and carbides with 12 flutes or medium to fine diamonds are most frequently used. Studies have shown that carbides have a tendency to gouge out the prepolymerized resin fillers in microfill composites, and thus diamonds may be a better choice for these materials. The surface roughness (i.e., basically the average height of the scratches) of the composite after either of these treatments is approximately 0.6 to 0.7 μm but may exceed 1.0 μm with medium diamonds.

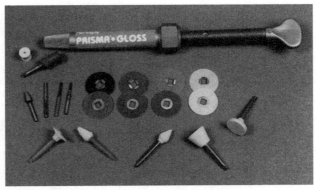

Figure 14–9 Various instruments used for finishing and polishing of composites. *Top row*, a polishing paste with prophylaxis cup and pad; *middle row* (*left* to *right*), green stone, medium diamond, 12-fluted carbide burs, and coarse to extra-fine sandpaper disks; *bottom row*, various abrasive-impregnated rubber points.

After the initial contouring is achieved, finer carbides (30 or 40 flutes) or diamonds (fine or extra fine) can be used to smooth the surface further (Fig. 14-9). A common protocol, however, is to use abrasive sandpaper disks on a slow-speed handpiece. These disks are rated coarse, medium, fine, and extra-fine and produce average roughness values on composites of 2.0, 0.6, 0.3, and 0.1 μm, respectively. These disks work on all surfaces but, owing to their thinness, are especially suited to interproximal spaces. Therefore, when finishing a surface that has already been contoured with a carbide or medium diamond, one would proceed to the medium, fine, and then extra-fine disks (Fig. 14-9). An alternative to the disks is to use rubber points containing abrasives. These instruments are used on the slow-speed handpiece and produce final roughness values of 0.1 μm or so.

Manufacturers now supply a paste, containing either aluminum oxide or diamond, for the final polishing of composites. The pastes contain the abrasives in an aqueous suspension. When composites contained large-diameter fillers, there was less of a need for such a paste, since the final smoothness usually was determined by the size of the largest particles. Along with the trend toward producing composites with smaller particles came the realization that these materials could be polished to produce smooth, shiny surfaces similar to those produced on microfills. Many studies have shown that the final smoothness of small-particle hybrid composites is very close to that of microfills. This final polish is achieved with polishing pastes used in rubber cups or on specially designed pads (Fig. 14-9). The polish produces surface roughness values of 0.1 μm or less and smears the material across to produce a scratch-free surface that has shine or gloss. The surface appears scratch free because the final scratches are smaller than the wavelength of visible light and, therefore, are imperceptible to the naked eye.

Amalgam

Amalgam is a mixture of several different metal phases having different compositions and, therefore, varying hardnesses. The overall hardness of amalgam is 4 to 5 on the Moh's scale, which is similar to that of most gold alloys used in inlays and onlays. Because of the relatively slow setting of amalgam, it is recommended that these materials not be finished until a later appointment, ideally within 24 or 48 hours. Although most modern high-copper amalgams harden more quickly than the older low-copper amalgams, marginal integrity is believed to be enhanced by delaying finishing. Therefore, the amalgam usually is carved and the occlusal surface is burnished with steel ball burnishers to improve adaptation to the margins and smooth the surface (see Fig. 6-10). As evidence for the importance of the burnishing step, the final roughness of the carved surface is approximately 4.0 to 5.0 μm, whereas that of the burnished surface may be less than 0.4 μm.

At a subsequent appointment, the amalgam is finished with stones, points, and disks and use of the slow-speed handpiece and water coolant (Fig. 14-10). The use of water is important because of the high thermal conductivity of the amalgam. In addition, mercury can be brought to the surface of the amalgam during heating, creating a mercury-rich layer that is weaker and more prone to failure than the original surface. Providing coolant during finishing prevents the formation of this surface. Contouring to produce the anatomic features of the restoration is performed under moderate pressure with a steel finishing bur, or a green or white stone. Care should be taken to rotate the bur from the amalgam to the tooth to avoid chipping the brittle margins. These initial contouring steps actually may roughen the surface to values of 0.5 to 1.0 μm.

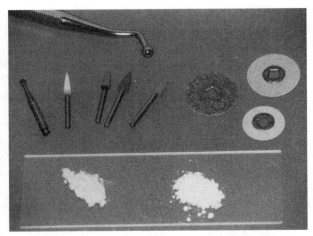

Figure 14–10 Various instruments used for finishing and polishing of amalgams. *Top row,* ball burnisher; *middle row (left* to *right),* steel bur, white stone, green stone, brown rubber point, green rubber point, and sandpaper disks; *bottom row,* pumice and tin oxide.

The next step is to smooth the surface with rubber points impregnated with abrasive particles (Fig. 14-10). Brown points ("brownies") are somewhat coarser than green points ("greenies"). Proximal margins on the lingual or buccal surfaces between teeth can be smoothed with abrasive disks and the use of light pressure. Interproximal strips are available to produce a final surface roughness of 0.1 to 0.3 μm in this region.

Final polish can be achieved with a rubber cup or brush, first with a slurry of pumice (with a roughness of 0.3 μm) and then a slurry of XXX Silex or tin oxide (one brand is Amalglos). These are used on the slow-speed handpiece with light pressure. The tin oxide produces the smoothest surface, with a roughness of 0.1 μm.

Alloys

Metals, such as the gold alloys used to make castings for inlays or onlays, have hardness values on the Moh's scale of 3 to 4. Some of the very hard metals used in partial dentures and porcelain-fused-to-metal applications have values of 5 to 6 on the Moh's scale and are similar to enamel. Most of these alloys can be finished with a combination of stones, disks, and wheels. A typical procedure is described next.

After the casting has been cleaned of investment debris with water and a toothbrush, it is often soaked, or **pickled**, in warm hydrochloric acid to remove the surface oxide layer. Any small nodules of metal can then be removed with a carborundum stone. Then casting is cut off from the sprue with a separating disk ("Joe Dandy"; Fig. 14-11).

While the casting is seated on the die, a carborundum stone is used with a slow-speed handpiece to provide the proper contour of the occlusal surface (Fig. 14-11). Next, a green stone (inverted cone shape) can be used to finish all the occlusal margins by rotating it from the surface of the inlay to the margins. This motion also tends to deform the metal slightly, drawing it to the margin and creating a closer adaptation of metal to tooth. For a class II inlay, the proximal margins can be finished with a medium cuttle disk, revolving from the inlay to the tooth surface. Care is taken to avoid disturbing the gingival margin, where only burnishing

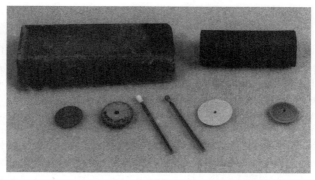

Figure 14–11 Various instruments used for finishing and polishing of dental alloys. *Top row,* bars of tripoli and rouge; *bottom row* (*left* to *right*): "Joe Dandy" disk, carborundum stone, white stone, green stone, cuttle disk, and burlew wheel.

is indicated. The surface has a final roughness of approximately 0.3 to 0.5 μm after the treatment with the disk, so many scratches may still be visible.

The surface of the casting can then be polished with a rubber wheel (Fig. 14-11). These rubber wheels are impregnated with abrasive particles (e.g., aluminum oxide or silicon carbide) of varying sizes and, therefore, vary from coarse to fine. This procedure reduces the surface roughness to a level of 0.10 to 0.15 μm. Essentially all of the scratches are removed, but the surface remains somewhat dull in appearance. Final polish can be achieved with tripoli and rouge on a rag wheel (Figs. 14-7 and 14-11). The final surface roughness of a casting polished in this manner would be on the order of 0.05 μm. This means that the scratches are an order of magnitude smaller than the wavelength of light and are imperceptible; thus, the surface has a high shine or luster.

After the inlay has been cemented in the tooth, a final finishing can be performed with a prophylaxis cup or bristle brush and the use of XXX Silex or flour of pumice.

Ceramics and Porcelains

The hardness of porcelain (with a Moh's value of 6 to 7) is greater than that of enamel. This creates the same problem with abrasion of opposing dentition that was discussed for certain composites. There are new ceramics that are reported to be kinder to enamel than porcelain, but often the benefit is lost because they must be glazed with porcelain to produce the proper esthetic effect. The benefit of glazing is that it produces a glassy surface on porcelain, which is the smoothest surface possible. Any instrumentation of a glazed surface removes the glaze and leaves the porcelain rougher and more abrasive. Polishing procedures have been developed for porcelain and ceramic restorations, however, that leave them with minimal surface roughness.

Adjustments to porcelain restorations can be made with fine diamonds in the high-speed handpiece. Finishing burs and sandpaper disks can also be used. After initial adjustments, rubber wheels and points impregnated with aluminum oxide or silicon carbide particles can be used to smooth the surface. Moving the wheel or point in a crisscross fashion produces the most lustrous surface. Final polishing is achieved with fine-particle diamond pastes. Research suggests that on certain types of ceramics, these pastes can produce a surface as smooth as the glazed surface.

Acrylics

Acrylics are the softest permanent restorative material and must be treated with care at all times. They have a Moh's hardness of 2 to 3 and can be abraded by gypsum. In addition, acrylics have low thermal stability. Very aggressive finishing and polishing procedures can build up sufficient heat within portions of an acrylic appliance to create significant distortions.

Acrylic appliances can be ground and contoured with steel burs in a handpiece or dental lathe. Smoothing is then performed with a slurry of pumice on a rag wheel mounted on a dental lathe. Final polishing to produce a surface with high shine is achieved with tripoli or tin oxide paste on a rag wheel on the lathe.

Summary

"Abrasion" refers to the process by which one surface or material erodes or wears another. Abrasion can be detrimental, as in the wearing away of tooth or restorative material surfaces, but it can also be useful, as in removing excess material for contouring or finishing to produce more natural and esthetically pleasing structures. The act of finishing is accomplished by proceeding from coarse- to fine-grained abrasives to remove material with each step, but to replace the larger scratches from the previous step with smaller ones in subsequent steps. Eventually the scratches become so small that they are imperceptible to the naked eye and the surface appears polished.

Abrasion depends on many factors, including the hardness of the abrasive (harder abrasives, such as diamond, are more efficient), particle size of the abrasive (larger particles remove more material), speed of the abrasion (faster speeds generally remove more material faster), pressure (more pressure means more material removed), and amount of lubrication (lubricants remove debris and limit temperature increases to enhance cutting efficiency). A variety of abrasives are used in dentistry, including diamond, emery, aluminum oxide, tin oxide, and pumice. The different abrasives vary in their abilities to wear surfaces and, therefore, are used for various stages in a finishing-polishing process. Different procedures are established for different materials.

STUDY QUESTIONS AND PROBLEM SOLVING

1. **In explaining to a patient the benefits of polishing a recently placed occlusal amalgam restoration, you would be correct to say all of the following except:**
   a. A polished restoration will feel more natural to the tongue
   b. Amalgam may show less tarnish and corrosion during aging
   c. Amalgam will be less likely to wear down the opposing teeth
   d. A polished restoration is better for oral hygiene
2. **Which of the following would *not* increase the rate of abrasion?**
   a. Increased pressure
   b. Use of a lubricant
   c. Increased speed
   d. Smaller particles

3. In the sequence, *carborundum stone → green stone → rubber wheel →* _____, what is the next abrasive to be used for polishing a crown made from a gold alloy?
   a. Diamond disk
   b. Aluminum oxide stone
   c. Tripoli
   d. Pumice

4. An abrasive material that would most efficiently abrade a surface with a hardness of 5 on the Moh's scale might be one with:
   a. Irregular particles of hardness 6
   b. Spherical particles of hardness 6
   c. Irregular particles of hardness 3
   d. Spherical particles of hardness 3

5. Why would it be inappropriate for a prophylaxis paste to contain diamond particles?
   a. It would be too expensive
   b. It would remove enamel
   c. It would not remove plaque
   d. It would not remove calculus

6. In the sequence, *12-fluted carbide →* _____ *→ fine rubber point → aluminum oxide paste,* what is the missing abrasive to be used for polishing the occlusal surface of a small-particle hybrid composite?
   a. Coarse sandpaper disk
   b. Rouge
   c. Tin oxide paste
   d. Fine diamond

7. The smoothest surface on amalgam is achieved with a final polish using:
   a. Pumice
   b. Brown stones
   c. Tin oxide
   d. Green points

8. Which of the following produces the smoothest surface on a dental porcelain?
   a. Aluminum oxide
   b. Tin oxide
   c. Rubber wheels
   d. Glazing

9. Patients with base metal-containing partial dentures should be instructed to clean their dentures with:
   a. Household bleaches
   b. Fine emery paper
   c. Detergent solutions
   d. Rouge

10. Which of the following would be least likely to scratch the surface of an acrylic denture?
    a. Quartz dust
    b. Talc powder
    c. Ground glass
    d. Pumice stone

SELECTED READINGS

Barbakow F, Gaberthuel T, Lutz F, Schuepbach P. Maintenance of amalgam restorations. Quintessence International 19:861–870, 1988.

This article provides a step-by-step procedure for contouring and polishing existing amalgam restorations.

Eide R, Tveit AB. Finishing and polishing glass-ionomer cements. Acta Odontologica Scandanavica 48:409–413, 1990.

Four different methods for finishing and polishing several glass-ionomer cements are compared by using profilometric tracings to determine average roughness. The results show that, like composites, Mylar strips produce the smoothest surfaces and that finishing with sandpaper disks is preferential to finishing with diamonds or stones.

Gladwin M, Bagby M. Clinical Aspects of Dental Materials. Philadelphia, PA: Lippincott Williams & Wilkins, 1999.

This text contains an excellent chapter on polishing materials and abrasives used in dentistry for restorations and tooth prophylaxis.

Goldstein RE. Finishing of composites and laminates. Dental Clinics of North America 33:305–318, 1989.

This article discusses the principles of finishing and polishing and provides a detailed description of the instruments available for finishing composites (and porcelains). The advantages and disadvantages of each system are discussed, and specific procedures are outlined.

Jefferies SR. The art and science of abrasive finishing and polishing in restorative dentistry. Dental Clinics of North America 42:613–627, 1998.

This review article presents a description of the abrasive instruments used in dentistry and describes in detail the procedure for finishing and polishing posterior composites.

Pratten DH, Johnson GH. An evaluation of finishing instruments for an anterior and a posterior composite. Journal of Prosthetic Dentistry 60:154–158, 1988.

This article compares the surfaces created on two types of composites by a variety of different finishing instruments and includes scanning electron micrographs and profilometric data to depict the average surface roughness. The data show that Mylar strips produce the smoothest surfaces on composites, followed by sandpaper disks. A 25-μm "fine" diamond produced the roughest surfaces.

Rosenblum M. Abrasion, grinding, and polishing. In: O'Brien WJ, ed. Dental Materials: Properties and Selection. Chicago: Quintessence Publishing, 1989;437–448.

This text contains a chapter on the theory of abrasion and the applications of abrasives in dentistry.

Small BW. Seating, finishing, and polishing of ceramic restorations. General Dentistry 47:560–562, 1999.

This article provides a section on the finishing and polishing of ceramic restorations.

Chapter **15**

Dental Implants

Uses of Implants in Dentistry

Types of Dental Implants

Composition of Implant Materials
Metals
Ceramics
Coated Metals

Clinical Factors Concerning Implants
Criteria for Patient Selection
Criteria for Clinical Success

Summary

Objectives

- Describe the three different types of dental implants and compare their uses.
- Explain what is meant by osseointegration and how it affects the success of a dental implant.
- Identify the composition and compare the properties of the various types of metals used in dental implants.
- Explain the rationale for applying a surface coating to a metallic dental implant.
- Explain what is meant by a "bioactive" ceramic.
- Identify the composition of the ceramics used for dental implants.
- Identify factors that can affect the success of dental implant therapy.
- Identify criteria for success of endosseous implants.

Uses of Implants in Dentistry

An **implant** is a device that is placed within the confines of the body tissue. Although most dental restorations reside within the mouth, they still are external to the body, like a ring on a finger. Any material that comes into contact with any bodily tissues must be biocompatible, but the requirements for a material that actually is inserted and enclosed within the tissues are more rigorous. Not unexpectedly, the testing required to prove the safety of such an implantable device is extensive, time consuming, and costly, but of obvious importance. Therefore, there are relatively few materials that have been shown to be safe and effective as implants.

Implants are used to replace missing teeth by anchoring a prosthesis to the mandible or maxilla. The prosthesis may be a single crown or an entire denture. For example, single-tooth implants can be used to place a porcelain crown between two adjacent teeth without using the two teeth as abutments for a bridge. In another example, patients with extensive resorption of the alveolar ridge, which makes it difficult for them to support a full denture arch, can, as an alternative, have implants placed to support the framework. Stability is one of the major benefits derived from the placement of an implant-supported prosthesis. In theory, the implant performs within the bone the way the tooth would, thus maintaining the health of the mandible or maxilla with minimal bone resorption. The cost of this type of therapy, however, is beyond the means of many patients.

This introductory chapter simply provides a background to the current types of implants available and their compositions. The technology is constantly changing and improvements are continual in the materials, their designs, and the clinical techniques.

Types of Dental Implants

Many different types of dental implants have been tried over the years. They have come in a variety of different shapes and have been made from a wide variety of materials. Many metals, such as platinum, silver, steel, cobalt alloys, and titanium, have been used, as have acrylic, carbon, sapphire, porcelain, alumina, zirconia, and calcium phosphate compounds. To date, the most successful single-tooth implant has been a screw-shaped device made from titanium. The device is placed into the bone by first drilling a hole and then tapping a screw thread into which the implant is fitted (Fig. 15-1). Because it resides partially within the bone but does not penetrate it completely, this type of implant is referred to as **endosseous**. Other shapes also have been used with success.

There have been three basic designs of dental implants. The endosseous implant was preceded by the **subperiosteal** and **transosteal implants**. Subperiosteal implants have metal frameworks that rest on the alveolar ridge (Fig. 15-2). The gingiva is reflected and the implant is placed on the ridge, with the abutments or attachments for the prosthesis protruding from holes in the gingiva after it is sutured shut. This design is less invasive than that of the endosseous implant because the metal does not penetrate the bone, but it is less stable. Subperiosteal implants have shown a success rate of approximately 55% survival after 15 years in clinical trials, which is not as good as the success rate of certain transosteal implants.

The transosteal is a design that can be used in the mandible only because it is

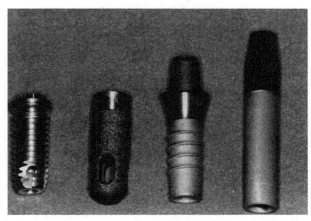

Figure 15–1 Several endosseous dental implants, including (from *left* to *right*) a pure titanium screw, a titanium cylinder sprayed with titanium, a titanium screw coated with hydroxyapatite, and a titanium cylinder coated with hydroxyapatite.

placed up through the bone. The bottom plate protrudes from the underside of the mandible, and the attachments for the prosthesis reside above the alveolar ridge, poking through the gingiva. Success rates with one type of transosteal implant, the transmandibular staple, have reached 90% over periods of 8 to 16 years.

The most successful and frequently used implant design is the endosseous type. Some of the initial endosseous implants were designed as blades. A groove was cut into the bony ridge, and the blade-shaped implant was fitted into the slot, leaving the attachments for the prostheses rising up above the gum line. The blade portion of the implant usually had holes or "cutout" regions so bone could grow through it and secure the implant for maximum stability (Fig. 15-3). Owing to the length of the blade, these implants were not used for single-tooth replacements.

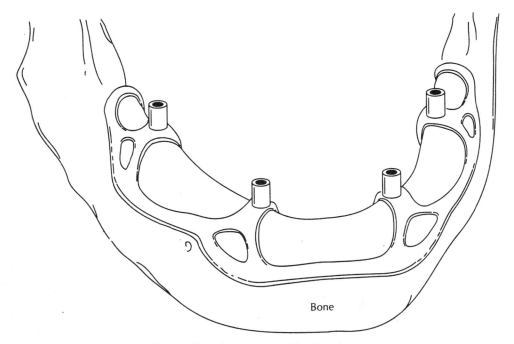

Bone

Figure 15–2 A subperiosteal implant design.

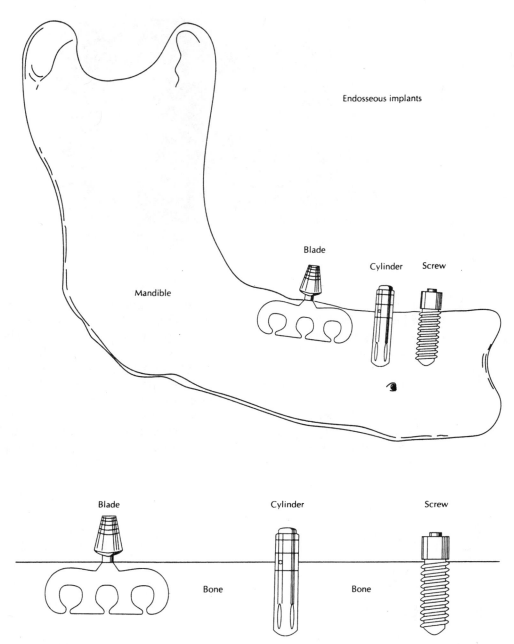

Figure 15–3 Several endosseous dental implant designs, including the blade, hollow cylinder, and screw.

Other designs were cylindrically shaped, with holes or cutouts (Fig. 15-3). A spiral shape was also used. The main purpose of having a complicated shape with holes was to provide sites for bone to grow into and anchor the implant, enhancing its stability as well as that of the prosthesis it supported. The screw design is perhaps the most effective because it is stabilized within the bone almost immediately, owing to the tightness of its custom friction fit. With time, bone grows up to and in contact with the implant, further stabilizing it within the cortical bone of the ridge. This process requires several months. Therefore, it is customary for an implant to be allowed to heal and stabilize for a period of 6 months before force is applied to it through a dental prosthesis. ***Can you imagine what would happen if the implant was subjected to stresses before it had completely stabilized within the bone?***

The success of the endosseous dental implant depends on the formation of a tight junction or interface between the bone and the implant. This junction is formed by the growth of new bone. Under the correct conditions, there appears to be an actual bonding between the new bone and the surface of the implant. Whether this adhesion is produced from a chemical union or a tight physical attachment is not completely clear, but the fact that a strong and intimate contact can be produced is certain.

This bonding has been called **osseointegration** because it represents an integration of the implant surface within new bone. The formation of this interface depends on the chemical composition of the implant, its surface characteristics, the care with which the surgical procedure was performed, the design of the prosthesis, and the follow-up hygiene care. Many of these factors are under intense study, with the goal of producing a successful and predictable biologic response to dental implants.

Another type of dental implant has been used to repair defects in the mandible or maxilla or to enhance or augment the quality of the bone. Ceramic blocks or particles that can be shaped or packed into a void in the existing bone have been used with much success. These materials fill in and enhance the ability of the bone to support prosthetic devices. Bone grows into and through these particular materials and secures them in place. One problem with the particulate types, however, has been their tendency to migrate from the site and become dislocated before the formation of the stabilizing new bone.

A new field of study, called **tissue engineering**, has been initiated. The goal of this field is to grow hard or soft tissue in situ (in the body) through a planned process. For hard tissue replacement, such as the repair of bony defects, a porous ceramic implant, such as a calcium phosphate or silicate, may be seeded with cells capable of developing into new bone with the help of added growth factors, such as bone morphogenetic protein, and surgically placed into the defect site. Other materials, such as freeze-dried bone, synthetic bone and collagen, and polylactic and polyglycolic acid copolymers, have been used as carriers of the growth factors. These materials have minimal strength, however, and do not provide structural support for the bone. They serve solely as space fillers or scaffolds into which new bone will grow. Although this field is in its infancy, future dental implants will most likely serve as intermediates that are used to produce engineered natural tissues rather than serve as final synthetic replacements.

■ Composition of Implant Materials

Metals

The first metals used as dental implants were surgical stainless steels. These metals were the same as those used for many years in orthopaedic surgery. A common type of steel is 316L, an alloy of iron and carbon (0.05%; this is a minimal amount of carbon, thus the designation "L," i.e., low carbon) with 18% chromium to provide corrosion resistance and 8% nickel to stabilize the particular steel structure. This composition is similar to that used in orthodontic wires except that the carbon concentration is lower for the surgical alloy. Another alloy commonly used for implants was based on an alloy of cobalt (65% Co) and chromium (30% Cr), which also contained a small amount of carbon. These two alloys are very hard, stiff, and strong and have excellent corrosion resistance, but they have not been as successful clinically as titanium.

Titanium is used as an implant metal, either in a pure form, such as commercially pure Ti (cpTi; 99.75%), or as an alloy with aluminum (6%) and vanadium (4%). Other titanium alloys containing zirconium and niobium are also being used to a lesser extent. Titanium is a strong, corrosion-resistant metal. It is lightweight, having a density only half as great as steel or Co-Cr. This characteristic is one reason it is a preferred metal for the aerospace industry, where the combination of high strength and lightweight are so important. The pure metal and its alloys are relatively flexible, possessing an elastic modulus only half that of stainless steel and Co-Cr. The stiffness of titanium is about 10 times greater than bone, however, so it is still adequate for use as an implant. The corrosion resistance of titanium is the result of its tremendous reactivity with oxygen. A freshly exposed titanium surface reacts with oxygen to form a tough, tenacious oxide film. This oxide film makes the metal passive in the same way chromium oxide passivates steel or cobalt alloys. It is believed this oxide film is responsible for the excellent biocompatibility of titanium implants. This favorable biologic response is the major driving force for the use of titanium in other areas of dentistry, as was pointed out in Chapter 13.

Ceramics

Perhaps the most biocompatible materials are the ceramics; hence, the choice of a ceramic for an implant would seem to be most logical. In this case, one structure, the bone, is replaced with something of similar composition. Because bone is composed of a calcium phosphate ceramic, **hydroxyapatite**, it would seem most reasonable to replace it with a synthetic hydroxyapatite. The problem is that as a pure ceramic and, therefore, not entirely mimicking bone, which also contains protein, hydroxyapatite is brittle and cannot support the same types of forces as bone or a metallic implant. This has led to the development of metallic implants containing calcium phosphate coatings.

Ceramic implant materials can be classified by the manner in which they interact with bone into two basic types, "nonreactive" and "bioactive." Typical nonreactive ceramics, such as aluminum oxide and sapphire, are well tolerated by bone tissue in much the same way as titanium. They have high strength, stiffness, and hardness. Their fracture resistance is poor, however, especially when they are subjected to bending forces.

The second type of ceramic implants is called bioactive because they react directly with bone tissue. The result of this reaction is the formation of hydroxyapatite or some other calcium phosphate compound on their surface. This reaction produces a direct chemical bond between the implant and the new bone. Synthetic hydroxyapatite is one example of a material with this quality; it is the same material used in bone augmentation surgery. Hydroxyapatite is a mineral rich in calcium and phosphate and thus is similar to teeth and bone. Although the material is strong, it is relatively weak in tension and bending and is not suitable for use in high-stress situations. Therefore, it works best as a coating for a titanium implant, as discussed in the next section.

Another bioactive ceramic is noncrystalline, or amorphous, calcium phosphate. This material is the precursor to the formation of the more stable apatite structure. Amorphous calcium phosphate and apatite are different, however. The amorphous material is very soluble in aqueous fluids and is much weaker than apatite; both characteristics are attributed to the lack of crystallinity. The solubility of calcium phosphate makes it readily resorbable by bone, however. One application for this material is as a bone cement that can be injected into the implant site, where it hardens around the implant, thus stabilizing it and possibly allowing early loading. In time, the material is resorbed and replaced by new bone.

There are other types of bioactive ceramics, such as Bioglass. This dense glass, which contains calcium, sodium, and phosphorus oxides as well as silicon dioxide, has properties similar to those of hydroxyapatite. The reaction at the surface of the implant is complex, involving ionic dissolution and changes in composition that provide a favorable environment for the adhesion and growth of new bone (Fig. 15-4). Although the material bonds strongly to bone through the formation of a calcium phosphate layer between the implant and bone, it does not have adequate strength to serve alone as a structural implant.

Coated Metals

Although implants with pure titanium surfaces appear to be well accepted by the body and often produce successful clinical results, many manufacturers and researchers have investigated ways to enhance the bond of bone to implants through the use of surface coatings. These coatings may be composed of titanium or a ceramic, which is sprayed or baked onto the metal implant during manufacturing. The ceramic coating is usually a calcium phosphate, such as tricalcium phosphate or hydroxyapatite. This design provides two benefits. First, the structural component of the implant is a rigid, high-strength metal with superior fracture characteristics, compared with that of an implant made entirely of ceramic. At the same time, the rationale for applying these coatings is to accelerate the rate

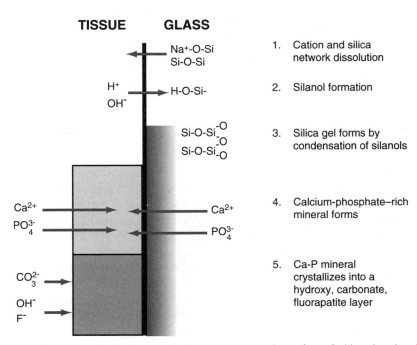

Figure 15–4 One possibility for the reaction that may occur at the surface of a bioactive glass implant in the body.

of formation of the bone-implant interface and to enhance its strength and stability. In theory, this could lead to the earlier placement of the functioning prosthesis on the implants.

One concern with these systems is that when a coating is applied, another interface is formed, one between the implant and the coating, and failure at this site could also cause failure of the entire implant. The long-term stability of this implant-coating interface is not known; a significant number of cases in which failure began in this region have been reported, however, causing considerable concern. The literature contains conflicting information about the stability of this ceramic-metal interface. Therefore, alternative ways of enhancing implant-bone contact through surface modifications of the titanium metal itself have proliferated. These methods include treatment with various acids and air abrasion (sandblasting) with calcium phosphate or titanium dioxide particulates.

■ Clinical Factors Concerning Implants

Criteria for Patient Selection

Correct patient selection may be as important to achieving a successful implant as the actual procedure or materials used. Patients must understand that the process will be lengthy and possibly painful, and they must be highly motivated for this type of therapy. Therefore, the clinician must assess the true wishes and psychological health of the patient before making a decision about implant placement. The patient should be healthy and free from systemic diseases that may retard or hinder the healing process after the implants are placed. Abnormal healing may predispose the endosseous implant to failure because it cannot become adequately anchored within the bone. Patients undergoing radiation therapy are often considered to be poor candidates owing to healing considerations and reduced salivary flow, which may affect oral hygiene. The patient must maintain a healthy oral environment and good hygiene practices to ensure successful implant therapy. Because the most common dental implants (i.e., the endosseous design) are positioned within the bone, sufficient healthy bone must be present to support the implant and, ultimately, the prosthetic appliance attached to it. All of these factors are considered by the clinician and discussed with the patient, along with the risks and benefits.

Criteria for Clinical Success

Various criteria have been developed to demonstrate the clinical success of implants. Most attempts have revolved around the endosseous implants because of the greater volume of available research data. Longitudinal clinical studies show that success rates of 81 to 85% for the maxilla and 98 to 99% for the anterior mandible at 10 years are possible. In general, successful implants have several characteristics in common. First, they are immobile. This usually is determined directly or by tapping on the implant with an instrument and listening for a solid ring, which denotes that osseointegration has taken place. Second, an x-ray film should show no radiolucency around the implant; radiolucency would suggest the presence of a fibrous capsule of connective tissue around the implant instead of a rigid and stable bone-implant contact. Mobility and radiolucencies are related, and their presence usually signals poor osseointegration and the ultimate failure of the implant. This is the most common cause of implant failure.

In addition to obtaining and maintaining osseointegration, marginal bone loss around the implant should be minimal. It is common for the bony ridge to resorb an average of 1.5 mm or so around titanium implants (the most common endosseous implants placed) within the first year, but subsequent resorption usually should be limited to less than 0.2 mm a year to ensure that adequate bone remains to provide stability. Although periodontal probing of sulcus depth is a common procedure for evaluating implants, the attachment often is not very strong and easily penetrated by the probe. In addition, there is not a good correlation between sulcus depth and success.

Another important criterion for success is that the patient should experience no persistent pain or discomfort from the implant or the prosthetic appliance it supports. Possible problems include the placement of an inadequate number of implants to successfully support the intended prosthesis or the placement of the implants at angles that make the restorative procedures difficult or impossible. When the number or orientation of the implants is incorrect, a disadvantageous distribution of loads to the implants and bone can be produced, leading to bone resorption or a loss of integration. Either would result in failure of the implant. Therefore, it is important to consider the implants and the prosthetics at all times. It also is important for the patient to be available for continued care and recalls to ensure that a stable, osseointegrated implant remains in such a condition. Oral hygiene is another problem associated with implant failure and must be taken very seriously.

The following recommendations are provided for follow-up of implant patients. Several can be designated to the dental hygienist. Frequent recalls of 3 months minimum will ensure that progress is followed closely. Periodontal indices, such as pocket depth and gingival bleeding, should be evaluated and recorded at each visit to ensure that the tissues are free of plaque and calculus. This is even more important for an implant patient than for other dental patients because infection could lead to complete implant failure, requiring removal. Radiographic evaluation is suggested at each recall to monitor the status of the bone. Soft tissues should be débrided with plastic curettes and/or plastic-tipped ultrasonic scalers. The latter ensures that the exposed implant surface will not be scratched or contaminated by other metals that would predispose it to corrosion and adverse tissue responses. Finally, topical and systemic antimicrobial drugs may be prescribed to minimize infections.

Implants are currently contraindicated for patients with osteoporosis and other bone diseases, as well as those with uncontrolled diabetes. Patients with low bone density are not good candidates because there is inadequate bone to stabilize the implant. Other factors that lead to implant failure and may serve as contraindications are smoking (leads to poor bone quality), parafunctional habits, poor home care, and progressing periodontitis.

Summary

Implants are materials placed directly on or within the bone to anchor prosthetic devices that replace a missing tooth or several teeth. They can provide more stability and improved hygiene, compared with fixed or removable appliances such as bridges and partial dentures. The most popular implants are called endosseous because they are submerged and integrated within the bone of the mandible or maxilla. Implants are made from metal or ceramic. The most popular implant metal is pure titanium or an alloy of titanium-aluminum-vanadium. Titanium is well tolerated by the tissues and, when placed and maintained properly with good oral hygiene, forms a stable link with bone. Stainless steel and cobalt-chromium alloys also have been used but with less success.

Ceramic materials used as implants have included hydroxyapatite (similar to bone), alumina (sapphire), and other calcium phosphate ceramics. Hydroxyapatite and other calcium phosphates are well tolerated by tissue and actually form chemical bonds with new bone, providing a firm anchor in the jaw. These materials have limited strength and structural stability, however. Therefore, a common procedure has been to coat titanium implants with ceramic to provide support and strong bonding to bone. The potential for instability at the interface between the ceramic and metal is of concern, however.

STUDY QUESTIONS AND PROBLEM SOLVING

1. **Which of the following is an acceptable definition of osseointegration?**
   a. Intimate contact between connective tissue and implant, resulting in bonding
   b. Placement of an implant directly within a bony structure
   c. Stabilization of an implant by the formation of new bone in intimate contact
   d. Bone growth through a hole in an implant to anchor it without adhesion
2. **Which of the following metals is *not* used as an implant material?**
   a. Stainless steel
   b. Pure titanium
   c. Nickel-chromium
   d. Cobalt-chromium
3. **Which of the following is (are) a good reason(s) to apply a surface coating of hydroxyapatite to a metallic implant?**
   a. It is the only way to ensure a strong union between the implant and bone
   b. The esthetic appeal of the metal implant is improved by the coating
   c. The metal would not be biocompatible without the coating
   d. The coating enhances bone growth at the surface of the implant
4. **A "bioactive" implant has which of the following characteristics?**
   a. Ceramic
   b. Stronger than steel
   c. Chemically bonds to bone
   d. Similar stiffness as bone
5. **The clinician checks the stability of an implant in a patient 6 months after placement. When tapping the implant with an instrument, a quiet, dull "thud" is heard, causing you to predict that the implant:**
   a. Has been anchored successfully within the bone
   b. Will demonstrate a radiolucency around a portion of its surface when filmed
   c. Will show mobility when pushed or pulled with the fingers
   d. Is ready to support prosthodontic treatment

6. **Which of the following patients would you consider to be a questionable candidate(s) for implant therapy?**
   a. A relatively active person with diabetes
   b. A person with cerebral palsy and minimal control of motor functions
   c. An otherwise healthy person with limited salivary flow
   d. A middle-aged woman with blood pressure at the low end of normal

SELECTED READINGS

Albrektsson T, Zarb G, Worthington P, Eriksson AR. The long-term efficacy of currently used dental implants: A review and proposed criteria of success. International Journal of Oral and Maxillofacial Implants 1:11–25, 1986.

   This article provides a well-documented review of many types of dental implants. Composition, indications for use, noted complications, and the results of clinical trials are presented.

Binon PB. Implants and components: Entering the new millennium. International Journal of Oral and Maxillofacial Implants 15:76–94, 2000.

   This comprehensive review of the design of current implant systems also contains information about surface coatings and quality control issues.

Brunski JB, Puleo DA, Nanci A. Biomaterials and biomechanics of oral and maxillofacial implants: Current status and future developments. International Journal of Oral and Maxillofacial Implants 15:15–46, 2000.

   This comprehensive review of the current status of dental implants provides an extensive review of the literature, specifically as it relates to bone/implant interfacial interactions and mechanics.

El Askary AS, Meffert RM, Griffin T. Why do implants fail? Part I and Part II. Implant Dentistry 8:173–183, 265–277, 1999.

   These two articles provide an excellent review of the factors that directly and indirectly are attributed to the failure of dental implants.

LeGeros RZ. Calcium phosphate materials in restorative dentistry: A review. Advances in Dental Research 2:164–180, 1988.

   This article provides a detailed report on the use, composition, development, and properties of many types of ceramics used in dentistry. Research data are presented, along with future directions of study.

O'Brien WJ (ed). Dental Materials: Properties and Selection. Chicago: Quintessence Publishing, 1989.

   This text contains a chapter summarizing the theory of osseointegration and describing the composition and properties of modern implant materials.

Parr GR, Gardner LK, Toth RW. Titanium: The mystery metal of implant dentistry. Dental materials aspects. Journal of Prosthetic Dentistry 54:410–414, 1985.

   This article provides an inclusive review of titanium, discussing its properties and characteristics as they relate to its use as an implant material.

Pilliar RM. Dental implants: Materials and design. Journal of the Canadian Dental Association 56:857–861, 1990.

   This article summarizes the factors that influence the success of dental implants, including the composition of the materials and the design of the implant.

Smith DE, Zarb GA. Criteria for success of osseointegrated endosseous implants. Journal of Prosthetic Dentistry 62:567–572, 1989.

   This article outlines the criteria for successful endosseous implants and reviews the basis behind their selection.

Glossary

Note: The number in parentheses represents the chapter in which the term receives its most complete coverage.

abrasion (abrasive) (14)—the act of producing scratches or gouges in a surface, resulting in the removal of material; the object causing the scratching is called the abrasive (e.g., sandpaper)

abutment (13)—teeth adjacent to an empty space in the mouth that will be used to support the prosthetic device that will fill the space

acid-etch technique (3)—treatment of tooth enamel with an acid to produce a microscopic roughening by dissolving the top layer, exposing the enamel rods and prisms

acrylic (12)—a family of organic molecules (containing a carbon-carbon double bond) that form polymers useful in many applications, such as making dentures or household paints

activator (12)—a chemical, usually an amine compound, used to cause an initiator molecule to become active and begin a polymerization reaction

adherend (2)—the surface with which an adhesive bonds

adhesion (adhesive) (2)—the forces of attraction existing between two different objects or surfaces that hold them together; the material causing the adhesion is called the adhesive (e.g., resin)

agar (8)—a polysaccharide seaweed derivative used to make an accurate, reversible hydrocolloid impression material suitable for crown and bridge dental work

air inhibition (3)—the top layer of a dental composite or sealant, which is exposed to the air, does not polymerize completely because of an inhibiting effect of oxygen

alginate (8)—a dental impression material made from a polysaccharide seaweed derivative that sets by a chemical reaction and is used for edentulous patients and on dentulous patients in cases in which accuracy is not essential

alloy (6, 7)—the combination of two different metallic elements (as distinguished from a pure metal)

aluminous porcelain (7)—a strong dental porcelain that is 40 to 50% by weight alumina, a crystalline material made of aluminum oxide (Al_2O_3)

amalgam (6)—a dental restorative material made when mercury is mixed with alloys of silver, tin, and copper

amorphous (2, 12)—a structure that has no regularity (i.e., noncrystalline)

anode (2)—the site in an electrochemical cell where oxidation reactions occur (i.e., the site where a metal is corroded)

APF (acidulated phosphate fluoride) (3)—a therapeutic agent usually delivered as a gel to increase the fluoride content of dental tissues

appliance (1)—a dental device used to position or maintain the position of teeth, such as space maintainers in orthodontics and pediatrics

armamentarium (1)—the materials and tools available to dental personnel for all types of dental procedures

articulator (8, 9)—a device that reproduces the hinge motion of the jaw; used in the production of dental restorations and devices to ensure correct occlusion

bacteriostatic (4)—maintaining bacteria in their current state without allowing them to proliferate and produce damaging by-products to further degrade sound tooth structure

base (4)—a cement material used in a thick layer (0.5 to 1.0 mm) under a restorative, such as an amalgam, to insulate the pulp of the tooth from thermal, electrical, and mechanical insult

base metal (13)—a non-noble metal, such as steel or nickel-chromium alloy, used to make dental instruments and restorations

biocompatible (1)—the ability of the material to perform with an appropriate host response in a particular situation; does not cause harm to the body; nontoxic (note that even biocompatible materials may cause allergic reactions in some people)

bioengineer (1)—a person who has knowledge of both engineering and biology and functions as a scientist or inventor in health care fields in which engineering principles and components are used

bite registration (8)—an impression of the occlusal surfaces of the teeth, taken with the upper and lower teeth in contact; used to orient casts accurately on an articulator

bridge (2)—a dental prosthesis used to restore a space where there is missing dentition; also known as a fixed partial denture because it is permanently attached to existing teeth to replace one or more missing teeth

brittle (2)—having the characteristic of fracturing before undergoing a significant amount of plastic or permanent deformation when placed under stress (i.e., having a low percent elongation)

bruxing (13)—excessive chewing or grinding of the teeth

burnish (6)—a procedure by which a dental instrument is forcefully rubbed over the surface of a metallic restoration, such as an amalgam or a gold inlay, to draw the metal out over a margin or smooth its surface

cast (9)—a plaster or stone model of a maxillary or mandibular arch, used for diagnostic purposes or to aid in preparing a restoration or appliance

casting (7, 11)—the process by which a metal is melted and poured into a ceramic mold to produce a dental restoration, machinery part, or piece of jewelry

catalyst (3)—a molecule that helps to speed up a chemical reaction

cathode (2)—the site in an electrochemical cell where reduction reactions occur (i.e., the site where corrosion products, such as rust, are deposited on a metal)

ceramic (7)—a class of materials composed of metallic oxides and minerals, having the characteristics of high stiffness and compressive strength, low thermal and electrical conductivity, brittleness, and low chemical reactivity

chroma (2)—the term used in the Munsell color system to describe the intensity or extent of saturation of a certain color

cohesion (2)—the forces of attraction within an object that hold it together (contrast with adhesion)

colloid (8)—a suspension of fine particles (less than 1 μm in size) dispersed throughout a liquid, such as water (i.e., hydrocolloid)

compomer (4)—a class of materials having composite- and glass ionomer-type characteristics that are mainly used as an anterior restorative; otherwise known as a polyacid-modified resin

composite (5, 6)—a class of materials produced by mixing two or more of the other three classes (metals, polymers, and ceramics); dental composites are mixtures of polymers and ceramic (glass) fillers

compressive (2)—a force directed down onto an object, causing it to be squeezed together

contact angle (2)—the angle that an adhesive liquid makes with a surface; used as a measure of wetting, where a low-contact angle signifies good wetting and enhances the potential for adhesion

copolymer (12)—a polymer made from the polymerization of two or more different types of monomers

core (5)—a preparation built up on a tooth on which a crown will be cemented; usually made from amalgam or composite but can be cast in metal or made of glass ionomer

corrosion (2)—an electrochemical process whereby oxidation and reduction reactions occur on a metal surface in the presence of an electrolyte (such as saliva); the reaction causes metal ions to be removed and often results in deterioration of the metal

covalent bond (2)—a strong, stable primary chemical bond characterized by the sharing of electrons between atoms

crazing (12)—the formation of fine cracks on the surface of a material as a result of stresses built up by dimensional changes within the structure; a common example is crazing of a denture base as a result of stresses produced by alternate drying and soaking

creep (2)—time-dependent deformation of an object subjected to a constant stress; related to marginal fracture of dental amalgams

crevice corrosion (2)—an accelerated corrosion caused by differences in the concentration of oxygen and pH levels within a groove or crevice compared with sites outside of the crevice; commonly found at the margins of metallic restorations, such as amalgams

cross-linking (12)—a molecular bridging structure formed by covalent bonds, connecting individual polymer chains to produce a giant polymer network (similar to a spider web)

crown (2)—a dental restoration made from metal, ceramic, or composite, which is cemented over the crown of a tooth and replaces the cusps

crystalline (2, 7)—a structure displaying a regular order or arrangement of atoms or molecules, often cubic; the opposite of an amorphous structure

custom tray (12)—a holder used to carry impression material into the mouth; the holder or "tray" is "custom" because it is fashioned on a model or cast of the actual patient's arch to fit perfectly and produce the most accurate impression

degree of conversion (12)—the percentage of carbon-carbon double bonds reacted or converted to single bonds during a polymerization reaction; abbreviated as DC; appropriate for describing the degree of polymerization of a cross-linked polymer

degree of cure (12)—the extent to which a polymer, such as a dental composite, has reacted; essentially the same as degree of conversion

degree of polymerization (12)—the average number of monomers that reacted to form each polymer chain in a linear polymer system

dental materials (1)—the science surrounding the study and development of the materials used to restore and replace oral tissues

dentifrice (14)—a paste used to clean the teeth; toothpaste

denture (2)—a prosthetic device containing a replacement for several or all of the teeth missing from an arch

diastema (5)—a space or separation between two teeth, most noticeably between the upper central incisors

die (9, 11)—a replica of a prepared tooth used to produce a wax pattern of a restoration for casting in metal or ceramic; usually made from gypsum or epoxy resin

direct gold (6)—a restoration made from essentially pure gold in the form of sheets or pellets; it is condensed directly into a cavity preparation

ductility (2, 7)—the characteristic of a material, allowing it to undergo significant plastic or permanent deformation under stress before fracturing; the opposite of brittleness

efficacy (1)—able to be used successfully and efficiently

elasticity (elastic) (2, 8)—the characteristic of a material allowing it to rebound to its original shape after being deformed

elastic limit (2, 7)—the maximum amount of stress that a particular material can withstand before undergoing a permanent change in shape

elastic modulus (2, 7)—the stress divided by the strain in the linear portion of a stress-strain diagram; a measure of a material's stiffness or flexibility

elastomer (8)—a material with a rubbery or elastic quality; usually refers to one of several types of dental impression materials

electrical conductivity (2)—a measure of a material's ability to transmit or conduct electricity; metals generally have high electrical conductivity

electrolyte (2)—a fluid that can carry ions to and from a corrosion site to maintain the oxidation and reduction reactions that produce corrosion; saliva is an electrolyte

electroplating (11)—an electrical process by which a metallic surface is "plated" or coated onto a substrate by applying electric current through a solution containing metallic ions

endosseous implant (15)—an implant placed directly within the maxilla or mandible

esthetic (2, 5)—the quality of being pleasing to look at

fatigue (2)—weakening of a material or device caused by repeated loading at a stress level below the fracture strength

finishing (14)—the process by which the surface of a restoration is contoured with abrasive instruments

fixed partial denture (2, 7)—a bridge replacing existing dentition that is permanently cemented to remaining teeth

fluorescence (7)—the characteristic of emitting light when stimulated by ultraviolet energy; teeth fluoresce, giving them a "vital" appearance

flux (11)—an oxide compound added to metal while it is being heated during the melting or soldering process to minimize oxidation of the metal itself and enhance the flow of the molten metal

force (2)—a load applied to an object in a tensile (pulling), compressive (squeezing), or shearing (sliding) direction, causing the object to be deformed

fracture toughness (2)—the ability of a material containing some type of flaw to resist propagation of a crack from the flaw; essentially, resistance to fracture

free radical (12)—a molecule (monomer) containing an unpaired electron, making it very reactive toward other molecules

galvanic cell (2)—the physical coupling of two different metals (like a battery), which causes the least noble of the metals to corrode at an accelerated rate

gel (8)—a solid or semisolid produced by a physical or chemical reaction in which large molecules are formed and become interlocked to provide some measure of rigidity and stability

glass ionomer (3, 4)—a dental material composed of an acidic polymer liquid and a fluoride-containing aluminosilicate glass, used as a restorative material, base, liner, and cement

glass transition temperature (12)—a characteristic temperature for certain types of materials, such as glasses and polymers, at which material physically transforms from a hard, glassy state to a soft, moldable state

glaze (7)—a smooth, shiny, glassy surface created on a porcelain restoration by heating; external glazes composed of low-melting porcelains also may be applied and baked onto a dental ceramic surface

gold foil (6)—a thin sheet (0.001 inch thick) of pure gold used to fill a tooth cavity by condensing it on itself, causing individual sheets to be welded together

grain boundary (7)—the boundaries separating individual metallic grains (crystals)

grains (7)—metallic crystals formed during the solidification of a metal that are visible during the examination of the microstructure of a piece of metal, such as a dental casting; grain size significantly influences the physical properties of the metal

gutta percha (1)—an isomer of natural rubber used as a filling material in endodontics

gypsum (9)—a mined mineral composed of calcium sulfate dihydrate, used to make models and dies for dental procedures

hardness (2)—a measure of a material's ability to resist a force of indentation on its surface

hue (2)—the term used in the Munsell color system to describe the dominant color of an object (i.e., red, yellow, blue)

hybrid composite (5)—a dental restorative combining a resin monomer with fillers of both a microscopic and submicroscopic (microfill) size

hydrocolloid (8)—a suspension of fine particles (less than 1 μm in size) dispersed in water to produce a viscous solution; reversible and irreversible types are used as dental impression materials (i.e., agar and alginate, respectively)

hydrodynamic theory (2)—a theory explaining the etiology of pulpal sensitivity, based on fluid flow through the dentinal tubules

hydrophilic (5)—having the characteristic of being "water loving"

hydrophobic (5)—having the characteristic of being "water hating"

hydroxyapatite (15)—a mineral or ceramic composing much of bone and teeth that contains calcium and phosphorus; a synthetic (artificial) form is used as an implant material

hygroscopic (11)—the characteristic of absorbing water from the atmosphere

implant (15)—a metallic or ceramic device that is placed on or within the jaw to provide a stable support for a dental prosthesis

impression (8)—a negative replica of a dental structure, usually a prepared tooth, used in the fabrication of a dental restoration or prosthesis; the impression material may be rubbery or hard and rigid

incipient caries (3)—caries in its early stages of formation

indirect pulp cap (4)—a cement or calcium hydroxide material placed over a deep suspected caries or possible exposure in order to "cap" and protect the pulp

inelastic (8)—the quality of not being elastic; a rigid, nonflexible material

inert (2)—the quality of being essentially nonreactive

inhibitor (5)—a molecule added to a material containing a polymerizing monomer to delay or prevent polymerization; provides shelf life and working time

initiator (12)—a molecule that causes or initiates a polymerization reaction

inlay (7)—a dental restoration made from metal, ceramic, or composite that is cemented within the crown of a tooth and does not include a replacement of any cusps

insulator (2)—a material that has a low thermal and electrical conductivity and, therefore, can be used to protect a sensitive structure from electric current or temperature changes

intermediary material (4)—a cement, lining, or base material placed between the tooth structure and a restorative material for a specific function, such as sealing the dentin or providing thermal, electrical, or mechanical protection under a restorative

investment (11)—a ceramic material used to create a mold for the casting process

in vitro (1)—literally, "in glass," i.e., not in the body but in the laboratory

in vivo (1)—in a living being; placed into the body or happening within a living subject

ionic bond (2)—a strong primary chemical bond characterized by the donation of an electron from one atom to another to make both atoms stable

leucite (7)—a crystalline potassium-aluminum-silicate component of dental porcelains

light-curing (5)—the process of applying light energy to a resin-based material containing specific light-sensitive initiators that cause polymerization of the resin

linear polymer (12)—a polymer with no chemical bonds between individual molecular chains

liner (4)—a cement-like material placed on the pulpal floor or dentinal walls of a cavity preparation in a very thin layer to seal the dentin from chemical or bacterial insult

lost wax casting technique (11)—the process by which metallic dental castings are made; a wax pattern of a restoration is invested in a mold and then burned out to leave a space; a molten metal is then thrust into the mold to fill the space and produce a metallic restoration on cooling

luster (2)—the characteristic of an opaque object reflecting light from its surface, causing it to look bright and shiny; a common appearance for polished metals

luting (4)—the process of attaching one structure to another with the use of an intermediate agent, such as a cement or wax; dental restorations are attached to teeth by this process

magnesia core porcelain (7)—a type of porcelain composed of up to 50% magnesia crystals; used to make a core or body on which an enamel layer will be fired; the benefit of this material is a much higher strength than conventional feldspathic porcelain

malleable (7)—a characteristic that allows a metal to be compressed and condensed on itself to change its shape without fracturing; similar to ductility, but specifically referring to compressive force applications

marginal leakage (4)—the movement of salivary components and bacteria toward the pulp along the interface or margin between a dental restoration and the cavity wall

maximum flexibility (2)—the maximum elastic strain an object can undergo before permanently changing its shape; the strain corresponding to the elastic limit on a stress-strain diagram

mercaptan (8)—a chemical compound or molecule having sulfhydryl groups (—SH); polysulfide impression material often is referred to as mercaptan

metal (7)—a crystalline material made up of metallic elements and having the characteristics of opacity, luster, high thermal and electrical conductivity, and high strength and stiffness

metallic bond (2)—the primary chemical bonds holding a metallic material together, characterized by rigid positive cores with loosely held electrons that can carry energy in the form of electricity and heat

microfill (5)—a type of highly polishable dental composite containing a polymer resin and submicroscopic silica filler particles of an average size of 0.4 μm

model (9)—a gypsum dental arch on which appliances are fashioned or used for diagnostic purposes, such as during orthodontic treatment

monomer (12)—a small molecule, usually of relatively low molecular weight, capable of reacting with similar molecules to produce giant polymer molecules

network (12)—a spider web-like arrangement of polymer molecules linked to one another through cross-links of covalent chemical bonds

noble metal (7)—a metal made predominantly from metallic elements that do not corrode, such as gold, platinum, and palladium

obtundent (10)—a chemical that has a sedative or numbing effect on a sensitive tooth; eugenol is a dental obtundent

onlay (7)—a dental restoration made from metal, ceramic, or composite that is cemented within the tooth and extends to include a replacement of one or more cusps

opacity (2)—having the characteristic of not transmitting light, such as a metal; being opaque

order-disorder transformation (7)—a change or rearrangement of the atoms produced in certain metals when they are heated above a specific temperature; the transformation results in a more regular atomic arrangement and affects physical and mechanical properties

osseointegration (15)—the process by which new bone forms at the surface of an endosseous implant, creating a strong adhesion to stabilize it within the tissue

passivated (2)—the process by which an oxide film forms on a metallic structure to make it less active in terms of corrosion (i.e., enhances corrosion resistance); chromium-containing alloys are passivated by chromium oxide film formation

pellicle (2, 14)—the invisible organic coating that forms on teeth and dental restorations as a result of their coming in contact with saliva

percent elongation (2)—the amount of permanent change in shape that an object may undergo before fracturing; a measure of ductility

permanent set (8)—the amount of change in dimension that an impression material undergoes when it is removed from an undercut; a measure of accuracy

PFM (porcelain-fused-to-metal) (7)—an esthetic dental restoration (crown, bridge, veneer, and the like) made by baking porcelain onto a metallic substrate used for support

phase (7)—a physically distinct, separable part of a system that has uniform composition and properties; a metal may be made from several different phases

pickling (11)—a process used to clean oxides from the surface of a cast metal by warming in an acidic solution

pitting corrosion (13)—a specific type of corrosion process that occurs on passivated metals as a result of a disruption of the oxide film, making the surface susceptible to localized and extensive electrochemical attack

plaster (9)—a calcium sulfate hemihydrate mineral powder produced by heating gypsum to eliminate water; used as a model material in dentistry by mixing with water to reform gypsum

plastic deformation (2)—a permanent strain or change in the shape of an object as a result of it being stressed beyond its elastic limit

plasticity (6)—having the characteristic of being moldable or deformable without breaking; for amalgams, this relates to their ability to be condensed

plasticizing (12)—usually relating to polymeric materials becoming more plastic or deformable as a result of having or acquiring molecules that tend to keep polymer chains separated and thus less rigidly entangled

polish (5, 14)—the act of producing a very smooth and shiny surface on an object through a process of abrasion with an abrasive consisting of very fine particles

polyacid-modified resin (4, 5)—a chemically descriptive term for a compomer

polycarboxylate cement (4)—a permanent dental cement made from a zinc oxide powder and a polyacrylic acid liquid

polymer (1, 12)—long, chain-like organic molecules used in a variety of applications in dentistry, such as dentures, composite fillings, and sealants

polymerization (12)—the chemical reaction that converts small, individual monomer molecules into long, giant polymer molecules

polymerization shrinkage (5)—a contraction that accompanies the polymerization reaction, often resulting in a loss of accuracy or a reduced fit

pontic (2)—an artificial tooth, usually made of metal, ceramic, or plastic, that is supported by a bridge to replace missing dentition

porcelain (7)—a ceramic material made from kaolin, feldspar, and quartz, used in dentistry as a restorative material

porosity (9)—an air bubble or void in a material

precious metal (7)—a dental metal or alloy usually containing gold, platinum, or palladium or a combination of these noble and noncorroding metals

prepolymerized resin fillers (5)—a reinforcing particle made from polymer and silica added to microfill composites to increase filler content

preventive resin restoration (3)—a restoration placed when there is a small occlusal lesion of a molar or premolar; caries is removed, and a small composite filling is placed and then sealed with a pit and fissure sealant by using the acid-etch procedure

propagation (12)—the stage of an addition (free radical) polymerization reaction in which the polymer chain actually is formed, or propagated, from the monomers

prophylactic paste (14)—a paste containing polishing agents that is applied to teeth with a rubber cup and handpiece for cleaning purposes

prosthesis (2)—an artificial part, such as a denture, used to replace missing tissues

prosthodontics (1)—the dental discipline dealing with the production of prosthetic devices to replace missing oral tissues; removable prosthodontics relates to dentures; fixed prosthodontics relates to crown and bridgework

pulp cap (4)—the process of placing a medicament, such as calcium hydroxide, over an exposure of the dental pulp

putty-wash (8)—an impression technique in which a putty-like material is first used to make an initial impression and then serves as a tray to carry a more fluid "wash" material, which more accurately reproduces the tissues

quenching (7)—the process of plunging a hot metal part (or dental casting) into cold water to cause a rapid cooling to room temperature

radiopaque (5)—the characteristic of scattering and only poorly transmitting x-rays; a radiopaque object thus appears white on a radiograph

reflection (2)—an interaction between some type of radiation and a surface that causes the radiation to be "bounced back" or off of the surface rather than penetrating it

refractory (7, 11)—ceramic-type materials with very high melting points used to provide thermal stability to investments and molds for dental casting processes

remaining dentin thickness (4)—the depth of dentin remaining between the pulpal floor of a cavity preparation and the pulp chamber

removable partial denture (2)—a denture that replaces several teeth (not an entire arch) and is not permanently attached to the remaining dentition, thus facilitating cleaning

replica (8)—a nearly exact copy of a part (or tissues); a dental impression is a negative replica of oral tissues

residual monomer (12)—monomers that did not react to form polymers during a polymerization reaction and, therefore, are left over or residual

resilience (2)—having the quality of a spring (i.e., elastic); being able to store energy to be used later; designated as the area under the linear region of the stress-strain diagram

resin (3)—a generic term for certain organic substances, either natural or synthetic, used in dental plastics

resin-modified glass ionomer (3)—a glass ionomer material modified by the addition of a resin monomer component to enhance its properties

restoration (1)—a device or component used to replace tooth structure

rigidity (2)—the quality of stiffness or resistance to deformation

rosin (10)—a natural resin material used as a filler in temporary dental cements

rubber dam (3)—a dental device made of a sheet of rubber that can be attached to teeth to provide isolation of a treatment area from the moisture and saliva of the oral cavity

scattering (2)—reflection of light as it penetrates through the surface and interacts with the interior of a substance

secondary bond (2)—bonds, such as van der Waals forces and hydrogen bonds, that usually are weaker and less stable than primary chemical bonds

secondary decay (2)—decay that forms at the site of an existing restoration

secondary (reparative) dentin (2)—an irregular type of dentin formed by the odontoblast cells as a result of some continual insult or stimulation; the secondary dentin is formed as a natural defense to "wall off" the pulp from the insult

self-curing (5)—a chemical polymerization or setting reaction that occurs through a chemical activation when two specific component systems are mixed; this is contrasted to materials cured by the application of heat or light energy; also called "auto-cure"

shape memory alloy (13)—alloys of nickel and titanium used in orthodontics that have the property of reverting to an original shape simply by being heated to a certain temperature

shear (2)—a force that tends to cause the top of an object to slide over the bottom

shelf life (5)—the amount of time a material can be stored before experiencing a significant change in handling characteristics or mechanical properties that causes it to be clinically useless

silane (5)—a molecule with silicon-oxygen groups at one end and methacrylate groups at the other, enabling it to couple or link ceramic materials (i.e., composite fillers and porcelain) to polymer resins

silicate cement (5)—a dental material made by mixing a fluoride-containing silicate glass powder with a phosphoric acid liquid; used as a restorative material before dental composites

sinter (7)—the process of heating a densely packed powder (i.e., porcelain) to a temperature just below its melting point, causing the edges partially to melt and fuse the individual particles together

smear layer (5)—a layer of debris containing mineral and protein, loosely adhered to the underlying dentin tooth structure and produced after the dentin has been abraded by a dental instrument, such as a burr

soft liner (12)—an elastic, resilient polymer containing plasticizers that is attached to the tissue-bearing surface of a denture base to improve the fit and comfort of the denture

sol (8)—essentially a solution or suspension of material in a liquid form; contrast with gel, which is the solid form the sol can be converted into

solder (2, 13)—the metallic material and procedure used to join two metal parts; solder is melted and flowed into a small space between the metal parts, joining them through the formation of a metallic bond on cooling

solid solution (7)—a solution in solid form produced by melting two completely miscible metals together

soluble (2)—the characteristic of being able to dissolve in a fluid

sorption (2)—the process by which an object or material takes up a solvent by diffusion of the solvent into its structure; a common example is water sorption of polymers

sprue (11)—a small tube of wax or metal used to connect a wax pattern to a crucible former, thus providing a channel for molten metal to flow through during the casting process

stainless steel (13)—steel containing at least 12% chromium that forms a protective oxide coating, keeping it from corroding in aqueous environments such as the mouth

stone (9)—a calcium sulfate hemihydrate mineral powder produced by heating gypsum to eliminate water; used as a die and model material in dentistry by mixing with water to reform gypsum; stronger and harder than plaster because of its greater density

strain (2)—the dimensional change produced in a material or object in response to the imposition of a force; a change in length per initial length (i.e., mm/mm), stated as a percent change in dimension

strain hardening (6, 7)—the process by which a metal becomes harder and more difficult to deform as a result of being strained beyond its maximum flexibility

stress (2)—the resistance built up within an object or material in response to the imposition of an external force; calculated as the force applied over a specific area, having the dimensions of kg/mm^2, MPa, or pounds/square inch

stress-strain diagram (2)—a plot of stress as a function of strain for an object being subjected to a deforming load or force

subperiosteal implant (15)—a metallic implant that rests on (not within) the bony ridge; usually covers the full arch and supports a denture prosthesis

surface energy (2)—the energy of a surface that determines how well it will be wetted by a liquid

surface tension (21)—similar to surface energy but particularly related to the surface of a liquid

surfactant (8, 11)—a molecule that reduces the surface tension of a solution, thus enhancing its capacity to wet another surface

tarnish (2)—a chemical interaction between a metal and its environment resulting in a discoloration of the metal surface

tension (tensile) (2)—a force tending to pull an object or material apart

thermal conductivity (2)—a property characterizing the rate at which heat is transferred through a material

thermoplastic (3, 8)—the ability to be reversibly transformed from a glassy, brittle solid to a softened, moldable plastic by heating beyond a certain temperature

tissue conditioner (12)—a rubbery material used on the tissue-bearing surface of the denture to cushion the gingiva from the hard denture base; a temporary material used when a denture wearer has severely irritated gums

tissue engineering (15)— an interdisciplinary field that applies the principles of biology and engineering to the development of viable substitutes that restore, maintain, or improve the function of human tissues

toughness (2)—the ability of a material to absorb energy without breaking; depicted as the total area under the stress-strain diagram

translucency (2)—the quality of partially transmitting and partially scattering light

transmission (2)—the passing of some form of radiation, such as light, through an object

transosteal implant (15)—a metallic implant that penetrates through both the lower and upper cortical plates of the mandible

transparent (2)—the quality of allowing light to pass through with minimal scattering or absorption; glass and air are transparent

triturate (4, 6)—the process of mechanically mixing a material in a device at high speeds (i.e., several thousand cycles per minute)

ultimate strength (2)—the maximum stress a material can withstand without fracturing; what is referred to as a material's "strength"

undercut (8)—an area like the cervical portion of a tooth that curves under and has a tendency to lock a material within it, making the material difficult to remove

unfilled acrylic (5, 12)—an esthetic dental restorative material made from polymethylmethacrylate, which preceded dental composites

value (2)—the term used in the Munsell color system to describe the lightness of an object on a scale of 1 to 10, where 10 equals white

varnish (4)—an organic substance used to coat a cavity or, as a restorative material, to seal it

veneer (2)—an esthetic metal-porcelain or ceramic dental restoration cemented onto the facial or labial portion of a tooth, usually through the acid-etch process

viscosity (2)—a fluid's resistance to flow; high viscosity results in low fluidity

wax pattern (11)—a replica of a dental restoration fabricated in wax; used to fashion a permanent metallic (or ceramic) restoration through the process of casting

weld (13)—the process of chemically joining two metal surfaces through the use of heat, pressure, or both

wear (2)—the process that results in the loss of material from surfaces whenever two surfaces come into contact with one another

wetting (2)—the interaction between a fluid adhesive and a substrate that determines the extent of the contact between the two; good wetting is essential for adhesion; water "balling up" on a wax surface is an example of poor wetting

working range (13)—similar to maximum flexibility; in orthodontics, the extent to which a wire can efficiently move teeth before needing reactivation

working time (3)—the time available to dental personnel for practical use of a setting material after it has been mixed

zinc oxide eugenol (ZOE) (4, 10)—a material made by mixing zinc oxide powder with eugenol liquid, used in dentistry as a cement, base, temporary restorative, impression material, and the like

Dental Materials Products

Alloys

High Noble Casting Alloys
B-2, JM Ney
Forticast, JF Jelenko
Modulay, JF Jelenko
Rajah, JF Jelenko

High Noble Porcelain-Fused-to-Metal Alloys
Artisan, JF Jelenko
Jelenko "O", JF Jelenko
Micro Bond 6, Nobelpharma
Olympia, JF Jelenko
Will Ceram Y-2, Williams Dental

Noble Casting Alloys
Maxigold, Williams Dental
Midas, JF Jelenko
Symphony, JF Jelenko

Noble Porcelain-Fused-to-Metal Alloys
Albabond 60, Degussa
Cameo, JF Jelenko
Olympia II, JF Jelenko

Palladium-Based Alloys
Jelstar, JF Jelenko
Naturelle, Jeneric/Pentron
Option, JM Ney
Tempo, JM Ney
Will Ceram W-1, Williams Dental

Nickel-Chromium Base Metal Alloy
Biobond C&B, Dentsply International
Ceramalloy, Ceramco
Micro Bond NP2, Nobelpharma
Rexillium III, Jeneric/Pentron
Ticonium, CMP Industries
Will-Ceram Litecast, Williams Dental

Cobalt-Chromium Base Metal Alloy
Genesis II, JF Jelenko
Neoloy, Neoloy
Nobilium, Nobilium Canada
Vitallium, Nobelpharma

Titanium
Titanium, Tanaka

Amalgams

Aristaloy CR Capsules, Baker Dental
Contour, Kerr
Dispersalloy, Dentsply/Caulk
Indisperse, Dental Management Services
Megalloy, Dentsply/Caulk
Original D, Wykle Research
SDI Logic Capsules, Southern Dental Industries
Tytin, Kerr
Unison, Dentsply/Caulk
Valiant and Valiant PhD, Ivoclar/Vivadent

Calcium Hydroxide Liners

Dycal, Dentsply/Caulk
Life, Kerr
Pulpdent, Pulpdent Corp.

Ceramics

Dicor; Dicor Plus, Dentsply International
Inceram; Inceram Spinell; Vita/Vident
IPS-Empress; IPS dSIGN, Ivoclar-Williams
Optec HSP; OPC, Jeneric/Pentron
Procera Allceram, Nobel Biocare

Compomers

Compoglass F; Compoglass Flow,
    Ivoclar-Vivadent
Dyract AP; Dyract Flow,
    Dentsply/Caulk
Elan, Kerr
F2000, 3M Dental Products
Hytac, ESPE

Composites

Microfills
Durafill, Kulzer
Epic TMPT, Parkell
Heliomolar, Vivadent
Renamel, Cosmedent
Silux Plus, 3M Dental Products

Hybrids
Aelitefil, Bisco
Bisfil-P, Bisco
Brilliant, Coltene
Charisma, Kulzer
Clearfil APX, Kuraray/J. Morita
Conquest, Jeneric/Pentron
Ful-fil, Dentsply/Caulk
Herculite XRV, Kerr
Pertac, ESPE
Point 4, Kerr
Prodigy, Kerr
Renamel Hybrid, Cosmedent
Tetric Ceram, Vivadent
TPH, Dentsply/Caulk
Vitalescence, Ultradent
Z-100, 3M Dental Products
Z250, 3M Dental Products

Flowable Composites
Aeliteflo, Bisco
Flow-It!, Jeneric/Pentron
Renamel Flowable, Cosmedent
Revolution, Kerr
Starflow, Danville Engineering
Tetric Flow, Ivoclar-Vivadent

Packable Composites
Alert, Jeneric/Pentron
P60, 3M Dental Products
Prodigy Condensable, Kerr
Pyramid, Bisco
Solitaire, Kulzer
Surefil, Dentsply/Caulk

Indirect Composites
Artlgass, Kulzer
belleGlass, Kerr
Concept, Vivadent
Gradia, GC
Sculpture, Jeneric/Pentron
Sinfony, ESPE
Targis 99, Vivadent

Composite Reinforcement Fibers
Connect, Kerr
Glasspan, GlasSpan
Ribbond, Ribbond
Splint-It!, Jeneric/Pentron

Dentin Adhesives

All Bond 2, Bisco
Amalgambond Plus, Parkell
Bond-It!; Bond One, Jeneric/Pentron
Clearfil Liner Bond 2V; Liner Bond SE,
    Kuraray/J. Morita
Denthesive II, Kulzer
Excite, Ivoclar-Vivadent
Gluma One Bond, Kulzer
Imperva Bond, Shofu
Optibond; Optibond FL, Optibond
    Solo, Kerr
Perma Quik; PQ1, Ultradent
Prime & Bond NT, Caulk/Dentsply
Prompt L-pop, ESPE
Scotchbond Multipurpose, 3M Dental
    Products
Single Bond, 3M Dental Products
Syntac SC, Ivoclar-Vivadent
Tenure; Tenure Quik, Den-Mat

Fluoride Gels and Rinses

Act Fluoride Anti-Cavity Dental Rinse,
    Johnson & Johnson
Fluorigard Anti-Cavity Dental Rinse,
    Colgate-Palmolive
Gel II APF Topical Gel, Oral-B
    Laboratories
Gel-Kam 0.4% Stannous Fluoride
    Home Fluoride, Scherer Laboratories
Luride 1.2% APF Topical Gel, Colgate-
    Hoyt Laboratories
Schein Home Care 0.4% Stannous
    Fluoride Gel, Henry Schein

Glass Ionomers—Conventional

Cements
Chemfil, Dentsply International
Fuji (Type I), G-C
Ketac-Cem, ESPE

Restoratives
Chemfill II, Dentsply International
Fuji (Type II); Fuji IX, G-C
Glass Ionomer Type II, Shofu
Ketac-Fil; Ketac-Molar, ESPE

Glass Ionomers—Resin-Modified

Liners
GC Lining Cement, G-C
Ketac-Bond, ESPE
Vitrebond, 3M Dental Products
XR Ionomer, Kerr

Restoratives
Fuji II LC, G-C
Photac-Fil, ESPE
Vitremer, 3M Dental Products

Cements
Fuji Plus, GC
Principle, Dentsply/Caulk
Rely-X Luting, 3M Dental Products

Gypsum Products

Type I, Impression Plaster
Plaster No. 2, Impression Type I, Kerr

Type II, Plaster Model
Kerr Snow White Plaster No. 1, Kerr
Laboratory Plaster, Whip Mix
Whip Mix Orthodontic Plaster, Whip Mix

Type III, Dental Stone
Coecal Buff-White, GC
Denstone, Miles Inc. Dental Products
Pemstone, Pemaco
Quickstone, Whip Mix
Rapid Stone, Kerr

Type IV, Dental Stone, High Strength
Die Keen, Modern Materials
Regal Die, Pemaco
Silky-Rock, Whip Mix
Vel Mix Stone, Kerr

Impression Materials

Agar
Dentloid, Keller Laboratories
Ruberloid Regular, Van R Dental Products
Supersyringe, Gingi-Pak Laboratories
Surgident Heavy Body, Lactona/Universal Dental

Alginate
Coe Alginate, GC-Coe
D-P Key to Alginates, Teledyne Getz
Healthco Alginate, Healthco International
Jeltrate Plus-Fast Set, Dentsply/Caulk
Super Gel Impression Material, Harry J Bosworth

Condensation Silicone
Accoe, GC-Coe
Citricon, Kerr
Rapid, Coltene

Impression Compound
Kerr Black-Grey-Perfection, White, Kerr
Mizzy Block Tray Compound, Mizzy

Polyether
Impregum F, ESPE
Permadyne, ESPE
Polyjel NF, Dentsply/Caulk

Polysulfide
Coe-Flex, GC-Coe
Healthco, Healthco
Omniflex, GC-Coe
Permlastic, Kerr

Polyvinylsiloxane
Aquasil, Dentsply/Caulk
Blu-Mousse, Parkell
Dimension, ESPE
Exaflex, GC-Coe
Express, 3M Dental Products
Extrude, Kerr
Hydrosil, Dentsply/Caulk
Imprint II, 3M Dental Products
Omnisil, GC-Coe
President, Coltene/Whaledent
Reprosil, Dentsply/Caulk
Take One, Kerr

Zinc Oxide Eugenol
Coe-Flo, GC-Coe
Luralite, Kerr
Superpaste, Harry J Bosworth

Investment Mateials

Gypsum-Based
Beauty Cast, Whip Mix
Kerr Cristabolite Inlay, Kerr
Luster Cast, Kerr
Novocast, Whip Mix

Phosphate-Based
Ceramigold, Whip Mix
Serafina, Whip Mix

Pit and Fissure Sealants

Concise White, 3M Dental Products
Delton Plus, Dentsply/Caulk
Ecuseal, DMG/Zenith
Helioseal; Helioseal F, Ivoclar/Vivadent
Prisma Shield; Fluroshield,
   Dentsply/Caulk
Ultradent XT Plus, Ultradent
Visio-Seal, ESPE

Porcelain

Biobond/Spectrum, Dentsply
   International
Ceramco II, Ceramco
Cerinate, Den-Mat
Crystar, Unitek
Duceram LFC, Degussa
Excelco Porcelain, Excelco
   International
Finesse, Ceramco
G-Cera, G-C
Microbond, Nobelpharma
Mirage II, Mirage Dental Systems
Vita, Vita-Vident

Provisional Resins

Acrylic
Jet Acrylic, Lang Dental
   Manufacturing
Scutan, ESPE
Snap, Parkell
Trim, Harry J Bosworth

Bis-Acryl
Iso-Temp, 3M Dental Products
Luxatemp, DMG/Zenith
Protemp Garant, ESPE
Provipont, Ivoclar/Vivadent
Temp-phase, Kerr
Triad—Dentsply/Caulk
Unifast LC, GC

Varnishes

Barrier, Teledyne
Copalite, Harry J Bosworth
Universal Dentin Sealant, Ultradent
   Products

Zinc Oxide Eugenol Cements

Temporary Cement
Teledyne Dental Products Trial
   Cement, Teledyne Getz
Temp Bond, Kerr

Permanent Cement
Alumina Super EBA Cement, Harry J
   Bosworth
Fynal, Dentsply/Caulk

Noneugenol Temporary Cements
Freegenol, GC
Nogenol, GC
Tempbond NE, Kerr

Zinc Phosphate Cements

Fleck's Extraordinary, Mizzy
Hy-Bond Zinc Phosphate Cement,
   Shofu Dental
Modern Tenacin, Dentsply/Caulk
Zinc Cement Improved, Mission White
   Dental

Zinc Polycarboxylate Cements

Durelon, ESPE
Hy-Bond Polycarboxylate Cement,
   Shofu Dental
PCA, Mission White Dental
Tylok Plus, Dentsply/Caulk

Dental Product Manufacturers

(Note: A full index of websites and phone numbers appears in the December 1999 *Dental Products Report*)

Apollo Dental Products
800-233-4151
559-292-1444
www.apollodental.com

Astron Dental Corp.
800-323-4144
847-726-8787

Austenal Inc.
800-621-0381
773-735-0600

Bisco, Inc.
800-BIS-DENT
847-534-6000
www.bisco.com

Harry J Bosworth Co.
800-323-4352
847-679-3400
www.bosworth.com

Brasseler USA Inc.
800-841-4522
912-925-8525
www.brasselerusa.com

Centrix Inc.
800-235-5862
203-929-5582
www.centrixdental.com

Colgate-Palmolive Co.
800-221-4607
212-310-3481
www.colgate.com

Coltene/Whaledent Inc.
800-221-3046
201-512-8000
www.coltenewhaledent.com

Cosmedent
800-621-6729
312-644-9586
www.cosmedent.com

Danville Engineering Inc.
800-827-7940
925-838-7940
www.daneng.com

Degussa Ney Dental, Inc.
800-221-0168
201-754-6300
www.degussa.com

Den-Mat Corp.
800-445-0345
805-922-8491
www.den-mat.com

Dentsply Caulk
800-532-2855
302-422-4511
www.caulk.com

Discuss Dental Inc.
800-422-9448
310-845-8200
www.discusdental.com

ESPE America, Inc.
800-782-1571
610-277-8000
www.espeusa.com

Essential Dental Systems Inc.
800-22F-LEXI
201-487-9090
www.edsdental.com

GC America, Inc.
800-323-7063
708-597-0900
www.gcamerica.com

Gingi-Pak Laboratories/A Division of
Belport Co., Inc.
800-437-1514
805-484-1051
www.gingi-pak.com

GlasSpan Inc.
800-280-7726
610-363-7583
www.glasspan.com

Healthco, Inc.
800-225-2360
www.healthco.com

Henry Schein, Inc.
800-D-SCHEIN
516-843-5500
www.henryshein.com

Heraeus Kulzer, Inc.
800-343-5336
219-291-0661
www.kulzer.com

Ivoclar North America
800-533-6825
716-691-0010
www.ivoclarna.com

JF Jelenko and Co.
800-431-1785
914-273-8600
www.jelenko.com

Jeneric/Pentron, Inc.
800-551-0283
203-265-7397
www.jeneric.com

Keller Laboratories, Inc.
800-325-3056
314-919-4000
www.kellerlab.com

Kerr (SDS Kerr)
800-537-7123
714-516-7400
www.kerr.com

Lactona Corp/Universal Dental Corp.
800-523-2559
215-368-2000
www.universaldental.com

Lang Dental Manufacturing Co., Inc.
800-222-LANG
847-215-6622
www.langdental.com

LaserMed Inc.
800-903-2873
801-256-0074
www.lasermed.com

Midwest Dental Equipment & Supply
800-766-2025
940-691-4102
www.mwdental.com

Mirage Dental Systems
800-366-0001
913-281-5552
www.miragecdp.com

Mission White Dental, Inc.
800-323-5087
201-544-0770

Mizzy, Inc.
800-333-3131
609-663-4700

J. Morita USA Inc.
800-831-3222
949-581-9600
www.jmorita.com

Neoloy, Inc.
800-628-7336

Nobel Biocare USA
800-993-8100
714-282-4800
www.nobelbiocare.com

Omnii Products
800-445-3386
561-689-1140
www.omniiproducts.com

Oral-B Laboratories/Braun
800-44O-RALB
650-598-5000
www.oralb.com
www.braun.com

Osteohealth
800-874-2334
516-924-1731

Parkell Inc.
800-243-7446
516-249-1134
www.parkell.com

Premier Dental Products Co.
888-670-6100
610-239-6000
www.premusa.com

Proctor & Gamble Professional Oral
  Care
800-543-2577
www.dentalcare.com

Pulpdent Corp. of America
800-343-4342
617-926-6666
www.pulpdent.com

Ribbond Inc.
800-624-4554
206-340-8870
www.ribbond.com

Scherer Laboratories, Inc.
214-233-2800

Shofu Dental Corp.
800-82S-HOFU
650-324-0085
www.shofu.com

Southern Dental Industries Inc.
800-228-5166
415-975-8060
www.sdi.com.au

Sulzer Calcitek Inc.
800-854-7019
760-431-9515
www.sulzercalcitek.com

Tanaka Dental
800-325-5266

3M Dental Products Division
800-634-2249
612-733-6216
www.3M.com/dental

Ultradent Products, Inc.
800-552-5512
801-553-4200
www.ultradent.com

Unitek Corp./3M
800-423-3748
818-574-4464

Van R Dental Products, Inc.
800-833-8267
805-488-1122
www.vanr.com

Vident
800-828-3839
714-961-6200
www.vident.com

Whip Mix Corp.
800-626-5651
502-637-1451
www.whipmix.com

Wykle Research Inc.
800-859-6641
775-887-7500

Zenith/DMG
800-662-6383
201-894-0213

Answers to the Study Questions

CHAPTER 2

1—b; 2—c and d; 3—c; 4—a, b, and d; 5—b; 6—b; 7—b and c; 8—a, b, c, and d; 9—b and c; 10—d; 11—a; 12—a; 13—a and b

CHAPTER 3

1—a and d; 2—a and d; 3—a, b, and c; 4—b; 5—b and c; 6—c and d; 7—b and d; 8—d; 9—b and c

CHAPTER 4

1—a; 2—b; 3—b; 4—c; 5—b and d; 6—a and d; 7—c; 8—c; 9—a; 10—b and c

CHAPTER 5

1—c; 2—b; 3—a; 4—d; 5—d; 6—b, c, and d; 7—c and d; 8—c and d; 9—a, b, c, and d; 10—a; 11—c

CHAPTER 6

1—b; 2—b and c; 3—c and d; 4—a and d; 5—a, b, and c; 6—a and c; 7—a, b, c, and d; 8—b; 9—a and c;10—a and b

CHAPTER 7

1—c and d; 2—a and b; 3—a and b; 4—a; 5—d; 6—c; 7—b; 8—b; 9—b; 10—c and d

CHAPTER 8

1—a and c; 2—b and d; 3—b; 4—b; 5—c; 6—b; 7—b; 8—c; 9—d; 10—d

CHAPTER 9

1—a and d; 2—b; 3—a, b, and c; 4—d; 5—b and c; 6—b

CHAPTER 10

1—c; 2—d; 3—a and b; 4—b; 5—d; 6—a, b, and d

CHAPTER 11

1—c; 2—b and c; 3—a and b; 4—b and d; 5—a and d; 6—a and b; 7—a; 8—b, c, and d; 9—a and d

CHAPTER 12

1—b; 2—a; 3—d; 4—c; 5—c; 6—b; 7—a

CHAPTER 13

1—a and c; 2—c and d; 3—a; 4—b; 5—b

CHAPTER 14

1—c; 2—d; 3—c; 4—a; 5—b; 6—d; 7—c; 8—d; 9—c; 10—b

CHAPTER 15

1—c; 2—c; 3—d; 4—a, c, and d; 5—b and c; 6—a, b, and c

Index

Page numbers in *italics* denote figures; those followed by a *t* denote tables; and those followed by a *b* denote boxes.